Diseases of the Heart and Blood Vessels

Nomenclature and Criteria
for Diagnosis

DISEASES

OF THE HEART AND

BLOOD VESSELS

NOMENCLATURE
AND CRITERIA FOR
DIAGNOSIS

by
The Criteria Committee
of the New York Heart Association

CHARLES E. KOSSMANN, M.D., *Chairman*

HERBERT CHASIS, M.D.   WILLIAM T. FOLEY, M.D.

CHARLES A. R. CONNOR, M.D.   RÉJANE M. HARVEY, M.D.

CLARENCE E. DE LA CHAPELLE, M.D.   EDWIN P. MAYNARD, JR., M.D.

JOHN B. SCHWEDEL, M.D.

Sixth Edition

LITTLE, BROWN AND COMPANY
BOSTON

Library of Congress Catalog Card No. 64–14260

SIXTH EDITION

Nomenclature and Criteria for Diagnosis of Diseases of the Heart and Blood Vessels

FIFTH EDITION, 1953

Nomenclature and Criteria for Diagnosis of Diseases of the Heart

FOURTH EDITION, 1939

Criteria for the Classification and Diagnosis of Heart Disease

THIRD EDITION, 1932
SECOND EDITION, 1929
FIRST EDITION, 1928

Published in Great Britain by J. & A. Churchill Ltd., London

PRINTED IN THE UNITED STATES OF AMERICA

Subcommittees of the Criteria Committee

Subcommittee on Criteria for Etiologic Diagnosis

RÉJANE M. HARVEY, M.D., *Chairman*

DAVID S. BALDWIN, M.D.
GEORGE E. BURCH, M.D.

HOWARD A. EDER, M.D.
EDWARD E. FISCHEL, M.D.

Subcommittee on Criteria for Anatomic Diagnosis

EDWIN P. MAYNARD, JR., M.D., *Chairman*

HOWARD G. BRUENN, M.D.
WILLIAM DRESSLER, M.D.

MARY ALLEN ENGLE, M.D.
DICKINSON W. RICHARDS, M.D.

ROBERT H. WYLIE, M.D.

Subcommittee on Criteria for Physiologic Diagnosis

HERBERT CHASIS, M.D., *Chairman*

SIDNEY BLUMENTHAL, M.D.
M. IRENÉ FERRER, M.D.

ALFRED P. FISHMAN, M.D.
BERTHA RADER, M.D.

JAMES V. WARREN, M.D.

Subcommittee on Criteria for Functional Capacity and Therapeutic Classification

CHARLES A. R. CONNOR, M.D., *Chairman*

LEWIS H. BRONSTEIN, M.D.
EUGENIE F. DOYLE, M.D.

S. CHARLES FRANCO, M.D.
HERMAN K. HELLERSTEIN, M.D.

Preface

The sixth edition of the *Criteria* has been written to integrate the ever-increasing profusion of new data on cardiovascular disease into a clinically usable set of terms and rules. These are the terms and rules necessary to further progress and essential to the achievement of the ultimate goal of all intellectual medical effort—the prevention and management of disease in man.

In the preparation of this new edition, many changes from the previous edition have been made. These changes simply reflect the numerous additions to the understanding of cardiovascular disease over the last decade. The volume has, as expected, grown in size, in spite of the omission of certain previously included portions such as the introduction to the section on Anatomic Diagnosis dealing with the physical examination of the heart. It has seemed that this had no rightful place in a nomenclature or in a set of criteria. The Criteria for Electrocardiographic Instruments have also been omitted because the field of medical instrumentation, especially electronic types, has moved forward so rapidly that the Committee considered the inclusion of such criteria to be beyond its sphere of competence.

The subject matter has been rearranged and divided into five principal parts: I. The Cardiac Diagnosis; II. The Vascular Diagnosis; III. The Pathologic Diagnosis; IV. The Roentgenologic Diagnosis; and V. The Electrocardiographic Diagnosis. These parts have in turn been subdivided into a total of thirty-three chapters. What might appear to be a major change is in reality only a rearrangement with the objective of increasing utility. A short chapter, Uncertain Diagnosis, has been included. Because the material for the Anatomic Diagnosis had become so long, it seemed desirable to divide it into two chapters: one on acquired and one on congenital heart disease. The former is an expansion of the old Anatomic Section; the latter is a greatly modified and enlarged version of paragraph 38, Congenital Anomaly of Heart or Great Vessels, in the Fifth Edition which was written for this new edition by Dr. Mary Allen Engle.

On many occasions in the past, complaints were registered against the Functional and Therapeutic Classifications. After long and considered deliberation, Dr. Connor's subcommittee decided that it could not devise anything that would better meet the special requirements of every investigative or clinical group. Accordingly, these classifications have been left unchanged but are set apart in a single chapter (Chapter 6).

The section on Vascular Diagnosis, which first appeared in the Fifth Edition, has been modified in accordance with new information. In addition, a means has been suggested by which the vascular diagnosis, like the cardiac diagnosis, can be subdivided into etiologic, anatomic, physiologic, and functional and therapeutic rubrics, but the section itself has not been rewritten on this basis pending further clinical experience.

Part III, dealing with the Pathologic Diagnosis, has been enlarged and brought up to date. Chapter 15, Congenital Anomalies of the Heart and Great Vessels, is exclusively the work of Dr. Jesse E. Edwards. As in the previous edition, Chapter 26, Diseases of the Conduction System, is the contribution of Dr. Maurice Lev. The Subcommittee on Pathologic Diagnosis again elected to use two frames of reference for presentation of its material. One is disease-oriented (Chapters 15–21), and the other is structure-oriented (Chapters 22–26). This decision has resulted in some unavoidable duplication and the creation of three new chapters, Atherosclerotic Coronary Artery Disease, Hypertensive Heart Disease, and Pulmonary Heart Disease.

There are difficulties encountered in trying to make a nomenclature and criteria into a classification as well. In the past, attempts to do this were made by placing rubrics in alphabetical order, so far as possible, and by including appropriate code numbers of the *Standard Nomenclature for Diseases and Operations* of the American Medical Association. The Criteria Committee has felt that the code numbers were not used a great deal. Furthermore, two other codification systems are now available. One is an adaptation of the *International Statistical Classification of Causes of Death and Morbidity*, the other is the *Current Medical Terminology* of the American Medical Association. Unfortunately, the *International Statistical Classification* is being revised rather radically, and the new fifth edition will not be released until 1965. The *Terminology* is in a trial period of general use. For these reasons no code numbers at all have been included in the Sixth Edition.

No attempt has been made to retain the alphabetical arrangement in sections new to the Sixth Edition, although it has been retained in sections that have not been completely altered for this edition. A simple numerical system has been included that makes it possible, with certain limitations, to codify cardiovascular and other diagnoses. Each chapter and paragraph bears an arabic number. In referring to a chapter and paragraph, two numbers are given: the first, in boldface, separated from the second by a period. Subparagraphs are represented by a third digit separated from the second by a period. This method is used for cross-referencing within the text. When, for example, (3.31.4) appears, it means that reference should be made to Chapter 3, paragraph 31, subparagraph 4.

If users of this book wish to utilize it both as a classification and as a numerical index, it can be used as is, or it can be adapted fairly easily to any digital system of classification preferred.

The Sixth Edition of the *Criteria* has been prepared by a

Committee of considerably different constitution than the Committees responsible for the earlier editions. Besides the loss, principally through retirement, of many members with long and distinguished service on the Committee and the addition of new members, an innovation has been made. At least one physician of national reputation who is not a resident of the immediate environs of New York City has been added to each subcommittee. In this way an attempt has been made to broaden the viewpoint and usefulness of the present edition.

The Chairman of the Criteria Committee, also new in that capacity, expresses the gratitude of the New York Heart Association and of cardiologists everywhere for the tireless efforts of former members, including those who for a variety of reasons are no longer able to serve. He also welcomes the new members and expresses to them the deep appreciation of all concerned for their generous and expert aid and advice in the accomplishment of the volume's objective.

The previous two editions of the *Criteria* were translated into Spanish by Dr. Pedro Cossio and published in Argentina under the auspices of the Argentine Society of Cardiology. The Fifth Edition was translated into Italian by Drs. A. Poppi and Vittorio Puddu and published in Bologna (Edizioni "Bologna Medica," 1959). In addition, the *Nomenclature and Criteria* was endorsed by the International Society of Cardiology at the First World Congress of Cardiology in Paris in 1950. Subsequently the present Chairman of the Criteria Committee was also appointed Cochairman (with Dr. Vittorio Puddu of Rome) of the Nomenclature Committee of the International Society of Cardiology. Such an arrangement has the advantage of insuring some continuity of viewpoints and uniformity of nomenclature and criteria for diagnosis on an international scale.

The Criteria Committee of the New York Heart Association has noted with interest and admiration the efforts of the Cardiovascular Committee of the World Health Organization along the lines of its own endeavors but with epidemiologic orientation. It is hoped that in the future the coordination of the activities of these committees may be closer, although the objectives of each are a little different. Actually, a step in the proper direction has already been taken: the former Chairman (Dr. Harold E. B. Pardee) and the present Chairman of the Criteria Committee are also members of the Subcommittee on Cardiovascular Disease of the United States Committee on International Statistical Classification of Causes of Death and Morbidity, United States Bureau of Vital Statistics.

A nomenclature and a set of criteria for diagnosis must of necessity be changed from time to time as new knowledge accumulates and new discoveries are made. Furthermore, it is probable that the present Committee has made errors of omission or commission that users of this book will detect. The Chairman will be most grateful for having his attention called to these in order to make future editions as accurate and as useful as the contemporary state of the science and the art will permit.

CHARLES E. KOSSMANN, M.D.
Chairman

Contents

*Part III | Nomenclature and Criteria
for the Pathologic Diagnosis*

Part IV | The Roentgenologic Diagnosis

Part V | The Electrocardiographic Diagnosis

List of Illustrations

The Pathologic Diagnosis
(Part III)

The Roentgenologic Diagnosis
(Part IV)

The Electrocardiographic Diagnosis
(Part V)

Part I | *Nomenclature and Criteria for the Cardiac Diagnosis*

1 / Nomenclature for the Cardiac Diagnosis

Diseases of the heart are considered to include not only abnormalities of structure which occur in the heart and coronary arteries, the pericardium, and the initial portions of the attached great vessels, but also disturbances of function which manifest themselves as an arrhythmia, abnormal cardiac sensations, or failure of cardiac output to meet bodily requirements.

A diagnosis should include one or more titles from each of the principal diagnostic rubrics of this nomenclature: etiologic, anatomic, physiologic, functional, and therapeutic. For example, a patient with advanced rheumatic heart disease might have the following diagnosis:

Cardiac
  (a) Rheumatic, inactive
  (b) Enlarged heart, mitral stenosis, mitral insufficiency, aortic insufficiency
  (c) Atrial fibrillation, congestive heart failure
  (d) Class IV D

As another example, a patient with anginal syndrome might have the following diagnosis:

Cardiac
  (a) Atherosclerosis
  (b) Coronary sclerosis, myocardial fibrosis
  (c) Normal sinus rhythm, anginal syndrome
  (d) Class II C

Certain patients may have symptoms, abnormal physical signs, or both which are referable to the heart but which after detailed study cannot be ascribed with certainty to structural or functional cardiac disease. These may be observed further with the diagnosis of No Heart Disease, Unexplained Manifestation. Patients who have a disease, such as essential hypertension, which can cause but which has not at the time of observation caused cardiac disease are to be diagnosed as No Heart Disease, Predisposing Etiologic Factor (Essential Hypertension).

2. The Etiologic Cardiac Diagnosis*

1. Acromegaly
2. Anemia
3. Atherosclerosis
4. Carcinoid
5. Congenital anomaly
6. Hypertension
7. Hyperthyroidism
8. Hypothyroidism
9. Infection
10. Neoplasm
11. Thiamine deficiency
12. Pulmonary disease
13. Rheumatic fever
14. Systemic lupus erythematosus
15. Toxic agent
16. Trauma
17. Unknown
18. Uremia

---

* To facilitate cross-referencing, the numbering of the section headings in the chapters on nomenclature conforms to the numbering of the corresponding chapters on diagnosis.

3. The Anatomic Cardiac Diagnosis: Acquired Disease

DISEASES OF THE AORTA AND PULMONARY ARTERIES

1. Aneurysm of the aorta (specify location)
2. Aneurysm of the pulmonary artery
3. Aortitis
4. Arteriosclerosis of the aorta
5. Arteriosclerosis of the pulmonary arteries
6. Dissecting hematoma of the aorta (dissecting aneurysm)
7. Embolism of the aorta
8. Embolism of the pulmonary arteries
9. Injury of the aorta or pulmonary artery
10. Other diseases of the aorta (specify lesion)
11. Other diseases of the pulmonary arteries (specify lesion)
12. Rupture of the aorta (spontaneous)
13. Thrombosis of the aorta
14. Thrombosis of the pulmonary arteries

DISEASES OF THE CORONARY ARTERIES

15. Arteritis of the coronary arteries
16. Atherosclerosis of the coronary arteries
17. Embolism of a coronary artery
18. Other diseases of the coronary arteries (specify lesion)
19. Polyarteritis nodosa (essential polyangiitis) of the coronary arteries
20. Stenosis of a coronary orifice
21. Thrombosis of a coronary artery
22. Trauma of a coronary artery (specify lesion)

DISEASES OF THE ENDOCARDIUM AND VALVES

23. Endocardial fibroelastosis
24. Endocarditis, bacterial (specify organism)
25. Endocarditis, indeterminate

5

26. Mural endocarditis
27. Mural thrombosis
28. Neoplasm of the endocardium
29. Other structural diseases of the endocardium or valves (specify location, if possible)
30. Rupture of valve or of chordae tendineae (specify valve)
31. Valvular deformity (specify valve)
32. Valvular sclerosis (specify valve)
33. Valvulitis, active (specify deformity, if any)
34. Valvulitis, inactive

DISEASES OF THE MYOCARDIUM

35. Aneurysm of the heart
36. Atrophy of the heart
37. Degeneration of the myocardium
38. Enlargement of the heart
39. Fibrosis of the myocardium
40. Infarction of the myocardium
41. Myocarditis, active
42. Neoplasm of the heart (specify type)
43. No structural disease of the heart
44. Other structural diseases of the heart (specify lesion)
45. Rupture of the myocardium (specify location)
46. Thrombosis within the heart (specify chamber)
47. Trauma of the heart
48. Undiagnosed structural disease of the heart (specify location, if possible)

DISEASES OF THE PERICARDIUM

49. Calcification of the pericardium
50. Hemopericardium
51. Hydropericardium
52. Neoplasm of the pericardium
53. Other structural diseases of the pericardium
54. Pericarditis, acute

55. Pericarditis, chronic
56. Pneumopericardium
57. Trauma to the pericardium

4. The Anatomic Cardiac Diagnosis: Congenital Disease

NONCYANOTIC GROUP

1. Coarctation of the aorta
2. Vascular ring
3. Right aortic arch
4. Right subclavian artery, anomalous origin
5. Aneurysm of the sinus of Valsalva
6. Coronary artery, anomalous origin
7. Aortic stenosis, congenital
8. Aortic insufficiency, congenital
9. Endocardial fibroelastosis
10. Glycogen storage disease of the myocardium
11. Mitral stenosis, congenital
12. Cor triatriatum
13. Pulmonic stenosis, congenital
14. Pulmonic insufficiency, congenital
15. Idiopathic dilatation of the pulmonary artery
16. Downward displacement of the tricuspid valve (Ebstein's anomaly)
17. Persistent left superior vena cava
18. "Corrected" transposition of the great vessels
19. Dextrocardia
20. Levocardia with situs inversus

POTENTIALLY CYANOTIC GROUP

21. Patent ductus arteriosus
22. Aortic septal defect (aorticopulmonary window)
23. Truncus arteriosus
24. Coronary arteriovenous fistula
25. Ventricular septal defect

7

26. Single ventricle (cor triloculare biatriatum)
27. Common atrioventricular canal
28. Atrial septal defect
29. Single atrium (cor triloculare biventriculare)
30. Total anomalous pulmonary venous connection
31. Partial anomalous pulmonary venous connection
32. Arteriovenous fistula of the lung

CYANOTIC GROUP

33. Pulmonic stenosis with patent foramen ovale or atrial septal defect
34. Downward displacement of the tricuspid valve (Ebstein's anomaly) with patent foramen ovale
35. Tetralogy of Fallot
36. "Pseudotruncus" arteriosus
37. Rudimentary right ventricle with tricuspid and pulmonic stenosis or atresia and defective atrial septum
38. Rudimentary left ventricle with mitral and aortic stenosis or atresia and defective atrial septum
39. Complete transposition of the great vessels
40. Incomplete transposition of the great vessels

5. The Physiologic Cardiac Diagnosis

DISTURBANCES IN CARDIAC RHYTHM AND CONDUCTION

1. Atrial arrhythmias
2. Atrioventricular (A–V) nodal rhythms
3. Atrioventricular (A–V) block
4. Escaped beats
5. Intraventricular conduction defects
6. Paroxysmal tachycardia
7. Premature contractions
8. Sinus rhythms
9. Undiagnosed arrhythmia
10. Ventricular fibrillation
11. Wandering pacemaker

DISTURBANCES IN MYOCARDIAL CONTRACTILITY

12. Cardiac insufficiency (heart failure)
13. Annular incompetency
14. Gallop rhythm
15. Pulsus alternans
16. Pulmonary hypertension

CLINICAL SYNDROMES

17. Anginal syndrome
18. Adams-Stokes syndrome
19. Carotid sinus syndrome
20. Wolff-Parkinson-White syndrome
21. Cyanotic crises
22. Cardiac tamponade
23. Intracardiac ball-valve obstruction

6. Physical Capacity with Heart Disease

1. Functional classification (I to IV)
2. Therapeutic classification (A to E)

7. Uncertain Diagnosis

1. No heart disease: predisposing etiologic factor
2. No heart disease: unexplained manifestation

2 / The Etiologic Cardiac Diagnosis

The causes of heart disease outlined in this section give recognition to the known major structural or functional disorders affecting the heart. Although the detailed mechanisms whereby these various disease processes ultimately lead to a disturbance in cardiac function are not completely understood, there is sufficient clinical, physiologic, or anatomic evidence to identify all of these causes and hence warrant their inclusion in this chapter.

The etiologic diagnosis may be derived from the patient's history, physical examination, and laboratory data, including the electrocardiogram, angiocardiogram, and cardiac catheterization. Both structural and functional disturbance should be considered in the determination of the cause of the heart disease. If two or more possible causes of heart disease are present, each should be mentioned.

Diseases which are rarely identified ante mortem will not be considered here but will be discussed in later chapters (Part III).

1. Acromegaly

Although most of the internal organs are enlarged in patients with acromegaly, when the heart is involved cardiac enlargement is out of proportion to the general splanchnomegaly. If the pituitary dysfunction is not corrected, cardiac insufficiency develops and is a frequent cause of death.

2. Anemia

Under certain circumstances anemia alone can cause structural heart disease (24.4.1)* other than dilatation. Most often its effects are physiologic with production of cardiac murmurs and a high cardiac output. In the presence of other types of heart disease, anemia may contribute to the production of cardiac insufficiency (5.12), anginal syndrome, and arrhythmias.

Criteria for the Diagnosis of Heart Disease Due to Anemia:
   The presence of significant anemia.
   Disturbances of cardiac function mentioned above.
   Disappearance of signs and symptoms following correction of the anemia.

2.1. SICKLE-CELL ANEMIA. In addition to disturbances of cardiac function attributable to anemia itself, sickle-cell disease may be responsible for occlusion of small pulmonary arteries and the production of pulmonary hypertension (5.16).

Criteria for the Diagnosis of Heart Disease Due to Sickle-Cell Anemia:
   The presence of sickle-cell anemia.
   Disturbances of cardiac function mentioned above.

3. Atherosclerosis†

3.1. CORONARY ARTERIES. Atherosclerosis may produce in the coronary arteries stenosing or occluding lesions which impair the supply of blood to the myocardium (3.39, 40; 16.1–10).

* Parenthetical cross references are given by chapter (**boldface**) and section numbers, and when applicable by subsection numbers.
† In certain vessels [e.g., aorta (3.4) and pulmonary artery (3.5)] it is not always possible from the clinical examination to say whether the lesion is intimal, medial, or both. In such instances the more general term *arteriosclerosis* (**21**.1–3) is preferred.

11

Coronary disease is usually a disease of middle or older age, but it may occur in younger age groups, particularly in the presence of familial hypercholesterolemia, idiopathic hyperlipemia, diabetes mellitus, hypertension, nephrotic syndrome, and myxedema.

When there is relative or absolute ischemia of the myocardium, one or several of the following may occur: anginal syndrome, infarction of the myocardium, cardiac insufficiency, disturbance of conduction, or abnormal rhythm.

Criteria for the Diagnosis of Atherosclerosis of the Coronary Arteries:
Anginal syndrome, or signs and symptoms of myocardial infarction.
In older age groups, the appearance of certain defects in conduction or certain arrhythmias.

3.2. AORTIC VALVE. Atherosclerosis may affect the aortic valve, thereby causing stenosis or insufficiency and calcification visible on roentgenologic examination (3.32). The absence of a history of rheumatic fever or deformity of other valves, and the older age of the patient may suggest atherosclerotic origin of the disease.

Criteria for the Diagnosis of Atherosclerosis of the Aortic Valve:
Evidence of aortic stenosis or insufficiency or both.
Absence of other than atherosclerotic cause for the valvular defect.

4. Carcinoid

Serotonin is produced in increased amounts and released into the circulation by carcinoid of the small intestine with hepatic metastases. In addition to the carcinoid syndrome, lesions of the pulmonic or tricuspid valves may develop with resultant cardiac insufficiency. The existence of carcinoid is established by the persistent presence of 5-hydroxy-indoleacetic acid in the urine.

Criteria for the Diagnosis of Heart Disease Due to Carcinoid:
   The presence of carcinoid.
   Evidence of a structural lesion of the pulmonic or tricuspid valve.

5. Congenital Anomaly

The diagnosis of congenital anomaly may be based on the finding of characteristic physical signs in association with electrocardiographic or roentgenographic abnormalities. In many instances additional data must be secured from angiocardiography or cardiac catheterization before a definitive diagnosis can be made (4.1–40).

6. Hypertension

When the level of diastolic blood pressure exceeds 90 mm Hg, systemic hypertension is considered to be present and may be an etiologic factor in heart disease. Systolic hypertension alone, such as that which occurs in hyperthyroidism, complete atrioventricular heart block, aortic insufficiency, and severe atherosclerosis of the aorta, is not considered an etiologic factor in heart disease.

Hypertension may be associated with most bilateral diffuse suppurative and nonsuppurative renal diseases as well as with unilateral renal disease such as that caused by renal arterial obstruction. Coarctation of the aorta, pheochromocytoma, aldosteronism, Cushing's syndrome, and toxemia of pregnancy may be accompanied by hypertension. In the absence of demonstrable underlying disease, the diagnosis of essential hypertension is made when persistent elevation of the diastolic blood pressure is found.

The primary manifestation of heart disease due to persistent hypertension is left ventricular hypertrophy, and persistent systemic hypertension should be considered a cause of heart disease only when left ventricular hypertrophy is demonstrated. When additional manifestations such as cardiac arrhythmias, cardiac insufficiency, or the anginal syndrome are present, another etiologic factor, atherosclerosis of the coronary arteries, for example, frequently coexists (16, 17.4).

Left ventricular failure may occur with acute or transient increase in the diastolic blood pressure, such as in the course of glomerulonephritis, toxemia of pregnancy, and pheochromocytoma. In such instances hypertension may be considered the cause of heart disease in the absence of left ventricular hypertrophy. Although hypertension is given as the etiologic diagnosis of heart disease in some patients with acute diffuse glomerulonephritis, hypervolemia may be responsible for many of the manifestations.

Criteria for the Diagnosis of Heart Disease Due to Hypertension:
   Persistent hypertension with left ventricular hypertrophy, or transient hypertension with left ventricular failure in the course of diseases known to cause hypertension.

7. Hyperthyroidism

The most common cardiovascular disturbances produced by hyperthyroidism are palpitation and sinus tachycardia. In addition, paroxysmal or permanent atrial fibrillation often occurs. In some patients with hyperthyroidism, cardiac enlargement and cardiac insufficiency appear. There is disagreement about whether hyperthyroidism per se is the cause of these manifestations or whether it is merely a precipitating factor in the presence of pre-existing heart disease. When cardiac insufficiency occurs in patients with hyperthyroidism, it is characterized by a high cardiac output, and the patient is cured by successful treatment of the hyperthyroidism.

Criteria for Diagnosis of Heart Disease Due to Hyperthyroidism:
  Evidence of hyperthyroidism associated with cardiac insufficiency or atrial fibrillation.

8. Hypothyroidism

In patients with myxedema, abnormalities of the heart are occasionally found. There may be enlargement of the cardiac silhouette, often in reality a manifestation of pericardial effusion, which can be reversed by the administration of thyroid hormone. In addition, there is usually bradycardia, and there may be a diminished cardiac output. There may be changes in the electrocardiogram, with low voltage of all deflections, sometimes inversion of T waves, and occasionally prolongation of the P–R interval. There may be an acceleration of atherosclerosis in patients with myxedema.

Criteria for Diagnosis of Heart Disease Due to Hypothyroidism:
  Evidence of hypothyroidism.
  Enlargement of the cardiac silhouette and electrocardiographic abnormalities which are decreased by administration of thyroid hormone.

9. Infection

Common forms of clinical heart disease rarely stem directly from infectious processes. Bacterial endocarditis may result from a variety of organisms, e.g., streptococci (*viridans, fecalis,* or *hemolyticus*), staphylococci, *Hemophilus influenzae,* pneumococci, gonococci, and meningococci. Syphilitic involvement of the aorta or heart, diphtheritic myocarditis, and tuberculous pericarditis are also encountered. Among certain populations, schistosomiasis may lead to pulmonary heart disease (**18.**2) and trypanosomiasis to chronic myocarditis and fibrosis.

Transient electrocardiographic abnormalities may be due to any systemic infectious agent, but these are rarely of clinical significance. Such infections include the acute exanthemata and infestation by such parasites as *Trichina, Plasmodium malariae,* and *Echinococcus.* Coxsackie virus has been reported as a cause of fatal myocarditis in the newborn. ECHO virus, influenza virus, and infectious mononucleosis may also be associated with myocarditis on rare occasion. Many other microorganisms may cause endocarditis, myocarditis, or pericarditis, e.g., *Pasteurella tularensis, Brucella,* various yeasts, and fungi.

The infectious agent should be specified in the diagnosis. Any acute infection may aggravate existing heart disease, but unless there is conclusive evidence that the infection has caused the heart disease, the primary etiologic diagnosis should be stated and the acute infection given as an "accompanying condition."

Criteria for Diagnosis of Infection of the Heart or Blood Vessels:

Demonstration of pathogenic organisms (bacterium, virus, spirochete, parasite, or fungus) by culture or smear from the blood or pericardial fluid, or inferential demonstration of their presence by serologic methods. In suspected diphtheritic myocarditis, a positive culture from the pharynx is sufficient to establish the diagnosis.

Signs and symptoms indicating involvement of the endocardium, myocardium, pericardium, or blood vessels by the infection.

10. Neoplasm

10.1. PRIMARY NEOPLASMS. These are rare and difficult to diagnose. Since the advent of angiocardiography and cardiac catheterization, some tumors have been diagnosed and have been treated successfully by surgery. They may be suspected in patients with otherwise unexplained signs and symptoms such as compression or thrombosis of the superior vena cava, pericardial effusion, intermittent and varying types of arrhythmias (especially atrial fibrillation), and cardiac insufficiency. The most common tumors, atrial myxomas, frequently produce emboli and murmurs suggestive of stenosis of the mitral or tricuspid valves.

10.2. SECONDARY NEOPLASMS. These are either metastatic or produced by extension of intrathoracic tumors, chiefly bronchial. The endocardium, myocardium, or pericardium may be involved.

The diagnosis of secondary tumor may be suspected whenever cardiac manifestations are present in a patient with an intrathoracic neoplasm.

Criteria for Diagnosis of Cardiac Neoplasm:
　Demonstration of neoplasm involving the heart by angiocardiography, or by pericardial biopsy or other surgical exploration.

11. Thiamine Deficiency

In patients with thiamine deficiency, cardiac insufficiency accompanied by a high cardiac output and peripheral vasodilatation may occur. A history of a deficient diet, the presence of peripheral neuritis or pellagra, and cardiac insufficiency may suggest this diagnosis.

Criteria for Diagnosis of Beriberi Heart Disease:
　Cardiac insufficiency which disappears upon treatment with thiamine.

12. Pulmonary Disease

Pulmonary heart disease (cor pulmonale) is the term used to define right ventricular enlargement or insufficiency resulting primarily from certain disorders of pulmonary function or structure. The basic mechanisms by which the right heart may be embarrassed are: (1) disturbance in exchange of pulmonary gases with resulting hypoxemia and hypercapnia leading to pulmonary vasoconstriction, hypervolemia, and increased cardiac output; (2) anatomic curtailment of the pulmonary vascular bed; (3) a combination of these factors. A variety of diseases may produce these alterations; the manner in which they do so may be fundamentally different, and the pulmonary parenchyma may not be directly involved by the pathologic process. For these reasons the responsible disease process should always be given when a diagnosis of pulmonary heart disease is made, e.g., pulmonary heart disease due to pulmonary emphysema. Impairment of gaseous exchange in the lungs may result from lesions that involve the nervous system, the thoracic cage, or, most frequently, the bronchopulmonary apparatus. Anatomic curtailment of the pulmonary vascular bed, as a primary cause of pulmonary heart disease, is rare but may be produced by multiple or massive pulmonary emboli, the pulmonary arteritides, or certain of the pulmonary fibroses, particularly those producing the syndrome of alveolar-capillary block.

The presence of pulmonary arterial hypertension per se does not constitute evidence of pulmonary heart disease. There are many conditions that produce pulmonary hypertension in which the primary abnormality is not a disturbance in pulmonary structure or function, e.g., congenital heart disease with left or right shunt, mitral stenosis, or left ventricular failure (5.16). These cardiac states should not be included under the heading of pulmonary heart disease, nor should the term *pulmonary heart disease* be utilized in patients with primary pulmonary disease in whom there is pulmonary hypertension, either transient or fixed, but in whom there is no evidence of right ventricular disease.

Criteria for the Diagnosis of Pulmonary Heart Disease:
The demonstration of right ventricular enlargement or in-

sufficiency in association with a disease process known to attack primarily the lungs or some aspect of breathing. Absence of heart disease of other etiology and absence of clinically detectable left ventricular enlargement.

13. Rheumatic Fever

Rheumatic fever is a generalized disease characterized by inflammatory lesions, which are usually found in the heart, blood vessels, and joints. It follows infection with a Group A hemolytic streptococcus and is a nonsuppurative and apparently sterile sequel. The manifestations and course of rheumatic fever are extremely variable. Certain of these are considered rather indicative of the disease and therefore classified as "major": carditis (murmurs, cardiac enlargement, pericarditis, or congestive heart failure), polyarthritis, chorea, subcutaneous nodules, and erythema marginatum. The first three manifestations, carditis, polyarthritis, and chorea, may occur independently of one another.

Other manifestations suggestive of rheumatic fever are less uniquely characteristic of that disease and are therefore classified as "minor": fever, arthralgia, prolongation of the atrioventricular conduction time, and increased erythrocyte sedimentation rate or other evidence of inflammatory reaction such as leukocytosis or an elevated C-reactive protein. Since rheumatic fever tends to recur, a previous history of rheumatic fever is also occasionally considered to contribute to the diagnosis. Evidence of a preceding hemolytic streptococcal infection by culture or by antibody response (antistreptolysin titer) is classified as a "minor" criterion because streptococcal infections may occur and not be followed by rheumatic fever. Rheumatic fever may also be accompanied by less specific symptoms and signs such as loss of weight, malaise, fatigability, tachycardia, pallor due to anemia, precordial or abdominal pain, and erythema nodosum.

19

Certain structural lesions are characteristic of rheumatic heart disease (**3.**31, 33, 34, 41). Whenever this diagnosis is made, the physician should state whether the rheumatic process is *active* or *inactive*. Patients with the major or minor manifestations noted above should be classified as active, provided that there is no other discoverable cause for these findings. If these features are not present, the patient should be considered to have inactive rheumatic heart disease.

Rheumatic heart disease may be encountered in individuals who have no history of any of the manifestations of acute rheumatic fever mentioned above. This occurs in about one-third of all adult patients with rheumatic heart disease.

Criteria for the Diagnosis of Rheumatic Heart Disease:
   History of rheumatic fever, as characterized above, accompanied by a characteristic structural lesion of the heart, or evidence of a characteristic structural lesion of the heart even in the absence of a history of rheumatic fever or of the above-mentioned manifestations.

14. Systemic Lupus Erythematosus

Cardiac involvement may occur in systemic lupus erythematosus but is not ordinarily a prominent feature of the disease (**3.**25; **9.**15; **23.**2.2). Pericarditis with effusion and fibrinous pericarditis are the most common manifestations, but myocardial lesions and nonbacterial verrucae (atypical verrucous endocarditis) may also occur. Cardiac insufficiency may occur late in the disease and is usually associated with renal involvement and hypertension.

Criteria for Diagnosis of Heart Disease Due to Systemic Lupus Erythematosus:
   Presence of systemic lupus erythematosus.
   Evidence of involvement of the heart.

15. *Toxic Agent*

The diagnosis of heart disease due to a toxic agent includes those instances of abnormal cardiac function clearly due to chemical substances. These toxic agents should be specified. Some commonly encountered industrial and pharmaceutical chemical substances which may produce toxic effects are phosphorus, nicotine, amphetamine, emetine, quinidine, and digitalis.

This etiologic diagnosis should not be made unless the particular agent is definitely identified. Toxic effects due to infection or to bacterial toxins, e.g., as in diphtheria, are regarded as a result of infection and should be recorded as such.

Criteria for the Diagnosis of Heart Disease Due to Toxic Agent:
Presence of a known toxic agent associated with abnormal cardiac function.

16. *Trauma*

Structural cardiac and abnormal cardiac function may occur as the result of penetrating wounds, severe blows upon the chest, crushing injuries of the chest, or the abrupt application of decelerative forces to the moving body. Injuries of peripheral vessels producing arteriovenous fistulas may have functional effects upon the heart.

Criteria for the Diagnosis of Heart Disease Due to Trauma:
The occurrence of exceptional trauma as described above.
Evidence of cardiac disease or dysfunction.

17. *Unknown*

The cause should be stated as "unknown" in those patients who present either definite structural changes in the heart or

21

evidence of abnormal cardiac function for which no definite cause can be determined. Those cardiac syndromes which can be recognized clinically because of characteristic patterns, e.g., idiopathic pericarditis, idiopathic ventricular hypertrophy, fibroelastosis, are to be included in this category since their etiology remains essentially unknown at present.

Criteria for the Diagnosis of Heart Disease of Unknown Etiology:
   Structural lesion of the heart without known cause, or abnormal cardiac function without known cause.

18. Uremia

Uremia may be associated with fibrinous pericarditis. Although disturbances in myocardial function may be seen in uremia, these can usually be related to hypertension, abnormalities of serum electrolytes, hypervolemia, or anemia.

Criteria for the Diagnosis of Heart Disease Due to Uremia:
   Presence of uremia.
   Evidence of pericarditis.

3 / The Anatomic Cardiac Diagnosis: Acquired Disease

A correct anatomic diagnosis can be made clinically in the majority of diseases of the heart. Of the various diagnostic methods available, the minimum that should be employed are: (1) history-taking and physical examination, including a determination of blood pressure with cuffs of appropriate size for adults and children, and a determination of the blood pressure in multiple extremities, if necessary; (2) electrocardiography; and (3) roentgenography, including fluoroscopy. In some instances the following may be necessary: (4) angiocardiography; (5) phonocardiography; (6) determination of venous pressure and circulation times; (7) catheterization of the right or left heart, or both; and (8) recording of indicator-dilution curves or their equivalents. Finally, a variety of tests may be required to support a diagnosis suspected on other grounds. These may include a complete blood count; a serologic test for syphilis; a urinalysis and estimation of renal function (blood urea nitrogen and others); a determination of the acute phase reactants (erythrocyte sedimentation rate, C-reactive protein), serum enzymes, and serum electrolytes; and performance of pulmonary functional studies. Although ordinarily used for appraisal of function, stress tests (e.g., electrocardiographic exercise or hypoxia test) may yield evidence in support of a specific anatomic diagnosis.

A compilation of a complete catalogue of the signs of the structural changes associated with different diseases of the heart is beyond the scope of this chapter. An attempt has been made to set down those features regarded to be of major diagnostic importance, together with a few such minor ones as may on occasion prove helpful.

Diseases of the Aorta and Pulmonary Arteries

1. Aneurysm of the Aorta (Specify Location)

The term *aneurysm* should be applied only to a saccular or sharply demarcated fusiform dilatation of the aorta (3.6, 12; 9.22.3; 20.2; 21.1, 4). In the thoracic aorta aneurysms are usually due to syphilis or arteriosclerosis, whereas in the abdominal aorta arteriosclerosis is the usual cause. Aneurysms due to acute infections are rare and usually too small to be diagnosed before death. Traumatic aneurysms of the aorta are uncommon.

Aneurysms of the aorta may remain latent without signs or symptoms. When present, these may be signs caused by a local change in dynamics (3.3), or signs and symptoms resulting from pressure on or erosion of adjacent structures. Pressure on a bronchus can result in bronchiectasis or pulmonary suppuration.

Symptoms and Signs:
Cough, hoarseness, and dysphagia.
Localized thoracic pain.
Inequality of the pulse and blood pressure in the two arms.
Tracheal tug.
Localized or diffuse pulsation at the point where the aneurysm impinges upon the chest wall.
Abnormal dullness over the manubrium sterni or in the first and second interspaces to the right or left of the sternum.
Recurrent laryngeal or phrenic nerve paralysis.

Roentgenography may reveal sacculation or a sharply demarcated fusiform dilatation of some part of the aorta.
Fluoroscopy may show increased pulsation of the vessel,
localized or diffuse. Angiocardiography, aortography,
roentgenkymography, or electrokymography may help to
differentiate an aneurysm from other intrathoracic tumors.
The more sensitive serologic tests will be positive in the
majority of cases when the aneurysm is due to syphilis.

2. *Aneurysm of the Pulmonary Artery*

This type of aneurysm may be encountered in patients with
congenital malformations of the heart associated with pulmonary hypertension or greatly increased pulmonary flow. It
must be differentiated from idiopathic dilatation in these
patients (4.15). On rare occasions aneurysm of the pulmonary
artery is due to syphilis. It usually can be diagnosed only by
roentgenography or angiography.

3. *Aortitis*

Aortitis usually is caused by syphilis, more rarely by rheumatic
fever or other infectious diseases. The form due to syphilis is
the only one, however, in which a clinical diagnosis can be
made with reasonable certainty. The diagnosis of uncomplicated syphilitic aortitis is especially difficult in patients over
40 years of age or in those with hypertension, arteriosclerosis,
or other lesions that may lead to dilatation of the aorta.

Syphilitic aortitis frequently escapes clinical recognition
since it may never produce symptoms. The appearance of
symptoms indicates that a complication, such as occlusion of
one of the coronary ostia or aneurysm of the aorta, has arisen.
Evidence of aortitis may be found within three to ten years
after the chancre. The blood Wassermann reaction is often negative, but more sensitive serologic tests for syphilis may be
expected to give a much higher percentage of positive re-

actions. In syphilitic patients under 40 years of age and with a normal blood pressure, the diagnosis may be suspected from the presence of a ringing aortic second sound, and more rarely from a systolic murmur over the aortic area; both signs are often associated with excessive systolic excursion of the ascending aorta, as demonstrated on fluoroscopy.

Although the demonstration of a widened aortic silhouette by radiologic techniques (13.10) is one of the most important aids in the diagnosis of uncomplicated syphilitic aortitis, its appearance may be simulated by the effects of hypertension or of arteriosclerosis of the aorta. A bulging and elongation of the ascending aorta in an individual of 40 years or less may indicate syphilitic aortitis, particularly if this portion shows exaggerated pulsation under the fluoroscope.

Syphilitic aortitis is frequently complicated by aneurysm, aortic insufficiency, or coronary ostial stenosis. The presence of one or more of these lesions facilitates the recognition of the underlying lesion.

In patients with syphilis who are over age 40 and in whom dilatation of the aorta has been demonstrated by the criteria listed below, a clinical diagnosis of "aortitis or arteriosclerosis" of the aorta should be made. In this age group it is not possible to state with certainty whether syphilis or arteriosclerosis, or a combination of the two diseases, has caused the aortic dilatation.

Symptoms:
    None.

Signs:
    Ringing quality of the aortic second sound, with or without increased intensity.
    A systolic murmur, heard loudest at the aortic area.
    Increase in width of the aortic silhouette as demonstrated on fluoroscopy, radiography, orthodiagraphy, or angiocardiography.
    Increased amplitude of pulsation in the ascending, trans-

verse, or descending thoracic aorta as demonstrated on fluoroscopy or electrokymography.

Elongation and localized convexity seen on the lateral or ventral aspect of the ascending aorta.

Calcification of the ascending aorta, which should make one suspect the presence of syphilitic aortitis.

4. Arteriosclerosis of the Aorta

This is usually minimal in the ascending portion, may be moderately severe in the arch and descending thoracic aorta, and is generally most severe in the abdominal segment (21.1). The condition is rarely found in young persons, but it appears to a significant degree after age 40. As a clinical disease it is seen chiefly in patients over 65 years of age.

Signs:
Systolic murmur, heard best over the second right interspace near the sternum.

Elongation, uncoiling, and increase in width and density of the aortic silhouette as demonstrated on fluoroscopy, radiography, or angiocardiography. The descending aorta becomes readily visible and often curves well to the left. Calcareous plaques may be demonstrated roentgenographically in the aortic knob and in the abdominal aorta.

5. Arteriosclerosis of the Pulmonary Arteries

This condition is usually associated with elevated pulmonary arterial pressure or increased pulmonary blood flow, or both, as, e.g., in mitral stenosis, pulmonary emphysema, silicosis, deformities of the thorax, recurrent pulmonary emboli, and congenital anomalies of the heart and great vessels (21.3). It may occur in the absence of any of these lesions.

This diagnosis is rarely made clinically because signs and symptoms are frequently lacking, and, when present, they are the result of the primary disease and its effects upon the right heart (2.12).

6. Dissecting Hematoma of the Aorta (Dissecting Aneurysm)

This condition results from rupture of the intima into the media (3.12; 9.23). Medial necrosis is usually the underlying lesion. At first, dissection occurs within the media, and an intramural hematoma may result. Later, rupture of the aorta through the intima into the media takes place, resulting in rapid extension of the intramural hematoma, which now communicates with the aortic lumen through the intimal tear. Individuals with Marfan's syndrome or with aortic coarctation, especially when complicated by pregnancy, are particularly prone to this disease. Rarely is the rupture through an intimal atheromatous area. Hypertension often plays a part in its production. The initial intramural rupture usually occurs in the ascending aorta or arch and more rarely in the descending portion. The hematoma may extend proximally and distally as well as circumferentially between the layers of the media. As it does so, it may occlude small arteries and compress the orifices of larger ones, such as the coronaries, as they leave the aorta. Death may ensue rapidly or after many hours and may result from hemorrhage into neighboring organs or from occlusion of important vessels, especially the coronary arteries. Death due to cardiac tamponade is not uncommon when rupture into the pericardium occurs. Spontaneous recovery is rare. Second or even third attacks may follow, ending in fatal hemorrhage. Dissecting hematoma occurs predominantly in males and in the middle or older age groups.

Symptoms and Signs:
    Sudden onset of severe, continuous tearing or crushing pain in the front or back of the chest, less often in the abdomen. The pain may be accompanied by extreme prostration, dyspnea, and loss of consciousness.

Symptoms resulting from the pressure of the hematoma upon, and stenosis or occlusion of, the branches of the aorta, such as the renal arteries (hematuria, anuria), the mesenteric arteries (acute surgical abdomen), or the iliac arteries (acute arterial insufficiency of the lower extremities).

Presence of hypertension in some instances.

Pericardial friction rub and enlargement of the cardiac silhouette if hemopericardium develops.

Abrupt appearance of a diastolic murmur at the base of the heart and peripheral signs of aortic regurgitation.

Roentgenographic evidence of widening of the aorta in certain instances.

7. Embolism of the Aorta

Emboli usually lodge at the bifurcation of the aorta. Large emboli usually come from the heart. In rheumatic heart disease they may arise from thrombi in the left atrium or its auricle. In atherosclerotic coronary artery disease (3.16; 16) they are derived from mural thrombi in the left ventricle after myocardial infarction, or more rarely from thrombi in the fibrillating left atrium or its auricle.

It may be difficult and at times impossible to distinguish between thrombosis and embolism as the cause of sudden occlusion of the aorta. However, in patients with rheumatic heart disease or recent myocardial infarction, embolism is the more probable cause.

Symptoms:

Sudden onset of severe pain in the legs, lower abdomen, or back (rarely pain may be absent).

Sudden onset of numbness, coldness, and tingling of both legs, usually asymmetric in severity.

Signs:

Pallor or mottled cyanosis of one or both legs.

Coldness of one or both legs.

Absence of arterial pulsation in all arteries of one or both of the lower extremities.

Collapsed superficial veins of the lower extremity.

Weakness in one or both legs.

8. Embolism of the Pulmonary Arteries

The common sites of thrombi which may give rise to pulmonary emboli are, in the order of their frequency, the deep veins of the feet and legs; the femoral, iliac, pelvic, and prostatic veins; the right atrium or its auricle; and the right ventricle (21.7).

Symptoms result from infarction of the lung and vary in degree with the size of the vessel occluded. If it is small, there may be no symptoms. The presence of embolism of a small pulmonary artery may be suspected when a rise in respiratory rate is followed by fever. A large embolus may, in addition, cause sweating, weakness, collapse, or sudden death, for the obstruction is large enough to cause acute pulmonary hypertension and impairment of output of the right heart (acute cor pulmonale). When pain in the chest occurs, it may be aggravated by deep breathing. It may be retrosternal or radiate to the left shoulder and may closely resemble the pain of acute myocardial infarction. Hemoptysis may occur soon after the onset of pain, but more commonly it is delayed for several hours or may not occur at all. Repeated episodes of pulmonary emboli may so reduce the pulmonary vascular bed as to produce chronic pulmonary hypertension and chronic cor pulmonale (3.12; 22).

Symptoms and Signs:
Sudden onset of rapid, shallow respiration.
Cyanosis.
Pallor, sweating, and syncope.
Dilatation of the cervical veins.
Hemoptysis.

Jaundice and fever.

Rapid, weak pulse.

Accentuation of the pulmonic second sound.

Pleural friction rub and evidence of pulmonary consolidation.

Pericardial friction rub.

Electrocardiographic abnormalities influenced by the extent of the pulmonary artery occlusion and by the nature of the electrocardiogram before the occlusion occurred. At times right bundle-branch block appears early, differing from the usual block in that the S–T segment is depressed in leads I and II and in the left precordial leads, and is elevated in lead aV_R and in the right precordial leads. The defect in intraventricular conduction usually disappears in 24 hours, and the S–T segment displacement disappears soon after. The features that remain are a prominent S_1 and Q_3, with inverted T waves in leads II and III and in the right precordial leads. Often the abnormalities of the curve are nonspecific in type, involving the T waves only, or there may be no deviations from normal.

Roentgenographic examination shows areas of increased pulmonary density. These are usually apparent two to four days after the acute episode.

9. Injury of the Aorta or Pulmonary Artery

Trauma due to compression, stab or bullet wounds, or the swallowing of foreign bodies may injure the aorta or pulmonary artery. The aorta may rupture as the result of crushing injuries to the chest. Bleeding into the pericardial sac, pleural space, or mediastinum usually occurs. Such injuries are usually rapidly fatal. The diagnosis depends upon the presence of a history of trauma or evidence of the same, and upon manifestations of intrathoracic bleeding.

10. Other Diseases of the Aorta (Specify Lesion)

Under this diagnosis may be listed diseases not included in the other categories. The various forms of infectious aortitis not due to syphilis, including those occurring in septicemia, in bacteremias with or without endocarditis, and in rheumatic fever, may be mentioned here. In this group should also be included medial necrosis, when suspected, and the arteritides (21.5), which may give rise to the "aortic arch syndrome."

11. Other Diseases of the Pulmonary Arteries (Specify Lesion)

Under this diagnosis may be listed diseases not previously mentioned, such as arteritis due to rheumatic fever, tuberculosis, polyarteritis nodosa, septic infections, and parasitic invasions. These diagnoses are rarely made except at necropsy.

12. Rupture of the Aorta (Spontaneous)

This may be partial or complete. It never occurs in a structurally intact aorta. Medial necrosis and degenerative and inflammatory processes are the most important predisposing lesions, especially when associated with arterial hypertension. Coarctation of the aorta and hypoplasia more rarely lead to rupture. A syphilitic aorta rarely ruptures unless an aneurysm is present. Complete rupture may be rapidly fatal, but with slow bleeding into the esophagus, pericardium, or pleural space, death may be postponed for hours or days.

13. Thrombosis of the Aorta

Mural thrombi of infectious nature are usually found in the ascending aorta. They may be associated with bacterial endocarditis of the aortic valve. The presence of such thrombi rarely produces symptoms. Thrombosis with gradual occlusion is encountered most frequently in the abdominal aorta near its bifurcation. The thrombus usually forms on an atherosclerotic plaque or atheromatous ulcer, rarely on a syphilitic lesion. At times a thrombus may occlude so abruptly that the symptoms may closely resemble those of embolism of the aorta, or so gradually that there are no symptoms.

Signs:
Diminished or absent pulsations in the femoral arteries.
Evidence of deficient arterial blood flow in both feet.

14. Thrombosis of the Pulmonary Arteries

Congestion of pulmonary circulation, especially when accompanied by stasis, may cause development of thrombosis of the pulmonary arteries. Occasionally the thrombus forms on an atherosclerotic or inflammatory lesion. Pulmonary thrombi may propagate from an initial embolus.

The onset of symptoms is not usually as abrupt as in embolism. Cardiac failure may ensue or be aggravated if it was present before the thrombosis. This may be the only manifestation, or the signs and symptoms may be similar to those described for embolism of the pulmonary arteries (3.8).

Roentgenographic examination may reveal infarcts of the lungs, often multiple and irregularly distributed, but these may be obscured by pulmonary congestion. When large branches of a pulmonary artery are thrombosed, they may be seen as large, gradually tapering densities emerging from the hilum of the lung.

Diseases of the Coronary Arteries

15. *Arteritis of the Coronary Arteries*

This unusual lesion is found occasionally in rheumatic fever, thromboangiitis obliterans (**9.9**), lupus erythematosus, and other rarer conditions. It is always part of a general disease. An acute inflammatory reaction involves the arterial coats and may lead to thrombosis.

16. *Atherosclerosis of the Coronary Arteries*

This is usually part of a general atherosclerosis, but the coronary arteries may be the only ones affected. Diagnostic signs and symptoms occasionally may be absent even when atherosclerosis is present to a marked degree. Atherosclerosis of the coronary arteries results in narrowing of the lumen and consequent reduction of blood flow (**16.1**). Coronary insufficiency is the usual result of this condition and indicates that coronary blood flow under certain circumstances fails to meet the myocardial needs. Myocardial ischemia results.

Symptoms may arise because of coronary insufficiency, which may come as a result of slowly progressive narrowing of the lumen or may be precipitated by an extracardiac event such as severe hemorrhage or exertion. It may be manifested by:

Anginal syndrome.
Cardiac arrhythmia.
Cardiac insufficiency (left ventricular failure).
Acute myocardial infarction.
Electrocardiographic abnormalities, as specified under infarction of the myocardium (**3.40**).

When sufficiently prolonged or severe, coronary insufficiency may give rise to sudden death.

Coronary occlusion often occurs during the course of coronary atherosclerosis. The signs and symptoms vary according to the abruptness of the event, the size and location of the affected myocardial area, and the effectiveness of the collateral circulation. With gradual onset symptoms may not appear; with abrupt onset they may be those of myocardial infarction.

Enlargement of the heart, if present, is due to a complicating factor such as hypertension or myocardial infarction with cardiac insufficiency.

17. Embolism of a Coronary Artery

This is a rare condition which occurs most often in the presence of acute or subacute bacterial endocarditis. The diagnosis may be considered when death or signs and symptoms of myocardial infarction occur suddenly in an individual with bacterial endocarditis.

18. Other Diseases of the Coronary Arteries (Specify Lesion)

Under this heading may be listed diseases not mentioned elsewhere, e.g., aneurysm of coronary artery, acquired coronary arteriovenous fistula, and the arteriolar lesions encountered in sickle-cell anemia and lupus erythematosus (22.1–6).

19. Polyarteritis Nodosa (Essential Polyangiitis) of the Coronary Arteries

This coronary disease is part of a widespread involvement of the smaller of the medium-sized arteries and is of unknown cause. The diagnosis may be suspected when the anginal syndrome or signs of myocardial ischemia or infarction appear in the course of the systemic disease (9.10).

20. Stenosis of a Coronary Orifice

This condition is most often the result of syphilitic aortitis (**20.**4) but may occasionally be found with atherosclerosis of the supravalvular aorta. The signs and symptoms are the same as those described for atherosclerosis of coronary arteries (3.16). When occlusion of an orifice occurs, sudden death may ensue or the signs and symptoms of myocardial ischemia or infarction may follow.

21. Thrombosis of a Coronary Artery

This condition may or may not give rise to signs and symptoms, depending upon the size and location of the vessel occluded and the state of collateral circulation. When it does give rise to symptoms, they are of myocardial ischemia or of myocardial infarction. Coronary thrombosis is not recommended as a clinical diagnosis.

22. Trauma of a Coronary Artery (Specify Lesion)

Trauma of a coronary artery may be due to a stab or bullet wound. It may also result from an accident in paracentesis of the pericardial sac, from crushing injuries of the chest, and during cardiotomy. It results in hemopericardium and rarely, as a later development, in a coronary arteriovenous or arterioatrial fistula (3.18).

Diseases of the Endocardium and Valves

23. Endocardial Fibroelastosis

This results from proliferation of endocardial and subendocardial fibrous and elastic tissue (**23.**7). It often occurs in infants as a congenital condition (4.9), but it may also affect older children and adults. The clinical features are not distinctive; they include cardiac enlargement, often in the absence of murmurs; congestive heart failure; systemic embolization; low-grade fever; gallop rhythm; aberrations of intraventricular conduction; and electrocardiographic abnormalities, particularly of the final ventricular deflections in leads from the left side of the precordium. Sometimes the clinical manifestations may resemble those of constrictive pericarditis ("constrictive endocarditis").

24. Endocarditis, Bacterial (Specify Organism)

This includes all forms of bacterial infection of the endocardium and valves (2.9). Acute and subacute forms of bacterial endocarditis are usually distinguished according to the cause and the pathologic effects produced by the infecting organism. If these effects are locally destructive and include abscesses in various organs, the course is rapid (acute bacterial endocarditis). If, on the other hand, the bacterial agent fails to produce significant destruction of the cardiac tissues or metastatic abscesses, the course is slower (subacute bacterial endocarditis). Although the clinical course, as far as the heart is concerned, is dominated by the endocardial involvement, almost all patients with bacterial endocarditis have myocarditis as well.

24.1. ACUTE BACTERIAL ENDOCARDITIS. The staphylococcus, pneumococcus, and streptococcus are the most frequent infecting organisms. The gonococcus is rarely encountered. Signs of sepsis usually outweigh those of cardiac involvement unless acute perforation of a valve occurs.

Signs:
   Evidence of sepsis.
   Embolic phenomena.
   Appearance of a significant cardiac murmur, especially if it

is diastolic, or a change in the character or intensity of a pre-existing murmur.

Positive blood culture.

24.2. SUBACUTE BACTERIAL ENDOCARDITIS (ENDOCARDITIS LENTA). This form is usually caused by the streptococcus viridans and more rarely by the staphylococcus, enterococcus, *Hemophilus influenzae,* or one of a variety of other bacteria. The infection is usually engrafted upon old rheumatic valvular deformities or congenital anomalies and more rarely upon sclerotic valves in instances of atherosclerosis or syphilis. Normal valves are said to be affected in 15 percent to 20 percent of cases.

Cardiac insufficiency, diffuse glomerulonephritis, and aseptic emboli may occur and cause death in patients who have been cured of the active infection.

Signs:
    Fever.
    Pallor due to anemia.
    Leukocytosis.
    Positive blood culture (the diagnosis occasionally has to be made on clinical grounds in the absence of a positive blood culture).
    Evidence of valvular deformity or congenital anomaly.
    Embolic phenomena (petechiae, Osler's nodes, hematuria, arterial occlusions).
    Enlarged spleen.
    Clubbing of fingers.

25. Endocarditis, Indeterminate

Several different types of endocardial lesions are included under this heading. Although the cause of these is unknown, they are probably not due to direct bacterial infection, for the lesions do not contain bacteria. They are mainly of pathologic interest. One type, atypical verrucous endocarditis, may occasionally be recognized clinically because of its frequent association with lupus erythematosus disseminatus (23.2).

26. *Mural Endocarditis*

This is a common finding in bacterial endocarditis, atypical verrucous endocarditis, and rheumatic endocarditis; it is less common in rheumatoid endocarditis and fibroelastosis. It may complicate a ventricular septal defect. It is chiefly of pathologic interest, for it cannot be recognized clinically.

27. *Mural Thrombosis*

Endocardial thrombi may form in any of the chambers of the heart but are most frequently found in the atria and their auricles. Among the causative factors are inflammation, necrosis, sclerosis, and especially retardation of blood flow as occurs with valvular stenosis, atrial dysrhythmia, or cardiac insufficiency with congestion.

Mural thrombi are often friable and produce emboli either in the lungs or in the systemic circulation. Rarely a portion or all of a thrombus may become detached from the wall of an atrium or be attached by a thin pedicle in such a way as to occlude the mitral or tricuspid orifice intermittently (ball-valve thrombus, 3.46; 5.23).

Atrial mural thrombosis is commonly encountered in rheumatic heart disease, particularly in association with active rheumatic infection, with atrial fibrillation, or with mitral stenosis. Ventricular mural thrombi are most often encountered in myocardial infarction involving the endocardium (16.2) but are also seen in endocardial fibroelastosis and in certain of the ventricular hypertrophies of unknown cause.

In the presence of atrial fibrillation, myocardial infarction, cardiac failure of any cause, mitral stenosis, or recurrent rheumatic activity with old valvulitis, the diagnosis is suggested by the following signs:

Embolic manifestations in the systemic or pulmonary circulation.

Angiocardiographic evidence of thrombi in the atria when they are large.

28. Neoplasm of the Endocardium

Myxomas arise from the endocardium most often in the region of the fossa ovalis of the left atrium, but sometimes they appear on the valves. They may vary from a few millimeters to as much as 6 cm in diameter, and are usually attached to a short stalk. These tumors are of clinical interest because their size, location, and pedunculated nature occasionally allow them to block an orifice of the heart, usually the mitral, and cause syncope. They may be accompanied by prolonged, low-grade fever, auscultatory phenomena resembling mitral stenosis, and systemic myxomatous emboli. Myxoma in the right atrium may imitate the clinical picture of constrictive pericarditis. The diagnosis can at times be confirmed by angiocardiography.

Fibromas and other endocardial tumors (sarcomas) of the heart are less frequent. They may be suspected if they alter the contour of the heart, obstruct blood flow through it, or alter the electrocardiogram.

29. Other Structural Diseases of the Endocardium or Valves (Specify Location, If Possible)

These include conditions not mentioned in any of the other categories, e.g., tuberculous endocarditis, endocardial blood cysts, and endocardial pockets (23.3, 10).

30. Rupture of Valve or of Chordae Tendineae (Specify Valve)

Valvular rupture is most frequently caused by bacterial endocarditis or trauma (accidental or surgical). Sudden compression of the thorax or a self-sealing penetrating wound may cause rupture or tearing of a valve or of the endocardium without cardiac tamponade. A tear in the atrial endocardium is usually diagnosed only at necropsy. Rupture of a valve or a chorda can be suggested by the following signs appearing in the course of bacterial endocarditis or following thoracic trauma:

Sudden pain in the chest and dyspnea.
Sudden development of a loud murmur, often musical, which may be accompanied by a thrill.
Rapid development of congestive heart failure.

31. Valvular Deformity (Specify Valve)

This condition is the result of acute or chronic disease affecting the valve. It is most often the sequel of rheumatic valvulitis and less frequently of syphilitic or bacterial valvulitis. It may be produced by atherosclerosis. Hemodynamic trauma from excess flow across a valve (as with arteriovenous fistula) may also be a cause, and there may be a possible chemical origin as in serotonin heart disease (2.4).

31.1.   AORTIC INSUFFICIENCY.   When the lesion is extensive, it may be associated with the anginal syndrome. The diagnosis of aortic insufficiency should be made only in the presence of a characteristic murmur.

Signs:
A diastolic murmur, high-pitched, blowing, decrescendo, occasionally musical, and rarely accompanied by a thrill. It may, if faint, be heard best with the ear directly applied to the chest. Audibility is better with the diaphragm type or shallow-chamber type of stethoscope chest piece than with the bell type. The murmur is usually loudest in the third or fourth interspace at the left border of the sternum or in the second or third interspace at the right border of the sternum; it is less often clearly heard in the apical

area. It is heard best with a relatively slow heart rate, with the breath held in expiration, and with the patient sitting or standing and leaning forward. When aortic insufficiency is marked, a systolic murmur or rarely a systolic thrill may be present in the aortic area, despite the absence of aortic stenosis.

Large pulse pressure, with lowered diastolic and elevated systolic pressures.

Collapsing pulse.

Apex beat heaving, displaced to the left and downward.

Roentgenographic examination shows enlargement of the left ventricle (**29.2**). The ascending aorta may be dilated and show pulsations of increased amplitude (**29.10**). Aorticoventricular regurgitation may be visualized on a selective aortogram.

Electrocardiographic evidence of left ventricular hypertrophy (**3.38.3**) in advanced cases.

31.2.   AORTIC STENOSIS.   This valvular lesion is usually associated with some degree of aortic insufficiency but may occur as an isolated lesion, especially in the older age group. It may be associated with the anginal syndrome. Attacks of syncope and sudden death may occur.

Signs:

Loud, harsh, systolic, crescendo-decrescendo murmur heard best in the first or second interspace at the right border of the sternum. The murmur and systolic thrill, if present, are transmitted to the carotid arteries. The murmur is often quite loud over the lower precordium and is easily confused with the murmur of mitral insufficiency. Both murmur and thrill are best observed in the expiratory phase of respiration with the patient leaning forward.

Systolic thrill, best felt in the first or second interspace at the right border of the sternum. The thrill, however, is neither characteristic of nor necessary for the diagnosis.

The second sound in the aortic area is usually faint or

absent with advanced obstruction to flow, but it may be
normal or even increased in intensity in the milder grades.
Occasionally the second sound displays paradoxical splitting in the pulmonic area, with the split becoming narrower or disappearing with inspiration.

Apex beat slowly heaving, displaced to the left and downward. In "tight" aortic stenosis, the heart rate is characteristically slow, the pulse is anacrotic and rises slowly to a
low, sustained plateau. Although the systolic blood pressure is low with a small pulse pressure, many exceptions
occur, especially in the presence of aortic insufficiency or
hypertension.

Roentgenographic examination reveals enlargement of the
left ventricle and often shows calcification of the aortic
valve and annulus. The ascending aorta may be dilated,
especially in the congenital types.

Electrocardiographic evidence of hypertrophy of the left
ventricle (3.38.3), frequently with widening of the QRS
interval but without deviation of the electrical axis of
QRS to the left.

Phonocardiography reveals the diamond shape of the systolic, ejection type murmur, which is midsystolic and
terminates in advance of a second aortic sound. The latter
is delayed and either fuses with the pulmonic component
or falls after it. These auscultatory features will vary with
the degree of stenosis.

Ventriculo-aortic gradient of systolic pressure across the aortic
valve as determined by catheterization of the left heart.

The aortic orifice must be reduced to approximately three-
quarters of normal to have an adverse effect on the circulation. A severe degree of aortic stenosis is indicated by changes
in the peripheral pulse, left ventricular hypertrophy (in the
absence of other causes), and by the finding, on left heart
catheterization or at operation, of a conspicuous systolic gradient of pressure across the aortic orifice in the presence of adequate forward flow.

31.3. MITRAL INSUFFICIENCY. Deformity of the mitral valve, caused by rheumatic fever and less frequently by atheromatous changes or bacterial infection, may give rise to mitral insufficiency. Dilatation of the mitral annulus due to myocardial disease may give rise to similar dynamics and signs (5.13.2).

Signs:

Pansystolic, loud, relatively high-pitched, blowing or musical apical murmur transmitted to the left axilla or back.

Loud pulmonic second sound.

A third sound often heard in early diastole which cannot be distinguished from a rapid-filling gallop sound.

The opening mitral snap present without accompanying mitral stenosis.

A short early diastolic murmur due to rapid filling of the left ventricle or to a minor degree of mitral stenosis.

Forceful apex beat displaced to the left and downward.

Roentgenographic examination reveals enlargement of the left ventricle and atrium, the latter grown occasionally to "giant" proportions and showing systolic pulsation.

Calcification of the mitral valve and, in the advanced stages, enlargement of the right chambers.

High V wave with rapidly descending limb terminating in an early and conspicuous "Y" trough may occur in the wedge pressure pulse or in the left atrial pressure pulse obtained by means of the cardiac catheter.

31.4. MITRAL STENOSIS. The underlying valvular deformity is most commonly caused by rheumatic fever.

Signs:

Apex impulse displaced to the left and brief, sharp, but not heaving.

Diastolic thrill in the apical area.

In "tight" mitral stenosis, a heaving systolic pulsation felt to the left of the sternum, caused by a hypertrophied right ventricle.

The characteristic murmur is a low-pitched presystolic or early diastolic rumble located at or just inside of the cardiac apex. The presystolic murmur is of crescendo character; in the presence of atrial fibrillation, the crescendo is absent, and only an early or prolonged diastolic murmur of decrescendo character is heard. At times the characteristic murmur can be elicited only after exercise or by having the patient lie on his left side, or both.

Loud, snapping first sound at the apex. The presence of such a sound together with the murmur of mitral insufficiency should arouse suspicion of mitral stenosis.

The second sound at the pulmonic area may be accentuated. It is often followed by a mitral opening snap best heard at the lower left sternal border, but occasionally audible over a wide area. There may be splitting of the second sound.

Roentgenographic examination reveals enlargement of the left atrium and right ventricle and often dilatation of the pulmonary artery (**29.3**, 14). Calcification of the mitral valve may be seen (**29.8**). There is little or no left ventricular enlargement.

The electrocardiogram shows a relatively vertical axis of QRS and less frequently a right deviation of the axis and signs of right ventricular hypertrophy. Large, broad, notched P waves are often seen, especially in leads I and II, and broad diphasic P waves are seen in lead V_1.

In the majority of cases of mitral valvular deformity, insufficiency and stenosis are combined, although one of the hemodynamic faults predominates. The presence of a presystolic or long diastolic murmur, a loud snapping first sound, and a mitral opening snap speak for predominant stenosis. On the other hand, the finding of a heaving apex beat, signs of left axis deviation or left ventricular hypertrophy in the electrocardiogram, and a rapid descent of the V wave in the left atrial pressure curve are in favor of mitral insufficiency. Although a loud, pansystolic, regurgitant type of murmur in the apical area usually indicates mitral insufficiency, this dynamic defect may also occur in the absence of such a murmur.

In a few cases of aortic insufficiency, there is heard at the apex a diastolic murmur simulating the murmur of mitral stenosis (Austin Flint murmur). If aortic insufficiency is of rheumatic origin, a rumbling diastolic murmur at the apex may be due to mitral stenosis.

31.5.   TRICUSPID INSUFFICIENCY ⎫
31.6.   TRICUSPID STENOSIS ⎬   At necropsy minor struc-
tural deformities of the tricuspid valve are not uncommonly seen in hearts displaying rheumatic disease elsewhere. Deformities severe enough to cause insufficiency or stenosis or both are not frequent. Invariably they are associated with other valvular deformities, especially mitral stenosis. Tricuspid insufficiency is more often the result of myocardial disease and consequent dilatation of the tricuspid annulus ("functional" tricuspid insufficiency or tricuspid annular incompetency [5.13]) than an effect of rheumatic valvular deformity. Bacterial endocarditis involving the tricuspid valve may occasionally produce tricuspid insufficiency or stenosis.

The presence of tricuspid valvular deformity may be suspected in a rheumatic patient with mitral stenosis who has recurrent ascites, a persistently enlarged liver, and engorged neck veins, but who may be free of orthopnea. Murmurs do not always contribute to the diagnosis of tricuspid deformity since they may be absent, or, if present, they cannot be readily distinguished from those of usually coexisting lesions of the mitral valve.

Symptoms and Signs of Tricuspid Valvular Disease:
   Cyanosis often combined with icterus.
   Recurrent ascites.
   Orthopnea is unusual and may be absent even with associated mitral stenosis.
   Roentgenologic examination shows enlargement of the right atrium and unexpectedly clear lung fields.

Right deviation of the axis of QRS is common with fibrillation of the atria.

Signs of Tricuspid Insufficiency:

Systolic pulsation of the cervical veins, of the liver, and sometimes of the veins of the extremities.

A large V wave in the right atrial pressure pulse, in the jugular phlebogram, and in the hepatogram.

Systolic depression of the precordial area. In the presence of advanced tricuspid insufficiency, the lower half of the chest moves briskly from left to right in systole.

A systolic murmur in the tricuspid area becoming louder during inspiration.

The signs of tricuspid annular incompetency ("functional" insufficiency) are almost identical to those of organic tricuspid insufficiency, and differentiation of the two by signs alone is not possible.

Signs of Tricuspid Stenosis:

Forceful, palpable, presystolic pulsation of the cervical veins, and a similar expansile pulsation of the liver.

Prominent A wave and slow descent of the V wave in the jugular phlebogram and in the right atrial pressure pulse.

A presystolic or early diastolic rumble, louder during inspiration, and a snapping first sound audible well to the right of the sternum.

A diastolic gradient of pressure across the tricuspid orifice.

32. *Valvular Sclerosis (Specify Valve)*

By valvular sclerosis is meant involvement and deformity of a valve by arteriosclerosis or other degenerative process (cf. Valvulitis, Inactive, 3.34). In the more advanced stages calcification is present. The aortic and mitral valves are most commonly affected. Occasionally the rings of these valves are also involved, producing rigid, collar-like lesions.

The mitral leaflets, especially the anterior one, are often calcified, but since only portions of the leaflets are involved, their function usually is not disturbed. The condition may be suspected clinically in the presence of a loud, harsh or musical systolic murmur in the apical area, with or without a palpable thrill except when aortic stenosis is also present, in which case the murmur is probably transmitted from the aortic area (3.31.2).

In elderly subjects, the aortic valve may be sclerotic, calcified, and deformed, the mitral valve frequently remaining normal. This may result in stenosis with or without insufficiency of the valve. The physical signs are commonly those of aortic stenosis rather than insufficiency. It is often difficult to decide whether the calcification is due to a degenerative process (principally the Mönckeberg type of arteriosclerosis) or is the result of an old rheumatic or bacterial valvulitis. In the former there usually are no signs referable to the mitral valve, and a history of rheumatic infection is lacking. The degree of deformity of the aortic valve determines the presence or absence of enlargement of the heart.

The presence of calcium in the valves may be demonstrated by appropriate roentgenologic techniques (**29.**8). Fluoroscopy is usually the most helpful.

33. Valvulitis, Active* (Specify Deformity, If Any)

Active valvulitis is most commonly observed as a part of rheumatic endocarditis (**19.**2), although bacterial endocarditis (3.24; **23.**1) and syphilis may also involve the valvular structure.

The process may be either acute or chronic, the differentiation being chiefly the duration of the inflammation. Chronic active valvulitis implies continued activity of the infection within the valve over a long period of time, the exact duration not being prescribed.

---

* *Active* and *inactive* refer to the etiologic agent. *Acute, chronic, healing,* and *healed* apply to the nature of the tissue response to this agent.

Acute rheumatic valvulitis is frequently part of a pancarditis in which the myocardium, endocardium, valves, and pericardium are involved.

Both the endocardium and the supporting tissues of the valves are affected. The valve most commonly involved is the mitral, less often the aortic, sometimes the tricuspid, and least frequently the pulmonic.

In the acute stage of rheumatic valvulitis, the inflammatory changes are not of sufficient degree to cause deformity or dysfunction of the valve. The associated myocarditis, however, may cause dilatation of the annulus with resulting valvular incompetency. Thus, at best, the diagnosis of acute rheumatic valvulitis is an inferential diagnosis made from certain physical signs which may have various causes and which may disappear with subsidence of the active stage. If the signs persist in the inactive phase, it may be concluded that valvular deformity has developed.

Acute active mitral valvulitis may be suspected in the course of a rheumatic infection when a systolic, apical murmur, usually blowing in character, can be heard. Occasionally, especially in children, a transient, low-pitched mid-diastolic murmur may be heard in the apical area.

In the presence of *acute active aortic valvulitis,* a high-pitched diastolic murmur like that of aortic insufficiency may occur. This murmur also is often transient and is more likely to occur in children.

In the presence of *chronic active valvulitis,* progressive valvular deformity of permanent nature usually develops. The murmurs described above become permanent and assume the characteristics that are mentioned under Valvular Deformity (3.31).

In most instances of active rheumatic valvulitis, clinical manifestations of disease of other cardiac tissues will be present, especially those due to inflammation of the myocardium (3.41). There will also be systemic and serologic evidence of activity of the rheumatic agent.

49

Signs:

Appearance of a murmur or murmurs, systolic or diastolic, in the apical or aortic area, during the course of rheumatic fever.

Enlargement of the heart.

Evidence of active myocarditis.

34. Valvulitis, Inactive

Recovery from acute valvulitis may occasionally be complete and without deformity; more often there is localized or extensive scarring (healed valvulitis or valvular fibrosis).

The clinical diagnosis of healed valvulitis is based on finding, in a patient known to have had rheumatic or bacterial infection in the past, the signs of valvular deformity, usually a systolic murmur, without evidence of activity of the etiologic factor and without evidence of a hemodynamic defect such as stenosis or insufficiency. If one of the latter defects has been produced, then the anatomic diagnosis is only of that defect (mitral stenosis, aortic insufficiency, or the like), the inactive valvulitis being implied.

Diseases of the Myocardium

35. Aneurysm of the Heart

The lesion in aneurysm of the heart is a localized bulge or outward protrusion of the wall of the heart. Of variable dimensions, the protrusion is usually in the left ventricle, and is the result of a transmural myocardial infarct (**16**.6). The area of scar tissue weakens and dilates with systole. Previous history, physical signs, and characteristic roentgenologic findings determine the diagnosis. The aneurysm may be more or less filled with thrombus, in which case it will show little or no systolic expansion. Although there are no characteristic symptoms, ventricular aneurysms may be associated with the following specific signs:

Small aneurysm: The only detectable change is roentgeno-graphic—on fluoroscopy a small outward bulging of the left ventricular wall during systole. Sometimes the altered contour can be detected in a roentgenogram of the heart in a suitable projection.

Large aneurysm: There may be an abnormal precordial systolic pulsation medial to and above the apex. On fluoroscopy the aneurysm may bulge further during sys-tole. The heart may become enlarged, effective cardiac output diminish, and congestive failure ensue. The elec-trocardiogram will usually show the changes of the old myocardial infarction. Persistent abnormal displacement of the S–T junction and segment, particularly in the thoracic leads, is not uncommon.

36. Atrophy of the Heart

Atrophy of the heart is usually recognized only at necropsy (24.7) but may be suspected in prolonged inanition. The heart is small and flabby, and shows brownish discoloration and in-dividual muscle fibers of abnormally small size. It is associated with chronic wasting diseases, and with old age. There is no cardiac insufficiency, and the condition is of no known clinical importance.

37. Degeneration of the Myocardium

Pathologically the parenchymatous degenerations which are recognized are cloudy swelling, fatty degeneration, and fatty infiltration.

In cloudy swelling the muscle is soft, flabby, swollen, gray or grayish brown and has a frosted glass appearance. This condition is sometimes found in infections with high fever (pneumonia, typhoid, diphtheria) and in metallic poisonings (mercury, copper).

Fatty degeneration, characterized by droplets of fat in the muscle fibers which often show as zigzag yellow lines (or "tigering"), is seen in severe anemia, in the infections at a somewhat later stage than that of cloudy swelling, and in poisonings (phosphorus, arsenic, chloroform, for example). Myocardial efficiency may be impaired, but this is not usually clinically detectable.

Fatty infiltration, which occurs infrequently in excessively obese individuals, is an infiltration and replacement of muscle tissue by fat, especially in the right ventricle (24.4). There may be cardiac enlargement and insufficiency of either or both ventricles.

There are no characteristic symptoms or signs of any of these degenerations. Physical signs, electrocardiographic abnormalities, and presence or absence of cardiac failure will depend upon the location, diffuseness, and severity of the lesions.

38. Enlargement of the Heart

Enlargement beyond normal limits in the size of one or more chambers of the heart (13.2) may be acute or chronic and may be caused by dilatation of the chambers, hypertrophy of their walls, or both.

38.1. DILATATION. Simple dilatation of the heart without hypertrophy is usually acute (16.10; 17.2). A normal heart exposed to extreme stress in an untrained subject may dilate, returning to normal shortly after cessation of stress. Acute right ventricular dilatation may occur in any individual with pulmonary embolism (3.8).

38.2. HYPERTROPHY. A "concentric" left ventricular hypertrophy with little or no enlargement of the ventricular chamber is seen in some cases of arterial hypertension (17.1) or aortic stenosis (3.31.2). Concentric hypertrophy of the right ventricle occurs with pulmonary stenosis.

38.3. HYPERTROPHY AND DILATATION

a. *Right atrium.* The most common causes of isolated or predominant right atrial hypertrophy and dilatation are those associated with congenital heart lesions (4). Rheumatic disease involving the tricuspid valve often results in right atrial hypertrophy and dilatation, which is sometimes extreme, especially with tricuspid stenosis. Rare conditions include right-sided bacterial endocarditis, massive thrombus or tumor in the right atrium, and malignant carcinoid with tricuspid lesions. Right atrial enlargement can usually be determined by fluoroscopy or roentgenography, although it is more precisely determined by angiocardiography (**39.5**). The electrocardiogram may show increased voltage of the P wave in leads II and III and in the right-sided precordial leads.

b. *Left atrium.* Mitral stenosis and mitral insufficiency usually of rheumatic origin are by far the most common causes of left atrial enlargement. Other causes are mitral valvular lesions of bacterial or congenital origin, thrombus or tumor of the left atrium, or left ventricular failure. An apparent enlargement backward of the left atrium may actually be a displacement caused by enlargement of other chambers. The electrocardiogram may show broad, notched P waves of increased duration, and in right precordial leads a diphasic P wave with a prolonged, late, downward phase. The most common cause of these effects is left ventricular insufficiency.

c. *Right ventricle.* Mitral stenosis and certain congenital cardiac malformations are commonly associated with hypertrophy or dilatation of the right ventricle. Right ventricular hypertrophy or dilatation that is secondary to diseases affecting the lungs is termed *cor pulmonale* (**2.**12).

Signs:

Forceful systolic (precordial) heave. If the chest is deep and emphysematous, the cardiac impulse is best palpated, and heart sounds are best heard just below the xiphoid.

53

The sound of pulmonic valve closure is characteristically accentuated.

On roentgenography the enlargement may be found chiefly at the base to the left (outflow tract) or at the inferior border of the cardiac silhouette (inflow tract). In the lateral view the heart tends to fill the retrosternal space. In the oblique projections the enlargement is seen to involve the anterior (right) ventricle (29.3).

In the electrocardiogram, leads to the right of the sternum will present a prominent R or R', a late intrinsicoid deflection, and occasionally a small Q wave or inverted T wave. Leads from the left side of the precordium will show a small R wave and a deep S wave. The unipolar right arm lead may have a large R deflection. The mean electrical axis in the frontal plane will usually be deviated to the right.

d. *Left ventricle.*   Left ventricular hypertrophy may be associated with arterial hypertension, mitral insufficiency, aortic valvular lesions, many forms of intrinsic myocardial disease, and some congenital anomalies such as those with a left-to-right shunt at the ventricular or aorticopulmonary level.

Signs:

The heart is enlarged downward and to the left with maximum impulse, usually strong and heaving, at the apex. Weakened, dilated hearts, however, may have a diminished apical impulse. The sounds, both at apex and base, vary greatly, depending upon the strength and quality of cardiac systole and upon attendant cardiac lesions.

Roentgenography shows enlargement to the left, downward, and backward.

The electrocardiogram shows: in the right precordial leads, a deep S wave and a large upright T wave; in the left precordial leads, a high R wave, a late intrinsicoid

deflection, and often a Q wave of conspicuous amplitude. The S–T segment may be depressed and the T
wave diphasic or inverted, although in certain dynamic
situations the latter may be unusually tall and peaked.
There is often left axis deviation of QRS.

e. *Generalized cardiac hypertrophy and dilatation.* Multiple
valvular lesions or diffuse myocardial disease of various origins leads to both left-sided and right-sided heart failure and
often results in generalized dilatation of all chambers. Physical signs, confirmed by fluoroscopy and roentgenography,
will give evidence of the latter. An electrocardiogram may
show a preponderance of one side or the other, or it may
show only evidence of a lesion such as old myocardial infarction.

39. Fibrosis of the Myocardium

In fibrosis the myocardium is replaced in variable degree by
fibrous tissue. The process may be local (healed myocardial
infarct) or diffuse. The latter is seen most often in patients
with impaired coronary arterial flow and in those with healed
myocarditis of rheumatic or other origin. The fibrosis may be
largely subendocardial, as in fibroelastosis, or subepicardial, as
in chronic pericarditis.

The signs and other manifestations are of the underlying
disease; there may be no clinical signs or symptoms of the
fibrosis. Suspicion of the entity, when there is no obvious clinical cause, may be raised by the presence of an enlarged heart,
especially when the electrocardiogram displays an arrhythmia,
unexplained abnormalities of QRS and T, or intraventricular
or atrioventricular block.

40. Infarction of the Myocardium

40.1.   ATRIAL INFARCTION.   This lesion occurs in conjunction
with approximately 10 percent of the cases of ventricular in-

55

farction. It may be suspected from a disturbance of atrial rhythm in the course of ventricular infarction. Rarely it may be recognized by electrocardiographic abnormalities. The apex of the P wave may be sharply pointed and of increased amplitude. The T_P wave may be altered in a manner similar to that of the ventricular S–T segment and T wave in ventricular infarction.

40.2. VENTRICULAR INFARCTION.   This lesion is the result of deficiency in coronary flow of a degree so advanced that the nutrition of a localized portion of the ventricular myocardium is affected. It may be due to thrombotic, atheromatous, embolic, or other occlusive disease of the coronary arteries (**16.**1–2). It may also occur in the distribution of a coronary artery with extreme narrowing of the lumen but without occlusion or thrombosis. The precipitating factor in such cases may be a temporarily increased demand for coronary blood due to prolonged and unusual effort or a diminished coronary flow due to shock, hemorrhage, or prolonged tachycardia. There may, however, be no obvious physiologic disturbance. In patients with hypertension and advanced cardiac hypertrophy, the disproportion between muscle mass and vascular supply may afford a basis for infarction without occlusion.

The location and extent of the infarction depend in part upon the position and caliber of the coronary arteries supplying the area and in part upon the adequacy of the collateral circulation to the area. Infarction may be localized in the anterior and apical portions of the left ventricle and in the adjacent portion of the ventricular septum. Infarction of the posterior and diaphragmatic portions of the left ventricle is also common and often includes the posterior portion of the septum. The right ventricle is infrequently affected by infarction except by extension from the adjacent septum.

The extent of infarction varies greatly. It is more commonly confined to the subendocardial region but may be transmural, intramural, or subepicardial.

Symptoms:

Upper retrosternal constriction usually present. It is of sudden onset, with radiation to a part or all of one or both arms, to the throat or lower jaw, or to the interscapular region. Most often it occurs while the patient is at rest, and occasionally during or just after severe effort or stressful emotions. The sensation is often described as pressing, squeezing, or crushing, and is usually not relieved by nitroglycerin. Constriction is usually prolonged for several hours but may be fleeting. At times the pain is mild or even absent. Occasionally it may be epigastric or low retrosternal. The pain is often accompanied by nausea, vomiting, and sweating. Rarely the onset is characterized only by dyspnea and a sense of suffocation.

Signs:

Weakness, sweating, collapse.

Pallor, with or without cyanosis.

Faint heart sounds.

Pericardial friction rub (delayed).

Cardiac arrhythmia.

Gallop rhythm.

Basal rales of pulmonary edema or other manifestations of cardiac failure.

Falling blood pressure, sometimes after an initial period of elevation.

Fever (delayed).

Leukocytosis (delayed).

Elevated sedimentation rate (delayed).

Elevated serum glutamic oxaloacetic transaminase.

Electrocardiographic records may reveal disturbances of rhythm and conduction. The effects of local necrosis and ischemia may be apparent in the QRS deflections, S–T segments, and T waves. The particular electrocardiographic features will be determined by the size, location (spatial and mural), and age of the lesion and by the degree of injury. Some characteristic changes are: The

57

QRS group may show low voltage in the limb leads. Often, with an infarct in the posterodiaphragmatic area, a large or relatively large Q_3 will appear; in the anterolateral area, a large Q_1 will appear. Lead II may also show a large Q wave in either case. In the precordial, extremity, and esophageal leads, the QRS group may show changes of three principal types: (1) an entirely negative deflection, QS, which may be notched or slurred to a variable degree (this may be called the central type QRS, for it is obtained when the electrode is placed directly over the center of an experimental infarct); (2) an abnormally deep or broad initial deflection, Q, followed by an R wave, usually smaller than normal, and occasionally also by an S wave (this may be called the marginal type QRS, for it is obtained when the exploring electrode is placed over the margin of an experimental infarct); (3) no characteristic changes in QRS or simply a change in the magnitude of the individual deflections, causing, often along with a minor prolongation of the QRS interval, deviation of the electrical axis to the left (anterior infarction) or to the right (posterodiaphragmatic infarction).

The S–T junction and segment may be elevated or depressed. This displacement is usually temporary. Reciprocal deviation of the S–T segment is usually encountered in leads I and III, lead I showing elevation with anterior and lead III with posterior infarction.

Subendocardial necrosis in the left ventricle may cause depression of the S–T segment of leads I and II and the left precordial leads, and elevation in lead V_R and the esophageal leads.

Deviation of the S–T segment usually gives way after a variable time to a T wave directed opposite to the original S–T displacement.

An abnormal form of the T wave may be the only evidence of recent myocardial necrosis. This abnormality may be transient or permanent. If transient, it remains for a longer time than do the S–T segment abnormalities when present. Since alterations in the S–T segment and T wave are initially rapidly progressive and then slowly regressive, serial electrocardiograms may be necessary to demonstrate them.

Although localization of the infarct in the heart can be made in a gross way from the electrocardiogram, attempts at exact anatomic definition may be quite inaccurate.

41. *Myocarditis, Active*

Active myocarditis, an inflammation of the myocardium in which the etiologic agent continues to operate, may be differentiated clinically into acute, subacute, and chronic forms depending upon an arbitrary duration of the inflammatory process (24.1). Chronic active myocarditis implies continued or frequently recurrent activity of the etiologic agent and the presence in the heart of all stages (acute, healing, healed) of inflammatory morbidity.

Myocarditis occurs most often in rheumatic fever (19.1) but may be encountered in a great variety of infections of bacterial, viral (including the acute exanthemata), and protozoal (Chagasic myocarditis) origin (24.1). It is common in the course of subacute bacterial endocarditis.

The clinical course may vary from mild, with the disease manifesting itself only by nonspecific, serial alterations in the electrocardiogram, to severe, often with rapid or sudden death.

Signs:

Sinus tachycardia (rarely bradycardia).

Abnormal rhythms, including gallop rhythm.

Enlargement of the heart.

Faint or snapping quality of the first heart sound.

Cardiac insufficiency.

Defective intraventricular or atrioventricular conduction and abnormal final ventricular deflections (S–T and T).

Increased serum glutamic oxaloacetic transaminase.

Constitutional and special manifestations of the basic infection (fever, leukocytosis, increased sedimentation rate, increased C-reactive protein, positive blood culture).

42. Neoplasm of the Heart (Specify Type)

Primary neoplasm is uncommon and is rarely diagnosed during life. Metastatic neoplasm may be suspected in the course of malignant disease elsewhere in the body if cardiac symptoms or signs develop, particularly atrial fibrillation or hemorrhagic pericardial effusion. Occasionally primary tumors (myxomas) or secondary neoplasms arising from the wall of the atrium may grow in a polyp-like fashion and obstruct the mitral or tricuspid orifice, thereby causing the signs of mitral or tricuspid stenosis (3.31.4, 5, 6). There may be acute respiratory distress and severe cyanosis when, in certain body postures, obstruction of the valvular orifice becomes nearly complete (5.23). Electrocardiographic abnormalities, especially inversion of the T wave and persistent displacement of the S–T junction and segment, are occasionally observed in the presence of tumors in the ventricular myocardium.

43. No Structural Disease of the Heart

44. Other Structural Diseases of the Heart (Specify Lesion)

This rubric includes conditions not mentioned in any other categories. It might include such lesions as those found in the myocardium with vitamin deficiency or electrolytic disturbances, or other specific metabolic cardiomyopathies (24.4.2).

45. Rupture of the Myocardium (Specify Location)

Rupture may follow myocardial infarction or injury of the chest, especially if the latter is of the crushing type. It usually gives rise to precordial pain and may be followed rapidly by pulmonary edema, which may be fatal. Rupture into the pericardial sac causes hemopericardium and cardiac tamponade; except in rare instances death follows immediately. Rupture of the ventricular septum secondary to recent infarction gives rise to a systolic thrill and to a loud, harsh systolic murmur which is loudest along the left border of the sternum in the fourth interspace. Rupture of a papillary muscle resulting in mitral insufficiency may cause a systolic thrill and a loud, often musical, murmur in the apical region.

46. Thrombosis Within the Heart (Specify Chamber)

This rubric applies to the rare thrombus occurring free in a chamber or attached to the endocardium by a thin pedicle. The specific syndrome which may result is ascribed to intermittent ball-valve action of the thrombus. Seen most often in mitral stenosis with atrial fibrillation, it is characterized by attacks of dyspnea, cyanosis, syncope, or abrupt exitus (5.23). There may also be intermittent emboli, to the systemic circulation particularly, which arise from the surface of the intracardiac thrombus as in mural thrombosis (3.27).

47. Trauma of the Heart

Clinical signs and symptoms vary with the nature of the trauma (e.g., bullet wound, stab wound, severe blow on the chest, fall, or crushing injury) and the extent and location of the lesion. In contusion of the heart as a result of crushing of the chest (e.g., steering-wheel accident), transient disturbances in rhythm may occur. Displacement of the S–T junction and segment and changes in the T wave in the electrocardiogram may serve as evidence of injury to the myocardium. Clinical and electrocardiographic findings may simulate those of myocardial infarction. Hemopericardium is a common sequel of severe injuries of the heart, often with acute cardiac tamponade. Rupture of the heart may occur (3.45).

61

48. Undiagnosed Structural Disease of the Heart (Specify Location, If Possible)

Diseases of the Pericardium

49. Calcification of the Pericardium

Occasionally calcium is deposited locally or diffusely in pericardial adhesions. Calcification of the pericardium may be present without apparent embarrassment of the heart, or it may accompany the clinical syndrome of chronic constrictive pericarditis (3.56). The diagnosis is made only by roentgenographic examination; the densities produced by calcium are best observed in the oblique or lateral views (**29.8**).

50. Hemopericardium

Hemopericardium refers to the presence of blood in the pericardial sac and does not include serosanguinous effusions. It usually follows injury or rupture of the heart or aorta (**3.6**). Clinically, it is marked by rapid progression of the diagnostic phenomena of cardiac tamponade.

Signs:
   Small pulse pressure and signs of shock.
   Faint or absent heart sounds.
   Increase in area of cardiac dullness, especially dullness to flatness over the lower half of the sterum.
   Increased venous pressure.
   Electrocardiographic abnormalities of the S–T segment and of the T wave.
   Roentgenographic abnormalities: see 3.54.2

51. Hydropericardium

Hydropericardium occurs as part of the anasarca of advanced cardiac insufficiency or renal failure; it may be produced by neoplastic infiltration and it may also be seen in myxedema. The fluid is a transudate. The physical signs are the same as those for serofibrinous pericarditis (3.54.2), except that no friction rub is audible.

52. Neoplasm of the Pericardium

Primary neoplasm of the pericardium is rare and is usually diagnosed only at necropsy. Benign cysts are not uncommon and may be diagnosed by roentgenologic techniques. Secondary invasion by neoplasm, especially from the lungs, may occasionally occur. It may be suspected if there is a persistent effusion, particularly if this be hemorrhagic, and sometimes a positive diagnosis can be established by demonstrating neoplastic cells in the pericardial fluid or in a pericardial biopsy. The electrocardiogram may display nonspecific abnormalities which direct attention to the heart.

53. Other Structural Diseases of the Pericardium

This rubric includes diseases not specified elsewhere.

54. Pericarditis, Acute

54.1. FIBRINOUS. This type of pericarditis is often part of the pancarditis of rheumatic fever or of various infectious diseases. It may sometimes occur following upper respiratory infections believed to be of viral origin (nonspecific pericarditis, 25.3). It occurs in myocardial infarction if the lesion reaches the epicardial surface, in the postmyocardial infarction syndrome, in the postcardiotomy syndrome, in acute pulmonary embolism, and in uremia. It may result from pericardial invasion by neoplasm.

Symptoms and Signs:

Precordial pain may be present, characteristically increased by deep inspiration, relieved by sitting up, and often referred to the left shoulder.

Pericardial friction rub, superficial and harsh, usually heard near the left border of the lower third of the sternum and often louder during inspiration. It may be limited to systole or diastole, but it may be continuous with a to-and-fro character. It may last for a few hours or for days.

Fever and leukocytosis, when present, occur early.

Electrocardiogram: Elevation of the S–T junction and segment usually in leads I and II and in those unipolar extremity and precordial leads which are semidirect leads from the area of the involved pericardium. This displacement is temporary, and as it disappears the T wave becomes diphasic or inverted in the same leads. In certain instances there may be nonspecific electrocardiographic abnormalities or none at all.

54.2. SEROFIBRINOUS. The causes of this type are usually the same as for the fibrinous type. An effusion, exudative in nature and variable in amount, occurs and may be sanguinous.

Signs:

Faint heart sounds.

Dullness and bronchial breathing in left infrascapular area with a large effusion.

Pericardial friction rub usually limited to the basal portion of the heart.

Paradoxical pulse.

Roentgenogram: Enlarged cardiac silhouette with a widened vascular pedicle and indistinct segmentation along the left contour, with diminished or absent pulsations.

Electrocardiogram: Abnormal S–T segment and T wave, as

described above (3.54.1). If a large effusion occurs, the voltage of the QRS complexes may be low.

54.3. SUPPURATIVE. The signs of this type are the same as those of serofibrinous pericarditis (3.54.2), plus evidence of sepsis. If the purulent effusion takes place rapidly, the signs of tamponade may occur (3.50).

55. Pericarditis, Chronic

The separation of pericarditis into acute and chronic types is made arbitrarily on the basis of the duration of symptoms and signs. Chronic pericarditis is frequently of rheumatic or tuberculous origin; less frequent causes are other infections and tumors. The formation of localized adhesions may be a sequel of chronic pericarditis and may also result from myocardial infarction or injury.

55.1. SEROFIBRINOUS. The signs are the same as those of serofibrinous pericarditis (3.54).

55.2. SEROUS. Tuberculosis is probably the most common cause of this form. The amount of effusion is usually considerably greater than in the serofibrinous form. The signs are the same as those of serofibrinous pericarditis (3.54), but a pericardial friction rub is usually lacking.

55.3. ADHESIVE WITHOUT CONSTRICTION. The diagnosis of this type cannot be made unless there is calcification of the adhesions between the pericardium and mediastinal structures shown by roentgenogram.

55.4. CONSTRICTIVE. This type is frequently of unknown cause but may be the sequel of viral, tuberculous, or septic infection, of rheumatic disease, or of the organization of a hemopericardium following trauma. The clinical picture may

65

vary with the site of the constriction, whether affecting chiefly the atria, the ventricles, the atrioventricular grooves, or the venous orifices. The heart may be enlarged but is often normal or even small. The adhesions may become calcified.

Signs:

Distended cervical veins with rapid diastolic collapse.

Increased venous pressure (250–400 mm H_2O).

Low arterial pressure with small pulse pressure in severe cases.

Diffuse systolic depression of the left side of the anterior chest wall (ribs and interspaces) followed by a palpable diastolic rebound and sound ("pericardiac vibration").

Roentgenography usually reveals a normal or small heart, small or absent pulsations of constricted areas (fluoroscopy or roentgenkymography), and calcification of the pericardium.

Low voltage of QRS complexes and low voltage or inversion of T waves.

Elevation of right ventricular end-diastolic pressure and right atrial mean pressure with early diastolic "dip" in the pressure pulse.

Recurrent ascites.

Enlarged liver.

56. Pneumopericardium

This disease is most often a result of injury and is often complicated by serous, suppurative, or sanguinous effusion. Instrumentation of the esophagus, direct diagnostic cardiac puncture, and surgical pericardiotomy are the most frequent causes. Tympany replaces the cardiac dullness, and, if fluid is present, splashing or churning sounds may be heard with systole. On roentgenologic examination, the air within the pericardium is apparent.

57. Trauma to the Pericardium

Bullet or stab wounds may involve the pericardium at times without injury to the myocardium. Instrumentation of the esophagus, particularly dilatation of strictures, may lead to perforation of the pericardium. Foreign bodies may also reach the pericardial sac through the esophagus or the bronchi and give rise to suppurative pericarditis. Severe trauma may rupture the diaphragm and pericardium and result in herniation of the stomach and colon into the pericardial sac.

The signs and symptoms will depend upon the character and extent of the injury and upon the occurrence of complications, e.g., hemorrhage or inflammation.

4 / The Anatomic Cardiac Diagnosis: Congenital Disease

Many congenital anomalies can be recognized on the basis of the history, physical signs, electrocardiogram, fluoroscopy, and roentgenogram. Most can be diagnosed when these data are combined with the results of cardiac catheterization and visualization of the entire heart (intravenous angiocardiography) or of selected portions (selective angiocardiography or aortography) by injection of contrasting substances (27.5). In the classification which follows, either isolated anomalies or common combinations of anomalies are described. Multiple malformations do occur, and each may modify the manifestations of the others.

Noncyanotic Group

As a solitary anomaly, each of the following malformations is characterized by the absence of an abnormal anatomic or functional communication between the systemic and pulmonic circulations.

1. Coarctation of the Aorta

A narrowing of the aorta sufficient to produce a systolic pressure gradient across the obstruction (15.64). Usually there is a diaphragm of tissue within the aorta at the coarcted site, and there is a poststenotic dilatation. The common location is just distal to the left subclavian artery at the level of the ligamentum arteriosum, but it may occur at any region in the thoracic or abdominal aorta and may be multiple. The narrowing may be localized or diffuse. If the ductus arteriosus should be patent, the coarctation is designated as either preductal or postductal, depending upon its relation to that structure.

Signs:
>   Pulse larger and blood pressure higher in vessels proximal to coarctation than in those distal.
>
>   Systolic murmur posteriorly overlying the narrowed site.
>
>   Forceful pulsation of a dilated aorta in the suprasternal notch.
>
>   Evidence of collateral circulation (beyond early childhood) as visible and palpable pulsations over the back.
>
>   Roentgenogram: The aortic knob is inconspicuous, but the ascending aorta and the innominate and left subclavian arteries are dilated. Poststenotic dilatation of the descending part is visible beneath the knob. In the frontal view these irregularities of the aorta cause impressions on the barium-filled esophagus simulating the letter E (E sign).
>
>   In the LAO projection there is anterior displacement of the barium-filled esophagus by poststenotic dilatation of the aorta and sometimes by dilated vessels of collateral circulation.
>
>   Notching of the inferior margins of the ribs and of the internal aspect of the sternum (rare in young children).
>
>   Left ventricular enlargement with rounding of apex; lesser degrees of left atrial enlargement.

2. Vascular Ring

A ring of vessels in the region of the aortic arch encircling the trachea and esophagus. Usually the ring is formed by a right and left aortic arch which unite and continue as the descending aorta.

Symptoms:

Often lacking, but may be present if the ring is small, especially in infancy.

Signs:

Stridor on inspiration and expiration.

Dysphagia.

"Brassy" cough.

Susceptibility to bronchitis.

Roentgenogram: Barium-filled esophagus is indented and may be constricted by a retro-esophageal vessel. The arch of the aorta and path of the descending aorta are outlined by the barium in the esophagus.

Angiocardiogram: Opacification of the patent vessels forming the ring may be displayed.

3. Right Aortic Arch

Persistence of the fourth right branchial arch. The major branches emerge in the same order but in mirror image fashion as compared with a left aortic arch. The aorta generally descends on the right to the level of the diaphragm and then crosses to the usual position of the abdominal aorta (right aortic arch with right descending aorta); occasionally the aorta crosses behind the esophagus high in the thorax (right aortic arch with left descending aorta). Unless it forms part of a vascular ring (4.2), it produces no symptoms.

Signs:

Roentgenogram: Aortic knob is absent on the left but is visible on the right within, and often displacing laterally, the shadow of the right superior vena cava. The right aortic arch indents the barium-filled esophagus toward the left in the frontal view and toward the back in the LAO view. There is no indentation in the RAO view. With a right descending aorta, the barium in the esophagus on frontal view descends to the left of the midline. With a left descending aorta, the barium-filled esophagus, on oblique projections, curves anteriorly around the aorta as the latter crosses behind it to descend on the left; in the frontal view, the barium column descends in the midline.

4. Right Subclavian Artery, Anomalous Origin

Occasionally the right subclavian artery takes its origin not from the innominate artery but from the descending aorta as the fourth major vessel. It courses obliquely upward behind the esophagus to the right arm.

Symptoms:
    Ordinarily lacking, but dysphagia lusoria may be produced.

Signs:
    Roentgenogram: The oblique views demonstrate an anterior displacement of the upper barium-filled esophagus by a small retro-esophageal vessel, and the frontal projection reveals an oblique filling defect, lower on the left side and higher on the right.

5. Aneurysm of the Sinus of Valsalva

Dilatation of one or more of the sinuses of Valsalva due to a developmental anomaly of the aortic media.

Symptoms:
    Lacking unless rupture occurs; then usually severe pain in the chest and development of a loud murmur which may be detected by the patient himself.

Signs:
    Angiogram or aortogram demonstrates aneurysm with or without rupture.

Other signs are determined by the site of rupture: (1) Into right atrium or ventricle: signs of arteriovenous fistula with murmurs; development of high ventricular systolic wave (C wave) in jugular and hepatic pulses; arterialization of right heart blood; sometimes rapidly progressive right heart failure. (2) Into left ventricle: signs simulating aortic insufficiency. (3) Into pericardium: cardiac tamponade. (4) Into pulmonary artery: signs of arteriovenous fistula (4.32).

6. Coronary Artery, Anomalous Origin

When the left coronary artery arises from the pulmonary artery, symptoms of coronary insufficiency and subsequent death in early infancy result (15.55).

Signs:

Electrocardiogram shows depression of the S–T segment and inverted T wave in the left precordial and other leads without characteristic changes in the QRS.

Roentgenogram shows left ventricular enlargement.

Angiocardiogram confirms enlargement and displays thinning of the left ventricle, when present. Selective injection of contrast medium into the main pulmonary artery opacifies the anomalous left coronary artery.

Selective aortography demonstrates a single coronary artery arising from the aorta.

7. Aortic Stenosis, Congenital

Obstruction to the left ventricular outflow which is commonly valvular but which may be subvalvular (subaortic membranous or muscular stenosis) or supravalvular as a constricting ring in the aorta (15.9).

Symptoms:

When stenosis is severe, symptoms may include syncope, fatigability, heart failure, or sudden death.

Signs:

Ejection-type systolic murmur in aortic area, transmitted to the neck vessels. (In infants and young children this murmur may be along the left sternal border.)

Narrow pulse pressure, if severe anomaly.

Electrocardiogram: Usually there is a normal QRS axis. In the left precordial leads the R wave may be high and, if stenosis is severe, the S–T segment is depressed and the T wave inverted.

Roentgenogram: Poststenotic dilatation of ascending aorta if the stenosis is valvular. An enlarged left ventricle and lesser degrees of left atrial enlargement are demonstrated.

In subaortic muscular stenosis the carotid arteriogram is characterized by a prominent reversal on its anacrotic limb and a pulse pressure inversely proportional to the duration of the preceding diastole.

8. Aortic Insufficiency, Congenital

As an isolated malformation congenital aortic insufficiency is rare, but it sometimes occurs with ventricular septal defect, aneurysm of a sinus of Valsalva, or aortic stenosis (4.7).

Signs:

Same as those of acquired aortic insufficiency (3.31.1) but usually associated with other evidence of congenital heart disease and without a history of an acquired etiologic agent.

9. Endocardial Fibroelastosis

Thickening of the mural and sometimes valvular endocardium, usually of the left side of the heart, associated with ventricular hypertrophy (3.23). The affected cardiac chambers are often dilated, sometimes contracted. The disease occurs as an isolated malformation or accompanies conditions such as mitral

73

or aortic atresia, anomalous origin of a coronary artery, or certain malformations which produce great dilatation of the cardiac chambers (15.44).

Signs:

Dilated type: Suspected in infancy on the basis of sudden heart failure, often in the absence of murmurs, and with great cardiac enlargement, especially of the left heart. The electrocardiographic signs are of left ventricular hypertrophy with unusually high voltage of the QRS deflections (3.38.3). Diagnosis is by exclusion of other causes of left-sided enlargement.

Contracted type: Signs of pulmonary hypertension and right-sided cardiac enlargement on roentgenography. The electrocardiogram may display a variety of abnormalities, including those ascribed to right ventricular hypertrophy (3.38; 30.8).

10. Glycogen Storage Disease of the Myocardium

An inborn error of metabolism in which excessive glycogen accumulates in the large myocardial fibers and sometimes in the skeletal muscles and in the tongue (15.42). Death usually occurs in the first year of life.

Signs:

Extreme cardiac enlargement and heart failure in infancy, often in the absence of murmurs.

Demonstration of excessive glycogen in biopsy of skeletal muscle.

11. Mitral Stenosis, Congenital

Obstructive malformation of the mitral valve which occurs in a variety of forms (e.g., thickening of leaflets with fusion of commissures, diaphragm formation with perforations, elongated "wind sack" with small orifice). Differentiation from rheumatic mitral stenosis is difficult except in infants and young children (15.33).

Signs:

> In infants or in young children without a history of rheumatic manifestations, signs are the same as those of acquired mitral stenosis (3.31.4).

12. Cor Triatriatum

Division of the left atrium by a diaphragm into an upper portion into which the pulmonary veins drain and a lower portion which communicates with the mitral valve. If the opening between the upper and lower chambers is restricted, pulmonary venous obstruction results (15.7).

Signs:

> Angiocardiogram demonstrates opacification of double chamber of left atrium.

13. Pulmonic Stenosis, Congenital

Obstruction to pulmonary blood flow, usually valvular due to fusion of valve leaflets, occasionally subvalvular or infundibular, and rarely supravalvular in the main pulmonary artery or its branches (15.6, 27). Symptoms and signs of an abnormal right ventricular burden are usually absent in patients with mild stenosis and right ventricular systolic pressure of 80 mm Hg or less.

Signs:

> Ejection-type systolic murmur and thrill in first and second left interspaces (valvular stenosis) or in third and fourth left interspaces (infundibular stenosis).
> Continuous murmur heard in region overlying a stenotic branch of the pulmonary artery.

Delay and often diminution in intensity of sound of pulmonic valve closure (valvular and subvalvular stenosis).

Roentgenogram: Poststenotic dilatation of main pulmonary artery (valvular stenosis) is seen and, if moderate or severe obstruction is present, enlargement of right ventricle and right atrium is evident.

Angiocardiogram: Region of obstruction may be visualized.

Electrocardiographic signs of right ventricular hypertrophy as severity increases (3.38).

Demonstration at cardiac catheterization of systolic pressure gradient across the site of obstruction.

14. Pulmonic Insufficiency, Congenital

In its isolated form a rare anomaly that results from absence or defective development of the pulmonic valve leaflets with consequent regurgitation (15.29). It may be secondary to surgery for valvular pulmonic stenosis. It should be distinguished from pulmonary incompetency (5.14) secondary to dilatation of the valvular ring associated with pulmonary hypertension and enlargement of the pulmonary artery.

Signs:

Decrescendo, blowing diastolic murmur along the left sternal border from the second to the fourth intercostal space.

Absence of peripheral physical signs associated with aortic insufficiency.

Pulmonary valvular insufficiency or incompetency can be demonstrated during cardiac catheterization by injection of indicator dye or contrast substance into the pulmonary artery.

15. Idiopathic Dilatation of the Pulmonary Artery

Unusual prominence of the main pulmonary artery in absence of signs of other cardiovascular or pulmonary anomalies (4.13).

Signs:

    Ejection-type systolic murmur in the pulmonic area.

    Unusual convexity of the main pulmonary artery on roent-
genography.

    Normal pressures in the pulmonary artery and right ven-
tricle, and absence of a left-to-right shunt.

16. *Downward Displacement of the Tricuspid Valve (Ebstein's Anomaly)*

Downward displacement of malformed tricuspid leaflets divides the right ventricle into a proximal atrialized portion and
a distal portion which functions as a ventricle (4.34; 15.25).

Signs:

    A superficial systolic and often a diastolic murmur low over
the precordium.

    Atrial gallop sound and third heart sound.

    Electrocardiogram may show an unusually high P wave and
an incomplete or complete right bundle-branch block
with low amplitude of QRS in right precordial leads. Occasionally, anomalous atrioventricular excitation occurs.
Arrhythmias are common.

    Roentgenogram displays an enlarged right atrium and an
"atrialized" right ventricle. The latter is often thin-walled
and pulsates poorly on fluoroscopy.

    Angiocardiography may demonstrate the abnormal division
of the right ventricle.

    Cardiac catheterization discloses a large right atrial cavity ex-
tending well to the left of the midline, and low systolic
pressure in the right ventricle and pulmonary artery. A
catheter-electrode in the right atrium may yield a ventricular type of "touch potential."

17. *Persistent Left Superior Vena Cava*

This vascular structure resembles the superior vena cava on
the right, with which it may be connected through an anasto-

mosis with the innominate vein (15.71). It customarily drains into the coronary sinus. The vessel may be inconspicuous in size or as large as the vena cava on the right.

Signs:
> Roentgenographic evidence of a straight, vertical shadow at the upper left border of the cardiac silhouette, lateral to the shadow cast by the aorta and the main pulmonary artery.

18. "Corrected" Transposition of the Great Vessels

Origin of the aorta as the anterior and lateral great vessel and of the pulmonary artery as the posterior and medial great vessel, usually in association with ventricular inversion (15.18). In the perfectly "corrected" transposition, the flow of blood is maintained in the physiologic direction. The right atrioventricular valve is bicuspid and communicates with the anterior, venous ventricle. This is an anatomic mirror image of the left ventricle and gives rise to the posteromedially placed pulmonary artery. The left atrioventricular valve is tricuspid and communicates with the posterior, arterial ventricle, which is a mirror image of the anatomic right ventricle and gives rise to the anterolaterally placed aorta. The aortic valve is more cephalad than the pulmonic valve. Often the "correction" is not complete, and there are associated lesions such as "mitral" insufficiency or ventricular septal defect.

Symptoms:
> Those that are apparent are due to the coexisting anomalies.

Signs:
> Loud second heart sound at left base (aortic valve closure), with splitting heard best in the second right intercostal space.
> Roentgenogram may show elongated convexity at left upper heart border due to the anterolateral aorta.

Angiocardiographic visualization of the relationship of the great vessels is the best diagnostic tool.

Electrocardiogram may indicate reversal of ventricular structures with Q waves and upright T waves in right precordial leads.

Cardiac catheter can be maneuvered into pulmonary artery with difficulty, but its posterior and medial course is diagnostic.

19. Dextrocardia

Presence of the heart in the right chest (15.3).

19.1. MIRROR IMAGE DEXTROCARDIA. Rotation of the primitive cardiac loop to the right instead of to the left so that the apex is on the right and there is a mirror image arrangement of normal chambers and vessels as visualized from the front. It occurs as an isolated anomaly or with intracardiac or extracardiac malformations with or without situs inversus.

Signs:

Roentgenogram: Configuration of the heart and vessels is a mirror image of the normally placed heart.

Electrocardiogram: inversion of lead I; leads II and III appear interchanged and the right and left precordial leads are reversed.

19.2. DEXTROROTATION OF THE HEART. Rotation of the heart on its axis so that the apex is toward the right and the venous atrium is on the right. The relationship of chambers and vessels to each other is similar to that in the normally placed heart. The degree of rotation varies.

Signs:

Roentgenogram: Atypical configuration and location of the heart in the right thorax due to rotation of portions of the cardiovascular silhouette.

79

Electrocardiogram: P wave is upright in lead I. The configuration of the precordial leads over the left and right chests will vary with the degree of rotation.

19.3. DEXTRODISPLACEMENT OF THE HEART. Displacement of the heart into the right thoracic cavity because of mediastinal shift, as, for example, from hypoplasia of the right lung, thoracic or skeletal anomaly, or eventration of the left diaphragm (15.2).

Signs:
Roentgenogram: Cardiac configuration is normal but displaced to the right.
Electrocardiogram: P and T waves are upright in lead I.

20. Levocardia with Situs Inversus

The heart is in the left chest although the thoracic and abdominal viscera are a mirror image of normal (15.4). Usually the heart is malformed and the patient cyanotic.

Signs:
Roentgenogram: Heart is on the left but the abdominal organs are reversed, confirmed by barium swallow.
Other signs depend on associated cardiac anomalies.

Potentially Cyanotic Group

In the following malformations, a communication exists between the systemic and pulmonic circulations, and under ordinary circumstances a left-to-right shunt of blood exists. Reversal of the shunt occurs chiefly as a result of obstruction to pulmonary blood flow. With extracardiac communications,

this obstruction is in the pulmonary vascular bed. With intracardiac communications, the obstruction may be in the pulmonary vascular bed or in the heart in the form of valvular
or infundibular pulmonic stenosis.

21. Patent Ductus Arteriosus

Persistence of a fetal channel between the descending aorta
(just distal to the left subclavian artery) and the main pulmonary artery (15.65).

Signs:

Continuous systolic and diastolic murmur, with late systolic
accentuation, in the second left interspace anteriorly.
Presence of a typical murmur usually suffices for diagnosis.
In infants and young children the diastolic component
may be absent.

If shunt is moderate to large, wide pulse pressure.

Radiologic evidence of enlargement of the left ventricle,
aorta, and main pulmonary artery.

Tall R and T waves in left precordial leads.

Catheter samples arterialized blood from the pulmonary
artery or its left branch and may traverse the ductus to
enter the descending aorta.

Selective retrograde aortography demonstrates opacification
of the pulmonary arteries when contrast material is injected into the descending aorta.

22. Aortic Septal Defect (Aorticopulmonary Window)

Communication existing between the ascending aorta and the
main pulmonary artery just distal to the semilunar valves
(15.60).

Signs:

Mimics patent ductus arteriosus (4.21). The diagnosis is suggested if, in addition, pulmonary hypertension is present

or if the continuous murmur is heard in the third or fourth left intercostal space.

Selective aortography demonstrates opacification of the main pulmonary artery when contrast medium is introduced into the root of the aorta.

23. Truncus Arteriosus

A single great vessel leaving the heart as a common trunk which gives off branches of the pulmonary artery and the vessels of the aortic arch and continues as the descending aorta (15.20). A common semilunar valve and a high ventricular septal defect or absence of the ventricular septum are integral parts of the anomaly. "True" truncus arteriosus, due to failure of partitioning of the pulmonary artery and the aorta, is associated with increased pulmonary flow unless there is pulmonary vascular obstruction, and is to be differentiated from "pseudo" truncus arteriosus with diminished pulmonary blood flow (4.36).

Signs:

Pansystolic murmur at base of the heart and along the left sternal border.

Single loud second sound.

Roentgenogram demonstrates a large vessel of same width in frontal and oblique projections; increased pulmonary vascularity.

Catheterization demonstrates shunt at ventricular and aorticopulmonic areas with systemic pressure in the right ventricle and distal vessels.

Systemic angiocardiography or aortography afford visualization of the common trunk.

24. Coronary Arteriovenous Fistula

Dilatation of a coronary artery which communicates with a cardiac chamber (usually the right atrium, coronary sinus, or right ventricle) or with the pulmonary artery (15.57).

Signs:

Continuous systolic and diastolic murmur of an arteriovenous fistula, located over the precordium; the murmur
is maximal near point of entry of the fistula.

Selective aortography may demonstrate origin and anomalous course of a coronary artery and its communication
with the right heart or pulmonary circulation.

25. Ventricular Septal Defect

A defect in the ventricular septum, usually occurring high in
the membranous septum but, in about 10 percent of the patients, occurring in the muscular septum. Symptoms and signs
depend on the degree of resistance to the shunting of blood
through the defect and into the lungs.

Signs:

Harsh holosystolic murmur and coarse thrill are heard along
the lower left sternal border.

Second sound of pulmonic valve closure varies directly in
intensity and lateness with size of shunt and pressure in
pulmonary circuit.

With a large left-to-right shunt, there is an overactive, enlarged heart and an apical diastolic murmur in addition
to the systolic murmur.

Radiography demonstrates enlargement of the left ventricle,
right ventricle, left atrium, and pulmonary arteries, but
not of the aorta.

Electrocardiogram is variable but often shows tall R and T
waves in the left precordial leads.

With a small shunt, the heart on the roentgenogram and the
electrocardiogram is essentially normal.

Cardiac catheterization reveals an increased oxygen content
of blood in the right ventricle and, when present, pulmonary hypertension.

26. Single Ventricle (Cor Triloculare Biatriatum)

Absence of the ventricular septum (15.14) and consequent complete mixture of arterial and venous blood. In the absence of obstruction to flow through the lungs, the proportion of oxygenated blood in the common chamber is so high that cyanosis is not observed. Often there is a rudimentary outlet chamber, and the arterial trunks are frequently transposed.

Signs:
   Progressive cardiac enlargement and heart failure may occur early in infancy.

   Holosystolic murmur is heard along the lower left sternal border.

   Cardiac catheterization: Diagnosis is suggested when a large increase in the oxygen content occurs at the ventricular level, when the oxygen content of the pulmonary artery and of a systemic artery is the same, and when the systolic pressures in the ventricle and in a systemic artery are the same.

   Angiocardiography shows spread of contrast medium throughout the region normally occupied by the right and left ventricles. A rudimentary outlet chamber, if present, can be delineated, and the relationship of the simultaneously opacified aorta and pulmonary artery can be determined.

27. Common Atrioventricular Canal

An endocardial cushion defect with complete and incomplete forms (15.11.2). In the complete form there is absence of the lower part of the atrial septum (ostium primum) and the contiguous ventricular septum with continuity of the septal leaflet of the tricuspid valve and aortic leaflet of the mitral valve, which are cleft. The most extreme form consists of total absence of the atrial and ventricular septa and a common atrioventricular valve (cor biloculare). In the incomplete form one or more of the above anomalies occur, most often as an ostium primum defect of the atrial septum with a cleft mitral valve (4.28). Occasionally a left ventricular–right atrial shunt occurs through a high ventricular septal defect and the cleft septal leaflet of the tricuspid valve.

Signs:

Complete form:

Holosystolic murmur and thrill over body of the heart.

Apical systolic murmur transmitted to the axilla as in mitral insufficiency.

Mid-diastolic murmur at the apex or lower left sternal border.

Enlargement of left ventricle in addition to that of the right atrium and ventricle and the main pulmonary artery and its branches.

Electrocardiogram: Left axis deviation, often with a prolonged P–R interval, tall R and T waves in the left precordial leads, and a late R′ deflection in the right precordial leads.

Cardiac catheterization: Arterialization of blood at the atrial and ventricular levels with pulmonary hypertension.

Selective injection of contrast material into the chambers of the left heart helps to define shunts and the structure of the septa and valves.

Incomplete form:

Findings as for atrial or ventricular septal defect (4.25, 28), often associated with mitral or tricuspid insufficiency and with electrocardiographic abnormalities as described for the complete form above.

28. Atrial Septal Defect

A defect usually in the mid or upper portions of the atrial septum (septum secundum defect) but occasionally in a lower portion of the septum just above the atrioventricular valves (ostium primum, 4.27). When the defect is high near the superior vena cava, some of the pulmonary veins drain anomalously into the right atrium or superior vena cava near the defect (15.11).

Atrial septal defect is to be differentiated from a patent foramen ovale guarded on the left atrial side by a flap. Although a foramen ovale may function under circumstances of elevated right atrial pressure to permit a right-to-left shunt (4.33, 34), it should not be regarded as a congenital anomaly since failure of anatomic sealing of the foramen ovale occurs in about 25 percent of the normal population.

Signs:

Septum secundum defect:

Left parasternal bulge due to right ventricular enlargement. Heaving precordial pulsation due to right ventricular enlargement is sometimes maximal in the left midclavicular line, thus simulating left ventricular enlargement.

Systolic ejection-type murmur, usually without a thrill, which is maximal in the second and third left interspaces.

Wide splitting of the second sound in the pulmonic area.

Short diastolic murmur along the lower left sternal border.

Electrocardiogram: Right axis deviation and a late R' deflection in the right-sided leads.

Roentgenogram: Enlargement of the right atrium, right ventricle, and pulmonary artery, with an aorta that is actually or relatively small. Fluoroscopy generally shows expansile pulsations of greater amplitude in the hilar arteries than in any of the lesions with increased pulmonary blood flow.

Cardiac catheterization: Arterialization of right atrial

blood. Pulmonary arterial pressure tends to be normal except in some adults.

Ostium primum:
　See above (4.7).

29. Single Atrium (Cor Triloculare Biventriculare)

Absence of the atrial septum and consequent existence of a common chamber for the receipt of systemic and pulmonic venous return.

Signs:
　Similar to signs of atrial septal defect (4.28) but often with greater cardiac enlargement and with pulmonary hypertension.
　Angiocardiography may demonstrate the common chamber.

30. Total Anomalous Pulmonary Venous Connection

Pulmonary venous drainage from both lungs into the right atrium or one of its tributaries (superior vena cava, innominate vein, left superior vena cava, coronary sinus, inferior vena cava, or hepatic vein). Admixed systemic and pulmonary venous blood then flows in two directions, the larger portion into the right ventricle and to the lungs again, and the lesser portion through a defect in the atrial septum into the left heart and systemic circulation (15.68).

Signs:
　Similar to signs of atrial septal defect (4.28).
　Roentgenogram demonstrates vascular collar around base of heart if drainage is into the left superior vena cava. The right superior vena cava is distended if that is the point of entry.
　Angiocardiogram may show "jet sign" of unopacified blood

from the pulmonary veins diluting the contrast material in the vessel or chamber into which they drain. At the time of pulmonary venous filling, the anomalous pulmonary venous channel and its course may opacify, especially if its connection is extracardiac.

31. Partial Anomalous Pulmonary Venous Connection

Drainage of pulmonary veins from one or more lobes, usually of the right lung into the right atrium or one of its tributaries. It is usually tolerated as a solitary anomaly, although it is often associated with a defect in the atrial septum secundum (4.28).

Signs:
  Similar to signs of atrial septal defect (4.28).

32. Arteriovenous Fistula of the Lung

A communication in the lung between a pulmonary artery and vein, sometimes multiple. When multiple, the fistulas may be associated with multiple telangiectasia of the skin (hereditary multiple telangiectasia). The patient may be asymptomatic, but if enough unoxygenated blood in a pulmonary artery flows through the fistula into the pulmonary veins and into the systemic circulation, cyanosis may appear.

Signs:
  Absence of heart murmurs.
  Continuous murmur may be present over the lung containing the fistula.
  Roentgenogram shows unusual vascular shadow in the lung.
  Angiocardiography may opacify the fistula at the time of pulmonary arterial filling.

Cyanotic Group

Cyanosis and the associated polycythemia and clubbing of fingers and toes are characteristic of this group of malformations. Fatigability, shortness of breath on exertion, and retardation of growth are common.

33. Pulmonic Stenosis with Patent Foramen Ovale or Atrial Septal Defect

When pulmonic stenosis is severe and right ventricular end-diastolic pressure and right atrial pressure rise, a right-to-left shunt occurs through a patent foramen ovale or through a true defect in the atrial septum.

Signs:
Same as those of severe pulmonic stenosis (4.13).

Electrocardiogram demonstrates high, late R waves with deeply inverted T waves in leads from the right side of the precordium, and small R waves and deep S waves in leads from the left side. The P waves may be high and peaked. The QRS axis in the frontal plane is usually deviated to the right.

Systolic pressure gradient between the right ventricle and the pulmonary artery is wide, and right ventricular systolic pressure usually exceeds 140 mm Hg and is higher than a simultaneously recorded peripheral arterial pressure.

34. Downward Displacement of the Tricuspid Valve (Ebstein's Anomaly) with Patent Foramen Ovale

In this anomaly of the tricuspid valve the foramen ovale usually is not sealed, and rarely is an atrial septal defect present.

If the valvular displacement is considerable and the partially atrialized right ventricle is distended, a right-to-left shunt occurs. Signs then depend on the degree of displacement and the volume of shunted blood.

Signs:
>   Same as those given in Section 4.16 plus evidence of arterial unsaturation and a right-to-left atrial shunt on angiocardiography or cardiac catheterization.

35. *Tetralogy of Fallot*

Four features constitute this malformation: (1) ventricular septal defect; (2) severe pulmonic stenosis, usually infundibular; (3) systemic pressure in the right ventricle; and (4) an aorta which receives blood from the right as well as from the left ventricle (**15.15**).

Symptoms and Signs:
>   Cyanosis and shortness of breath, increased by exertion and relieved by squatting position.
>
>   Precordial bulge overlying the right ventricle.
>
>   Systolic thrill and murmur of pulmonic stenosis along the left sternal border. Decrease in or absence of the sound of pulmonic valve closure. With an overriding aorta, the second sound may be louder in the second left interspace than in second right interspace and is the sound of aortic valve closure.
>
>   Roentgenogram and fluoroscopy: Small or average-sized, boot-shaped heart with concavity in the region of the main pulmonary artery and often with a bulge in the outflow tract of the right ventricle (due to the infundibular chamber). The aorta is wide, the branches of the main pulmonary artery small, and the peripheral lung fields excessively clear.
>
>   Electrocardiogram: Right axis deviation of QRS, peaked P

waves of right atrial enlargement, and reversal of normal R and S relationship in the precordial leads.

Angiocardiogram: Possible abnormal configuration of the infundibulum, the pulmonary valve, or both, and premature opacification of the overriding aorta.

Cardiac catheterization: Systolic pressure in the right ventricle equal to that in the aorta, low pressure in the main pulmonary artery, often with intermediate systolic pressure in the infundibulum. Bidirectional shunt at the ventricular level may be evident.

36. "Pseudotruncus" Arteriosus

Anatomically, this condition resembles a tetralogy of Fallot except that there is pulmonary atresia. Life is sustained by collateral circulation from vessels leaving the aorta and anastomosing with small pulmonary arteries in the lungs. Thus it functionally resembles a truncus arteriosus in that a single great vessel leaves the heart and supplies both the systemic and pulmonic circulations (4.23). Unlike a true truncus, the pulmonary blood flow is not increased.

Signs:

In a cyanotic patient, continuous murmur over the lung fields with radiologic evidence of a boot-shaped heart and diminished pulmonary blood flow and lacy hilar markings.

37. Rudimentary Right Ventricle with Tricuspid and Pulmonic Stenosis or Atresia and Defective Atrial Septum

Underdeveloped right ventricle with obstruction to inflow and outflow. Course of circulation is: systemic venous return to right atrium, through defect in atrial septum to left atrium, where it is mixed with oxygenated blood from lungs. Admixture in the left ventricle passes out of the aorta to the body and, by way of a patent ductus, to the lungs, or through a ventricular septal defect to a small right ventricle and the lungs.

Signs:
Cyanosis from birth.
Systolic murmur of pulmonic stenosis or absence of a cardiac murmur.
Absent or quiet sound of pulmonic valve closure.
No cardiac enlargement or precordial bulge over right ventricle.
Electrocardiogram: High peaked P waves of right atrial enlargement, left axis deviation, and left ventricular dominance in precordial leads.
Roentgenogram: Small or average-sized heart with concave main pulmonary artery segment and excessively clear lung fields. On fluoroscopy right atrial contractions may be seen in the LAO projection in the region normally occupied by a right ventricle.
Angiocardiogram: Contrast medium passes from the right to the left atrium, to the left ventricle, to the aorta, then to the pulmonary arteries.

38. Rudimentary Left Ventricle with Mitral and Aortic Stenosis or Atresia and Defective Atrial Septum

Venous outflow from the lungs is obstructed and passes through a defective atrial septum to the right atrium, where it mixes with systemic venous return. From the right ventricle admixed blood enters the pulmonary artery where it divides, part going into the pulmonary circulation and the remainder through a patent ductus arteriosus into the descending aorta and in retrograde fashion into the ascending aorta. If the ventricular septum is defective and the aortic valve stenosed rather than atresic, mixed blood may reach the body by this route. If the mitral valve is stenotic rather than atresic, some blood returning from the lungs may enter the rudimentary left ventricle directly.

Signs:

Systolic murmur at base or no murmur.

Loud sound of pulmonic valve closure.

Roentgenogram: Enlargement of right side of heart and engorgement of pulmonary circulation.

No evidence of left ventricular enlargement.

Electrocardiogram: Right axis deviation and greater dominance of right ventricular potentials than expected for the age of patient.

Angiocardiography: Contrast medium follows the abnormal circulatory course described. Opacification of the left atrium following pulmonary venous filling differentiates it from anomalous pulmonary venous connection.

39. Complete Transposition of the Great Vessels

The aorta arises from the right (venous) ventricle and the pulmonary artery arises from the left (arterial) ventricle (15.17). Intermixing of venous and arterial blood occurs through a patent foramen ovale or atrial septal defect, a ventricular septal defect, or a patent ductus arteriosus.

Signs:

Accentuation of a single second sound (the aortic) in the second left interspace.

Usually progressive cardiac enlargement and insufficiency.

Roentgenogram: In infancy, a narrow vascular pedicle at base of the heart in frontal view, wider in oblique projections. Although the pulmonary artery segment is concave, lung vascularity is increased unless there is coexistent pulmonic stenosis.

Angiocardiogram: Demonstration of the anterior origin of the aorta from the right ventricle. If contrast medium is injected into the left side of the heart, the posterior origin of the main pulmonary artery from the left ventricle is seen. The site of the shunt sometimes is visualized, especially if there is a patent ductus.

Electrocardiogram: Effects of right ventricular hypertrophy (3.38).

40. Incomplete Transposition of the Great Vessels

Morphologically, various degrees of incompleteness of transposition of the great vessels can occur (15.17, 18, 19). One clinically recognizable form consists of a ventricular septal defect, an overriding pulmonary artery in its usual anatomic position, and a transposed aorta (Taussig-Bing malformation).

Signs:

> Similar to those of complete transposition, with the following exceptions:
>
> Roentgenogram shows prominently convex main pulmonary artery in addition to enlarged branches.
>
> Angiocardiography demonstrates simultaneous opacification of an anterior aorta and an anterolateral pulmonary artery following right ventricular filling.

5 / The Physiologic Cardiac Diagnosis

Clinical manifestations of physiologic disturbances in cardio-dynamics may be classified thus: (1) Disturbances in cardiac rhythm and conduction (e.g., arrhythmias, intraventricular block); (2) disturbances in myocardial contractility (e.g., heart failure, pulsus alternans); (3) clinical syndromes (e.g., anginal syndrome, Adams-Stokes syndrome).

The physiologic diagnosis should include a title from one or more of these categories if the criteria for the disturbance are met. If no disturbance is present, the physiologic diagnosis is normal sinus rhythm.

Disturbances in Cardiac Rhythm and Conduction

The diagnosis of the basic cardiac rhythm or any disturbance of it is usually made by combining data obtained by the physical examination and by instrumental methods. Of the latter, the electrocardiogram is the most useful (see Part V).

1. Atrial Arrhythmias

1.1. ATRIAL RHYTHM. An atrial focus other than the sino-atrial node assumes the pacemaker function and discharges regularly.

1.2. ATRIAL FLUTTER. An ectopic atrial focus arises and initiates a sequence of stimuli faster than in atrial tachycardia; these stimuli occur at a rate usually between 200 and 380 per minute (33.2.3). This arrhythmia has been attributed by some to a circus movement around the orifices of the great veins, and by others to a single repetitive focus. The ventricular rate is rarely the same as the atrial rate; more often it is one-half, one-third, or one-fourth of that rate, depending upon the facility of atrioventricular conduction. The ventricular rate may be irregular when there is variation in the ventricular response, e.g., 2:1, 3:1, 4:1 in successive intervals. In atrial flutter there is a discrete and effective mechanical atrial systole following each atrial excitation wave.

Atrial flutter should be suspected clinically when the ventricular rate is regular and around 150 per minute (the atrial rate being 300 with a 2:1 atrioventricular response). This rate is unaffected by change in position, by rest, or by exercise. Carotid sinus pressure may increase the delay at the atrioventricular node and will then cause a change to a slower ventricular rate or a change from a regular to an irregular ventricular response because of varying atrioventricular conduction. Atrial flutter is usually transient but rarely may be a fixed or chronic arrhythmia of many months' duration.

1.3. ATRIAL FIBRILLATION. The atrial rate is the fastest of all atrial rhythms, ranging between 400 and 600 and even reaching 1000 impulses per minute. It is usually ascribed to a circus movement within the atrial musculature which follows an irregular pathway. The resultant chaotic excitation of the atria permits no discrete mechanical contraction and the atria remain as hemodynamically passive pools. Only a limited number of atrial stimuli reach the ventricles and do so in an irregular fashion. Hence the ventricular rate is totally irregular. Without treatment, the ventricular rate is generally between

90 and 160 per minute but may occasionally reach 200 per minute (33.2.4). Rates as low as 50 to 60 per minute may be observed when the patient has received adequate digitalis. When a patient known to have chronic atrial fibrillation demonstrates a slow but regular ventricular rate, the onset of complete atrioventricular heart block should be suspected.

Atrial fibrillation is one of the common causes of an irregular heart beat and certain characteristic features of the arrhythmia can be sought clinically. When the ventricular rate is unusually slow or unusually rapid, the irregularity may escape clinical detection. Exercise increases the ventricular rate and accentuates the irregularity, whereas an arrhythmia due to premature contractions interrupting a regular sinus rhythm may decrease or disappear with an increased heart rate. This arrhythmia may be transient or paroxysmal, and often is persistent or chronic when associated with heart disease.

2. Atrioventricular (A–V) Nodal Rhythms

The atrioventricular node can discharge impulses sporadically (A–V nodal premature contractions), at a regular but relatively slow rhythm (40 to 60 and occasionally up to 80 per minute), or at a fast pace (A–V nodal tachycardia with rates between 100 and 270 per minute). The diagnosis can be made with certainty only from an electrocardiogram (33.3).

3. Atrioventricular (A–V) Block

The conduction of impulses from atria to ventricles is impaired (33.7).

3.1. INCOMPLETE A–V BLOCK (PROLONGED A–V CONDUCTION TIME). This is simple prolongation of the atrioventricular conduction time above the normal limits for the age of the patient. It can be detected only by a graphic record.

3.2. INCOMPLETE A–V BLOCK WITH DROPPED BEATS. When conduction is more markedly impaired than indicated in Sub-section 3.1, some supraventricular beats never penetrate through to the ventricles, and there are one or more dropped beats. This may be suspected when auscultation reveals a regular rhythm interrupted by pauses which are approximately double the normal cycle. When the P–R interval gradually lengthens until one P wave is not conducted at all (Wencke-bach's phenomenon) and a ventricular beat is thus dropped, the ventricular rate may become totally irregular. A single dropped beat due to incomplete A–V block may be confused with the long pause which may follow an early premature contraction. These may be differentiated by the absence of any sound of the premature beat following shortly after the pre-ceding normal beat as when the arrhythmia is due to premature systoles. Dropped beats due to sinus arrest, to blocked atrial premature contractions, or to incomplete A–V block are best differentiated by the electrocardiogram.

3.3. COMPLETE A–V BLOCK. No impulses from the atria reach the ventricles and an idioventricular rhythm arises with a focus either in the bundle of His or in the ventricle. Atria and ventricles beat independently of each other, a phenomenon which can be seen by comparing jugular atrial pulsations with the apical or carotid beat. The idioventricular rhythm is regular and slow, usually ranging from 25 to 40 beats per minute in adults and usually faster (60 to 80) in children. Atrial systolic sounds may be heard, and the first heart sound will vary in intensity. The ventricular rate varies little if at all with changes in position or activity. Occasionally an idioventricular focus fails to discharge at the onset of or during complete block; ventricular arrest follows.

When transient periods of complete A–V block occur, there may be a sharp decrease in cardiac output and cerebral blood flow during the transitional phase of fast to slow rate; hence symptoms of syncope or convulsions may appear. When com-plete block is fixed and unchanging with ventricular rates above 25 to 30 per minute, the patient is usually asymptomatic at rest but may have symptoms of dizziness or momentary mental lapses during any effort. When the ventricular rate falls below 20 to 25 per minute, as it may do spontaneously or as a complication of a febrile episode or vascular accident, symptoms of decreased cerebral and visceral flow may appear at rest. Occasionally the patient with complete A–V block is subject to short attacks of ventricular tachycardia or fibrillation and during these has symptoms of decreased cerebral blood flow. Regardless of the mechanism responsible for them, these symptoms in the patient with heart block are grouped together as the Adams-Stokes syndrome (5.18).

4. Escaped Beats

When the sinus pacemaker is slow in initiating an impulse, as in sinus bradycardia, in sinus arrhythmia, or following a premature systole, or when it fails entirely to discharge (sinus arrest) or to reach the ventricle (A–V block), any lower rhythmic center may release an impulse. This is conducted to the ventricles if it is supraventricular, or through the ventricles if the escaped beat can be identified by the electrocardiogram (33.3, 4). It comes after a pause in the heart beat which is longer than normal.

5. Intraventricular Conduction Defects

Failure of conduction of a supraventricular impulse to the ventricles over the normal pathways below the bifurcation of the bundle of His. This includes right or left bundle-branch block and more distal blocks. The differentiation of these blocks is made electrocardiographically (33.8). There are no absolute physical signs of intraventricular block.

6. Paroxysmal Tachycardia

The rate may vary between 100 and 200 or more in adults and

is even faster in infants and children (200 to 300 per minute). Unless the arrhythmia is due to atrial fibrillation or atrial flutter with varying ventricular rate, the regular rapid heart beat is fixed and does not vary with position, exercise, or vagal stimuli. Carotid sinus pressure may abruptly terminate atrial tachycardia (5.1.2). The exact site of origin of the tachycardia may be determined by the electrocardiogram.

7. Premature Contractions

The basic rhythm of the heart may be interrupted by a stimulus originating prematurely outside the sino-atrial node, thus producing a premature cardiac contraction. Any part of the atria, A–V node, bundle of His, or ventricles may initiate this premature beat (33.2.1; 33.3.1; 33.4.3). The interruption of cardiac rhythm may be regular or irregular. If a premature contraction reaches the ventricles, it may be recognized as a beat falling before the next expected normal beat when the basic rhythm is regular. A pause which is longer than the interval between normal beats may, but does not always, follow premature contractions. These features are absent when the premature beat is completed without disturbing the next normal beat (interpolated premature contraction). When there is a basically irregular rhythm, it may be impossible to uncover premature beats without the aid of an electrocardiogram. Depending upon the size of the pulse wave generated by the premature contraction, the peripheral pulse may mirror the cardiac action or may, if stroke output and pulse waves are small, fail to register the beat. There will be no pause corresponding to the ventricular contraction (frustrane beat, pulse deficit).

Exercise may abolish these beats in the normal heart, but in an abnormal myocardium the beats may increase with exertion.

The site of origin of the premature beats can best be determined by the electrocardiogram.

8. Sinus Rhythms

8.1. NORMAL SINUS RHYTHM. The normal rhythm of the heart which originates in the sino-atrial (S–A) node. The rate is arbitrarily defined as 60 to 100 beats per minute.

8.2. SINUS ARREST. One or more impulses from the S–A node fail to reach the atria, either because the pacemaker failed to discharge or because the impulse was blocked from leaving the S–A node and penetrating the atrial tissue (33.1.5). The result is a dropped heart beat and the interval between the previous and subsequent contractions is two, three, or four times the usual interval between sinus beats, depending on whether one, two, or three successive sinus beats fail to materialize. Occasionally a lower pacemaker may escape during the period of sinus arrest. Sinus arrest must be distinguished from periods of incomplete A–V block with dropped beats and from blocked atrial or A–V nodal premature contractions. The electrocardiogram is the best means of diagnosis.

8.3. SINUS ARRHYTHMIA. A common variant of regular sinus rhythm that is characterized by fluctuations in the rate of impulse formation which often but not always coincide with the phases of respiration (33.1.4).

8.4. SINUS BRADYCARDIA. A slow sinus rhythm with a rate of less than 60 beats per minute, varying with exercise and often with position. Sinus arrhythmia often accompanies it.

8.5. SINUS TACHYCARDIA. A rapid sinus rhythm with a rate faster than 100 beats per minute.

9. Undiagnosed Arrhythmia

A short-lived arrhythmia which cannot be subjected to analysis.

10. Ventricular Fibrillation

An irregular, disorganized spread of impulses throughout the ventricles and virtual mechanical paralysis of them due to ineffective contractions. This arrhythmia is often a terminal event, although transient attacks with survival may occur. The diagnosis is made from the electrocardiogram (33.4.5).

11. Wandering Pacemaker

This term is limited to the progressive shift of the pacemaker, from one beat to the next, either within the S–A node or from the S–A node to the A–V node and the reverse. It is not used to designate shifts of pacemaker to the atria or A–V node which take the form of premature atrial or nodal contractions. Wandering pacemaker is often associated with sinus arrhythmia; it can be diagnosed only by means of the electrocardiogram (33.2.5).

Disturbances in Myocardial Contractility

12. Cardiac Insufficiency (Heart Failure)

When manifestations of inadequacies of the circulation (limited flow or congestion) can be attributed to impaired cardiac function, cardiac insufficiency is said to exist. When the pathologic physiology is known, more definite terms such as diminished cardiac reserve, congestive heart failure, right heart failure, or left heart failure may be employed.

Symptoms of heart failure are fatigue, dyspnea, and orthopnea.

Signs of heart failure include cyanosis, dilated neck veins, moist or dry rales, pleural effusion, tachycardia, gallop rhythm, pulsus alternans, hepatomegaly, splenomegaly, ascites, and edema. Objective findings that confirm heart failure include elevated venous pressure, prolonged circulation time, and hypervolemia.

Acute left ventricular failure is characterized by sudden dyspnea occurring typically at night and may be associated with sweating, coughing, prolonged expiration and wheezing, hemoptysis, frothy sputum, moist or dry rales.

There are clinical states (acute nephritis, severe anemia, pregnancy, and steroid administration) in which congestive phenomena are not due to failure of the heart. In such patients there may be paroxysmal nocturnal dyspnea, peripheral edema, decreased circulation time, and increased venous pressure.

13. Annular Incompetency

Incompetency is the result of dilatation of the annulus of the valve to a degree permitting regurgitation. It is distinguished from valvular deformity with insufficiency (3.31) in that there is no structural alteration in the leaflets. Annular incompetency is most often the result of cardiac insufficiency with congestion. Under these reversible circumstances it is regarded as a physiologic rather than an anatomic diagnosis.

In certain situations a disease process may involve the annulus itself and make it incompetent. The dynamic fault is then defined as *annular insufficiency* and should properly appear in the anatomic rather than the physiologic diagnosis.

13.1. AORTIC ANNULAR INCOMPETENCY. Dilatation of the aortic ring producing an early diastolic blowing murmur heard most often along the sternal border and sometimes transmitted over a wide area. The regurgitation may be sufficient to produce peripheral manifestations of aortic insufficiency. Aortic annular incompetency may occur in patients with any disease in which left ventricular hypertrophy with dilatation is present. The types which occur with arteriosclerosis, cystic degeneration of the aorta, and deforming spondylitis are probably organic in origin and should more properly appear in the anatomic diagnosis as *aortic annular insufficiency*.

13.2. MITRAL ANNULAR INCOMPETENCY.   Dilatation of the mitral ring associated with a loud harsh systolic murmur at the apex, radiating to the axilla and to the back. Mitral annular incompetency may occur in left ventricular hypertrophy or dilatation from any cause. Certain types may be organic in origin.

13.3. PULMONIC ANNULAR INCOMPETENCY.   Dilatation of the pulmonic ring giving rise to a diastolic blowing murmur at the left sternal border (Graham Steell murmur), usually heard at the second intercostal space but often heard over a much greater area. This murmur may simulate one due to aortic insufficiency or aortic annular incompetency. Pulmonic annular incompetency is most often present when heart failure is severe or when the pulmonary artery pressure is high.

13.4. TRICUSPID ANNULAR INCOMPETENCY.   Dilatation of the tricuspid ring giving rise to a systolic murmur along the right as well as the left lower sternal border. The presence of right heart dilatation from any cause tends to produce it. The diagnosis is almost certain when there is systolic pulsation of the neck veins, of the liver, or of both.

14. Gallop Rhythm

The auscultatory finding of an additional cardiac sound which, falling either before the first (presystolic or atrial gallop) or after the second (diastolic or ventricular gallop) heart sound, results in a triple arrangement of sound in each cardiac cycle. Although the presystolic gallop may be innocent and the diastolic most often implies functional disturbance of ventricular filling, it is best to evaluate gallop rhythm in relation to the other physiologic features of the clinical state with which it is associated. Diastolic gallop rhythm may be the earliest physical sign of ventricular failure. In left ventricular failure it is heard best at or near the cardiac apex, whereas in right ventricular failure it is heard best near the ensiform cartilage. Gallop may be absent at rest but appear during exercise. The ventricular gallop sound must occasionally be distinguished from the physiologic third heart sound, a split second heart sound, or the opening snap of the mitral valve.

15. Pulsus Alternans

The alternating magnitude of the arterial pulse due to alternating size of the ventricular pressure pulse. It can be observed only during regular rhythm. Although palpation of the peripheral pulse can elicit this sign, it is noted best when taking the blood pressure by the auscultatory method. At the upper limits of systolic pressure, the beats are heard at one-half the heart rate; when the pressure in the cuff is permitted to fall, the rate doubles and the large and small beats may be heard at varying intensities.

Although pulsus alternans often indicates serious abnormality of myocardial function, the prognosis depends on the associated cardiac disease. Pulsus alternans and acoustical alternans do not necessarily accompany electrical alternans (**33.11.13**).

16. Pulmonary Hypertension*

Pulmonary hypertension exists when the pressure in the pulmonary artery is above 30 mm Hg systolic pressure, 10 mm Hg diastolic pressure, or 15 mm Hg mean pressure. At birth an infant normally has a moderate elevation of pressure in the

* Included here because disturbance of myocardial contractility (left ventricular failure), although not its only cause, is probably its most common cause.

pulmonary artery, but this disappears in the early weeks of life. The causes of pulmonary hypertension include left ventricular failure, obstruction at the mitral valve (mitral stenosis, left atrial myxoma), pulmonary vascular disease (including pulmonary emboli, arteritis, pulmonary lymphohematogenous metastases), hypoxia (including pulmonary emphysema), and increase in pulmonary blood flow due to a left-to-right shunt. The diagnosis of pulmonary hypertension can be made with certainty only by direct measurement. Clinically, the presence of an adequate predisposing cause (see above) and evidence of right ventricular hypertrophy represent strong evidence for a presumptive diagnosis. No other clinical findings afford a reliable sign of pulmonary hypertension. Sequential observations of increasing intensity of the pulmonic second sound suggest the appearance or aggravation of pulmonary hypertension.

Clinical Syndromes

17. *Anginal Syndrome*

Pain in the chest produced in patients with organic heart disease by effort, excitement, ingestion of a heavy meal, or exposure to cold. It is characteristically relieved by rest and nitroglycerine. The pain is typically upper retrosternal, rarely epigastric, but may be localized in the interscapular region, the throat, the lower jaw, the teeth, the shoulders, or the arms. It often consists of or is accompanied by a sense of choking or inability to breathe. The quality of the sensation may be constricting, burning, or pressing. The intensity varies from a mild sense of heaviness to severe pain. The patient will often complain of flatulence as well. The duration of the sensation is relatively short. The pain of myocardial infarction in any particular patient may be identical with the pain of the anginal syndrome; only the precipitating factor and the subsequent course will establish the diagnosis.

Anginal syndrome is a physiologic diagnosis and is not synonymous with coronary atherosclerosis. The underlying mechanism is ischemia of the heart muscle; thus any factor which invokes this mechanism can initiate the anginal syndrome.

Anginal syndrome is the cardinal symptom of coronary artery disease, but may be present in hypertensive heart disease uncomplicated by coronary atherosclerosis, in aortic insufficiency, in aortic stenosis, in mitral stenosis, or in cor pulmonale.

18. Adams-Stokes Syndrome

Episodes of unconsciousness often accompanied by muscular twitchings and convulsions due to atrioventricular block, ventricular fibrillation, or asystole. The duration and severity of the episode depend upon the duration of decreased cerebral flow. These episodes may occur and their causes be unsuspected in patients in whom complete A–V block alternates with either normal conduction or incomplete A–V block.

19. Carotid Sinus Syndrome

Episodes of dizziness, fainting, and sometimes convulsions due to abnormal irritability of the carotid sinus. During an episode there is usually a fall in arterial blood pressure and a slowing of the heart rate. Episodes may occur without apparent cause. They may follow an emotional upset, result from pressure over the carotid sinus, or be produced by swallowing.

20. Wolff-Parkinson-White Syndrome

Episodes of paroxysmal tachycardia occurring in patients with anomalous atrioventricular excitation (3.8.10). In these individuals the heart is usually normal or only coincidentally diseased. If only the electrocardiographic anomaly exists (anomalous atrioventricular excitation), it alone is to be noted in the physiologic diagnosis.

21. Cyanotic Crises

Crises occurring in cyanotic individuals characterized by a sudden increase in cyanosis, restlessness, and dyspnea often accompanied by an expiratory grunt. These "spells" may progress to loss of consciousness, convulsions, and death. The phenomenon occurs most commonly in patients with tetralogy of Fallot with advanced pulmonary stenosis or atresia.

22. Cardiac Tamponade

Impairment of cardiac function by the presence of excess pericardial fluid. The fluid may be a simple transudate, a sterile or purulent exudate, or blood. Pain in the chest, dyspnea, peripheral congestion, and shock may appear, depending on the character, volume, and speed of accumulation of the effusion. A pericardial friction rub, muffled heart sounds, distended jugular veins, high venous and low arterial blood pressure, sinus tachycardia, low voltage of QRS and T waves in the electrocardiogram, and an enlarged and sometimes quiet cardiac silhouette may be present. The interference in cardiac function produced by elevated pericardial pressure due to tamponade causes an increase in ventricular filling pressure and hence high pulmonary venous and peripheral venous pressures, and a decrease in stroke output with a small arterial pulse pressure. Occasionally there may be a paradoxical pulse.

23. Intracardiac Ball-Valve Obstruction

Episodes of syncope and acral cyanosis due to intermittent obstruction to flow of blood within the heart caused by an intracardiac foreign body such as a thrombus or myxoma. The signs and symptoms depend on the location and size of the obstruction and are affected by change in the patient's posture. A left intra-atrial mass must at times be differentiated from mitral stenosis. The diagnosis is made by angiographic demonstration of a persistent intracardiac filling defect.

6 / Physical Capacity with Heart Disease

At the present time there is no clinical test which will measure accurately the functional capacity of the heart. For the purpose of this classification this capacity is to be estimated by appraising the patient's ability to perform physical activity. The estimate is only approximate, for it is derived largely by inference from the history, by observation of the patient in certain forms of physical activity, and occasionally by direct or indirect measurement of cardiac function in response to standardized exercises. It represents an expression of opinion concerning the functional capacity of the patient as modified specifically by cardiac disease. The presence of active disease in the heart, acute infectious diseases, convalescence, muscular weakness, anemia, arthritis, pulmonary disease, chest deformity, obesity, and psychogenic disability may interfere with judging the cardiac functional capacity by imposing limitations from these causes. For example, functional capacity is not to be regarded as limited, even though cardiac disease may be present, when it is clear that the patient's incapacity is due to a psychoneurotic state.

The diminution in functional capacity which results from cardiac disease may be accompanied by discomfort or by signs of impaired circulation, or both. The extent to which physical activity is thereby curtailed and the severity of the symptoms caused by effort are used in estimating the degree of reduction of functional capacity. Functional capacity is often limited because of cardiac insufficiency. Physical signs then may be present. Usually structural changes are present in the heart. Occasionally, as, for instance, in certain cases of atrial fibrillation or of paroxysmal tachycardia, or in certain patients suffering from the anginal syndrome, no anatomic lesions can be detected.

In the estimation of cardiac functional capacity, the term *ordinary physical capacity* is used to describe the actual physical performance of which each patient was capable prior to the onset of manifest cardiac disease, or such activity as would be normal for an individual of the same age, sex, and physical development. When cardiac disease exists from birth, a patient's functional capacity can only be estimated by comparison with that of normal persons. A parent's comparison of a child's activity with that of normal siblings or playmates is frequently helpful. Infants pose a special problem. Since an infant's activity is necessarily limited in type, other factors must be considered in evaluating functional capacity. These include fatigue with feedings, prolonged feedings, undue respiratory distress or cyanosis after crying or straining, and delayed motor development. Older children with congenital heart disease may disclaim any symptoms with *ordinary physical activity*. Careful questioning may reveal, however, that they have learned to limit their own activity so that the low-exertion program of living they have adopted as "normal" reflects a considerably reduced functional capacity.

In estimating a patient's response to effort, a comparison must be made between his ordinary physical activity and his present capacity for physical exertion. Usually this estimate is based upon the history, with particular reference to the patient's symptoms on effort or with emotional stress. A careful history is needed to determine, as accurately as possible, the rate at which an individual walks compared with others and compared with the way he walked before his heart trouble, as well as the number of yards (or miles) he can walk comfortably and how many stairs he can climb without noticing symptoms. It is also helpful to learn whether the patient needs to rest during the day or to get added rest at night or on week-ends. If there is difficulty in deciding on the proper rating by this method, direct observation of a patient during and after the performance of a moderately strenuous exercise may be helpful. This is particularly true when the patient restricts himself below the level of symptoms or gives a poor history. More detailed information may be obtained from the performance of standardized exercise tests with known energy requirements. The occurrence of undue dyspnea, exhaustion, or cardiac pain, or of changes in blood pressure, in heart rate, or in the electrocardiogram is of special significance. As was indicated in the opening paragraph, a test is not a substitute for but may be a helpful supplement to the clinical determination of cardiac function by history.

In general, the more intensive the subjective symptoms (or the objective findings), the more likely that there will be physical signs of cardiac disease, cardiac insufficiency, or both. Discrepancies often exist between the number and intensity of physical signs and the degree of subjective distress on effort. This is particularly so in patients suffering from the anginal syndrome in whom objective evidence of disease may be slight or absent. With dyspnea on exertion, special care should be taken to rule out or to evaluate the role of the pulmonary causes of dyspnea such as obstructive emphysema, bronchial asthma, and pulmonary fibrosis.

The classification of patients according to their cardiac functional capacity gives only a part of the information needed to plan the management of the patient's activities. A recommendation or prescription regarding physical activity should be based on information derived from many sources (see **6.2**). The functional classification is an estimate of what the patient's heart will allow him to do and should not be influenced by the character of the structural lesions nor by an opinion as to treatment or prognosis.

1. Functional Classification

CLASS I. Patients with cardiac disease but without resulting limitations of physical activity. Ordinary physical activity does not cause undue fatigue, palpitation, dyspnea, or anginal pain.

CLASS II.   Patients with cardiac disease resulting in slight limitation of physical activity. They are comfortable at rest. Ordinary physical activity results in fatigue, palpitation, dyspnea, or anginal pain.

CLASS III.   Patients with cardiac disease resulting in marked limitation of physical activity. They are comfortable at rest. Less than ordinary physical activity causes fatigue, palpitation, dyspnea, or anginal pain.

CLASS IV.   Patients with cardiac disease resulting in inability to carry on any physical activity without discomfort. Symptoms of cardiac insufficiency or of the anginal syndrome may be present even at rest. If any physical activity is undertaken, discomfort is increased.

2. Therapeutic Classification

The therapeutic classification is intended as a guide to the management of the activities of cardiac patients. It gives a prescription for the amount of physical activity which is advised for those in each functional class. From a practical point of view, it should be translated into terms of daily physical activity, such as walking a certain number of yards, climbing a specified number of stairs, lifting a certain number of pounds, and standing for an unlimited or limited part of the working day. For children it is necessary to individualize with permissible play programs, specifying the type and duration of outdoor and indoor activity which may be performed.

The functional capacity of the patient does not always determine the amount of physical activity that should be permitted. For example, although a child at the onset of active rheumatic carditis may not experience discomfort on playing baseball, rest in bed is imperative. Such a patient would be designated as Class I (Functional), E (Therapeutic). There is frequently a difference between the amount of activity which a patient can undertake in terms of his functional capacity and that which he should attempt in order to prevent aggravation of his disease. The recommendation of physical activity is based not only upon the amount of effort possible without discomfort but also upon the nature and severity of the cardiac disease. This is illustrated in the case of a patient convalescing from a myocardial infarction. Two months after his attack the patient may be free of symptoms on ordinary physical activity and may even be capable of heavy work, including lifting 40 pounds or doing repeated stair or ladder climbing. Such a patient would properly be designated as Class I (Functional), C (Therapeutic). If the patient continues in good health at a later time, the functional and therapeutic classifications would be changed to IB or even IA. On the other hand, if his cardiac condition deteriorates, the classifications would be downgraded to IID or lower.

It should be stressed that in prescribing activity for the cardiac patient an excessively conservative attitude is as harmful to the patient as an overpermissive attitude.

The therapeutic classification is as follows:

CLASS A. Patients with cardiac disease whose physical activity need not be restricted in any way.

CLASS B. Patients with cardiac disease whose ordinary physical activity need not be restricted, but who should be advised against severe or competitive efforts.

CLASS C. Patients with cardiac disease whose ordinary physical activity should be moderately restricted, and whose more strenuous efforts should be discontinued.

CLASS D. Patients with cardiac disease whose ordinary physical activity should be markedly restricted.

CLASS E. Patients with cardiac disease who should be at complete rest, confined to bed or chair.

7 / Uncertain Diagnosis

1. No Heart Disease: Predisposing Etiologic Factor*

Patients in whom no cardiac disease is discovered but whose course should be followed by periodic examinations because of the presence or history of an etiologic factor which might cause heart disease. These should be recorded as No Heart Disease: History of (*stating the etiologic factor*).

2. No Heart Disease: Unexplained Manifestation

Patients with symptoms or signs referable to the heart but in whom a diagnosis of cardiac disease is uncertain at the time of examination. These cases should be recorded as No Heart Disease: Unexplained Manifestation, with a further recommendation that re-examination be performed after a stated interval.

When there is a reasonable probability that the symptoms or signs are not of cardiac origin, the diagnosis should be No Heart Disease.

---

* Some patients in this category may also have symptoms or signs suggestive but not diagnostic of heart disease. The diagnosis in such cases should be No Heart Disease: History of _____ and unexplained manifestation; re-examine on _____.

Part II | *Nomenclature and Criteria for the Vascular Diagnosis*

8 / Nomenclature for the Vascular Diagnosis

The diagnosis of a vascular disease, as that of a cardiac disease, may be made in terms of the cause, the morbid anatomy, the functional circulatory disturbance, and the physical incapacity of the patient. Although the criteria for the vascular diagnosis have not been subdivided into these rubrics in the present edition, it is hoped that the practice of using these rubrics will become sufficiently prevalent and experience sufficiently great to justify such a subdivision in future editions. Although it is recognized that differences from cardiac disease may make the use of multiple diagnostic criteria difficult or impossible in some vascular conditions, they can be employed with advantage in the diagnosis of most vascular diseases. The method will usually be found helpful in the orderly formulation and recording of the thoughts and opinions of the examiner in the diagnosis of specific conditions. It should also aid in the extension of knowledge concerning the various significant aspects of vascular diseases. The method permits a broader, more inclusive diagnostic approach, one which is of particular importance in arterial occlusive disease where cerebral, coronary, renal, peripheral, and other vessels may be involved in the same individual.

It is suggested that the specific vascular condition be indicated as one of the broad subdivisions to which it belongs—arterial, venous, or lymphatic—and be further amplified by etiologic, anatomic, physiologic, and functional and therapeutic descriptions, the last defined as are those used in cardiac diseases (6.1, 2). Examples are given below.

An organic occlusive arterial disease combined with heart disease:

1. Arterial disease (atherosclerosis obliterans)
   a. Atherosclerosis
   b. Occlusion of left superficial femoral artery
   c. Intermittent claudication, left calf (150 yards)
   d. Class IIIC
2. Cardiac
   a. Hypertension and atherosclerosis
   b. Enlarged heart, coronary sclerosis, myocardial fibrosis
   c. Normal sinus rhythm, anginal syndrome
   d. Class IIIC

A vasomotor type of arterial disease:

1. Arterial disease (primary Raynaud's disease)
   a. Unknown
   b. Occlusion of distal digital arteries, both hands, necrosis of tips
   c. Digital artery spasm, fingers and toes (with cold or emotional stress)
   d. Class IIC

A disease of the veins:

1. Venous disease (thrombophlebitis, secondary)
   a. Mechanical injury (pelvic surgery)
   b. Left iliofemoral vein thrombosis with phlebitis and periphlebitis
   c. Edema, pain, limitation of motion
   d. Class IVE

A lymphatic disease:

1. Lymphatic disease (lymphedema, secondary)
   a. Surgical excision of lymph nodes (right radical mastectomy)
   b. Lymphatic obstruction, right axilla
   c. Edema, right arm
   d. Class IB

As in the diagnosis of cardiac diseases (7.1, 2), the terms No Vascular Disease, Unexplained Manifestation, or No Vascular Disease, Predisposing Etiologic Factor should be used when it is not possible to make a structural or recognized functional vascular diagnosis in the presence of symptoms suggestive of vascular disease or when there is a significant factor which may predispose to vascular disease and no vascular condition can be clearly identified.

9. Diseases of the Arteries and Arterioles*

FUNCTIONAL

Vasoconstrictor:
1. Raynaud's disease (primary or idiopathic Raynaud's phenomenon)
2. Raynaud's syndrome (secondary Raynaud's phenomenon)
3. Acrocyanosis
4. Cutis marmorata (marble skin)
5. Vasospasm, secondary

Vasodilator:
6. Erythermalgia, primary (erythromelalgia)
7. Erythermalgia, secondary

ORGANIC

Occlusive:
8. Arteriosclerosis
9. Thromboangiitis obliterans (Buerger's disease)
10. Polyarteritis nodosa (essential polyangiitis, periarteritis nodosa, panarteritis nodosa, essential periarteritis)
11. Cranial arteritis (temporal arteritis)
12. Ergotism

* To facilitate cross-referencing, the numbering of the sections in the chapter on nomenclature conforms to the numbering of the corresponding chapters on vascular diagnosis.

13. Arteritis, secondary
14. Hypertensive vascular disease
15. Arteriolitis, secondary
16. Arterial thrombosis
17. Abscess of wall of artery
18. Frostbite
19. Pernio (chilblain)
20. Idiopathic livedo reticularis
21. Arterial embolism

Nonocclusive:
22. Aneurysm
23. Dissecting hematoma (dissecting aneurysm)
24. Arteriovenous anastomosis (arteriovenous fistula)
25. Congenital anomalies of artery (other than aneurysm or fistula)
26. Trauma to artery
27. Scalenus anticus syndrome
28. Rupture of artery
29. Exposure to radiation

10. Diseases of the Veins

FUNCTIONAL

1. Venospasm
2. Venoparalysis

ORGANIC

Occlusive:
3. Superficial and deep thrombophlebitis and venous thrombosis (phlebothrombosis)

Nonocclusive:
4. Varicosities
5. Phlebectasia (venous anomalies)

6. Phlebosclerosis
7. Periphlebitis and phlebitis without thrombosis
8. Rupture of vein
9. Congenital hypoplasia of veins

11. Diseases of the Lymphatics

FUNCTIONAL
ORGANIC

Obstructive:
1. Noninflammatory lymphedema
2. Inflammatory lymphedema

Nonobstructive:
3. Lymphatic fistulas causing lymphedema
4. Other conditions causing lymphedema (specify condition)

Lymphatic Tumors:
5. Lymphangioma
6. Lymphangiosarcoma

12. Diseases of the Minute Vessels

INCREASED FRAGILITY OF VESSELS

1. Infectious (bacterial) purpura
2. Toxic purpura
3. Allergic purpura
4. Purpura due to avitaminosis
5. Von Willebrand's disease
6. Idiopathic purpura

INCREASED PERMEABILITY OF VESSELS

7. Sensitivity to physical agents
8. Purpura secondary to increased venous pressure

9. Hematogenic purpura
10. Frostbite

PURPURA SECONDARY TO DEFICIENCIES IN THE CIRCULATING BLOOD

11. Platelet deficiencies
12. Disturbances in the clotting mechanism

13. Neoplasms of the Blood Vessels

1. Capillary hemangioma
2. Cavernous hemangioma
3. Hypertrophic hemangioma
4. Racemose (cirsoid) hemangioma
5. Hemangioendothelioma (benign, malignant)
6. Hemangiopericytoma
7. Systemic hemangiomas
8. Congenital neurocutaneous syndromes associated with angiomatosis
9. Hemangiomas of organs other than the skin
10. Telangiectasis*
11. Angiosarcoma†
12. Kaposi's sarcoma‡

---

* Standard Nomenclature uses *Hemangiomatosis.*
† Standard Nomenclature uses *Hemangiosarcoma.*
‡ Standard Nomenclature uses *Multiple Hemorrhagic Hemangioma of Kaposi.*

9 / Diseases of the Arteries and Arterioles

Functional

VASOCONSTRICTOR

1. Raynaud's Disease (Primary or Idiopathic Raynaud's Phenomenon)

A vasospastic condition beginning usually in early adulthood and affecting women about three times as commonly as men. It is often symmetrical. The small arteries and arterioles of the fingers and occasionally of the toes, ears, nose, or cheeks become constricted upon exposure of the body (not just the hands) to cold or under the influence of emotion. The affected acral parts become pale or cyanotic and numb. Upon cessation of the stimulus, rubor may develop with tingling or burning lasting 15 to 20 minutes. Oft-repeated attacks may induce trophic changes and painful ulcers of the finger tips or other parts of the body. Extensive gangrene never develops. In a few cases scleroderma confined to the fingers (sclerodactylia) may eventuate; the skin becomes shiny, tense, hard, and pigmented, and the joints of the fingers ankylosed. Calcinosis is a rare sequel.

2. Raynaud's Syndrome (Secondary Raynaud's Phenomenon)

2.1. TRAUMATIC VASOSPASTIC SYNDROME (PNEUMATIC HAMMER DISEASE). Raynaud's phenomenon may result from the use of vibrating tools. It is usually unilateral at first, involving the hand nearest to the vibrating part of the tool. Thereafter both hands become involved. As in the idiopathic variety, an attack is always precipitated by exposure to cold and not by the use of the tool, unless the tool is cold when it is being handled. Recovery is not common even when the occupation is abandoned.

2.2. NEUROVASCULAR MECHANISMS

a. *Cervical rib.* Cervical ribs arising from the seventh, sixth, or less commonly the fifth cervical vertebra may exert pressure on the subclavian artery, brachial plexus, or sympathetic fibers and produce Raynaud's phenomenon, paresthesias, coldness, and cyanosis on abduction, and in rare cases enough persistent impairment of arterial circulation to cause gangrene. Roentgenograms are confirmatory. A fibrous band representing a residual cervical rib may cause the syndrome and yet not be visible roentgenographically.

b. *Scalenus anticus syndrome.* A neurovascular syndrome produced by contraction, spasm, and hypertrophy of the scalenus anticus muscle so that the subclavian artery, brachial plexus, or sympathetic fibers become pinched between the scalenus anticus and the medius muscles. Frequently there is tenderness on pressure over the scalenus muscle.

c. *Hyperabduction syndrome.* Circumduction which brings the arms together above the head with the elbows flexed, or with the plane of their long axes corresponding to that of the body as in sleeping with the arms behind the head, may cause compression and at the same time torsion of the subclavian artery and brachial plexus, resulting in paresthesias and obliteration of the radial pulses. In extreme cases pain and gangrene may result.

d. *Spondylitis.*   Cervical spondylitis or ruptured nucleus pulposus may produce vasospasm with resulting color and temperature changes in the hands and fingers, accompanied by paresthesias and often by severe pain. Aggravation is produced by extension or twisting of the neck, straining, and coughing. Roentgenographic examination, including myelography, is helpful in the diagnosis.

e. *Neuritis with secondary vasospasm.*   Any neurologic condition that results in long-standing disuse may result in a disturbance of the circulation, with changes in color and temperature. Examples include peripheral neuritis, chronic anterior poliomyelitis, progressive muscular atrophy, syringomyelia, causalgia, spina bifida, and monoplegia. The vascular manifestation may cause persistent cyanosis, pallor, coldness, or Raynaud's syndrome.

2.3.   RAYNAUD'S SYNDROME SECONDARY TO ORGANIC VASCULAR DISEASE

a. *Atherosclerosis.*   Raynaud's phenomenon occurs in about 10 percent of cases of atherosclerosis obliterans. In these pallor or cyanosis or both are produced by cold but usually not by emotion. Numbness and aching occur during pallor, burning and tingling during recovery. The advanced age of the patient and evidence of occlusive atherosclerotic disease suggest the primary process.

b. *Thromboangiitis obliterans.*   Raynaud's phenomenon may accompany thromboangiitis obliterans, at first affecting one or more digits.

c. *Syphilitic arteritis.*   Raynaud's phenomenon has been reported to accompany syphilitic arteritis of the acral parts. For a diagnosis positive serologic tests should be fortified by histologic examination.

2.4.   RAYNAUD'S SYNDROME SECONDARY TO INTOXICATION

a. *Arsenic.*   To prove the relationship, the vasomotor symptoms and other evidence of arsenical poisoning must clear up when the arsenic is discontinued.

b. *Ergot.*   Ergot will produce extensive vasospasm with resultant secondary Raynaud's syndrome and even gangrene of acral parts when hemostasis results in thrombosis. Coldness, cyanosis, and burning pain precede the dry gangrene and eventual mummification. Other symptoms of ergotism, involving the functions of many organs, may occur. Personal susceptibility to the drug varies greatly.

c. *Lead.*   Lead poisoning has been reported to produce Raynaud's phenomenon.

2.5.   SCLERODERMA (DIFFUSE SCLERODERMA, SYSTEMIC SCLERODERMA).   This is a diffuse collagen disease with vascular manifestations in many but not all cases. Frequently the earliest sign of its presence is the development of Raynaud's phenomenon in the fingers. This may be present many months before the signs of diffuse disease, such as thickening of the skin, are recognized by the patient and before telangiectases, bone absorption, calcinosis, and collagenous changes in the gastrointestinal tract, lungs, and heart occur.

2.6.   MISCELLANEOUS MECHANISMS.   Some of these may be temporary and some chronic, but any of them may sometimes be associated with Raynaud's syndrome. They include dermatomyositis, polyarteritis nodosa (essential polyangiitis), cryoglobulinemia, advanced pulmonary tuberculosis, leukemia, lupus erythematosus, cold allergy, paroxysmal hemoglobinuria, syphilis, malaria, polycythemia vera, and arthritis.

3. Acrocyanosis

Acrocyanosis is characterized by persistent coldness and cyanosis of the distal parts of the extremities. It is often associated with profuse sweating of the volar surfaces and occasionally with local edema. Pressure produces a white spot which slowly disappears. Spontaneous blanching, ulceration, and gangrene do not occur. In most cases symptoms begin between the ages of 20 and 45, and the sex ratio is about equal. Usually the color changes persist throughout life, but in later years they may lessen.

4. Cutis Marmorata (Marble Skin)

A mild form of livedo reticularis (9.20) unassociated with any other disease. Bluish-red mottling of the skin appears on exposure to cold and disappears in a warm environment. It is most common in girls and young women. The arterioles become spasmodically narrowed and the capillaries and venules dilated. Most frequently the feet and legs but occasionally the palms, forearms, arms, and pectoral regions are affected. Coldness, numbness, and aching may occur.

5. Vasospasm, Secondary

5.1. LESIONS OF THE PERIPHERAL NERVES. Vasospasm may occur secondary to peripheral neuropathy.

5.2. LESIONS OF THE BRAIN AND SPINAL CORD. Vasospastic states sometimes follow cerebrovascular and other lesions of the central nervous system.

5.3. THROMBOPHLEBITIS. Arteriospasm occasionally accompanies acute thrombophlebitis and may be severe enough to produce temporary absence of arterial pulsations with some lowering of the cutaneous temperature. Unlike simple arterial occlusion, the leg is swollen and cyanotic rather than pale, and the superficial veins are usually distended rather than collapsed.

5.4. EMBOLISM. Arteriospasm is a common accompaniment of embolism to peripheral arteries and is frequently responsible for severe pain. Both the artery containing the embolus and the neighboring arteries may be affected.

129

5.5. THROMBOSIS.   Acute arterial occlusion due to thrombosis may give rise to vasospasm in other arteries supplying the same region. Coldness, pallor, pain, and other evidences of ischemia are present. In an extreme case this may lead to additional thrombosis in the original or in the nearby blood vessels.

5.6. TRAUMA.   Reflex vascular spasm may result from trauma, producing the condition known as post-traumatic reflex sympathetic dystrophy. Osteoporosis may develop (Sudeck's atrophy, or painful osteoporosis). There must be a history of trauma (although this may have been relatively mild) or of an operation preceding the appearance of symptoms. In early phases there may be Raynaud's phenomenon. Frequently, after a suitable time has elapsed, the skin becomes tender, edematous, painful, cold, moist, and cyanotic, and there is roentgenographic evidence of osteoporosis.

VASODILATOR

6. Erythermalgia, Primary (Erythromelalgia)

In erythermalgia the extremities, especially the palms and soles, are red, hot, painful, and often somewhat swollen. Vasodilatation is the characteristic feature. The symptoms are aggravated by dependency and warmth, and moderately relieved by elevation and cooling. The disease usually occurs in middle or late life, and is chronic in the primary form. Arteries pulsate unusually well unless there is associated occlusive arterial disease. Ulceration and gangrene do not occur.

7. Erythermalgia, Secondary

7.1. IN POLYCYTHEMIA VERA

7.2. MISCELLANEOUS FACTORS.   Erythermalgia may be secondary to fever; hyperthyroidism; alcoholism; neurocirculatory asthenia; menopause; hypertension; diabetes mellitus; gout; rheumatoid arthritis; organic neurologic disease; poisoning by thallium, mercury, or arsenic; pellagra, especially in the early stages; beriberi; and the wearing of nylon hose. Many of these conditions clear up if the primary factor is relieved. With the exception of thallium poisoning, most of the cases reported as "erythermalgia" in these conditions have actually been burning paresthesia rather than true erythermalgia.

Organic

OCCLUSIVE

8. Arteriosclerosis

8.1. ATHEROSCLEROSIS OBLITERANS. Pain is the chief complaint, either (1) intermittent claudication, typified by fatigue and by tightness or cramps in the calves of the legs or the muscles of the thighs which develops after walking a limited distance and which is relieved by rest, or (2) pain at rest, which may be of an aching character when ulcer or gangrene is present, or of a shooting, stabbing, and burning nature when ischemic neuropathy is present. Temperature of the skin may be decreased. Atrophy of the muscles and skin with retarded growth and brittleness of the nails is a sign of severe and usually prolonged ischemia. Arterial insufficiency is confirmed by the development of persistent pallor on elevation of the involved extremity and a delayed venous filling time on dependency, often prolonged beyond the normal of 10 to 15 seconds. The pulsations in the accessible arteries in the involved extremity are diminished or absent, and hardening and tortuosity of the arteries may be noted on palpation. Ulcers, often precipitated by trauma, may develop on the toes, heels, or elsewhere. They are usually dry, but secondary infection may cause them to become moist. Gangrene may appear. The involved portion may become mummified. Oscillometric readings help in determining the patency of major vessels and the level of their occlusion. Studies of the surface temperature that may be made include vasomotor (reflex vasodilatation) tests, which are of value in determining the presence and degree of vasospasm. Roentgenograms may show atheromatous calcification, and arteriograms, necessary in some instances, will give information as to points of occlusion and extent of collateral circulation. The disease may, however, be confused with thromboangiitis obliterans or embolism.

8.2. MEDIAL (MÖNCKEBERG'S) ARTERIOSCLEROSIS.   The media of the main arteries is calcified but the lumen is uncompromised. Pulsations are maintained. Ulcers and gangrene do not occur unless atherosclerosis obliterans is also present. The diagnosis is usually made by palpation of the hardened, tube-like but pulsating vessels and by means of roentgenograms, which show the typical medial calcification in the wall of the arteries.

8.3. COMBINED.   The two forms of arteriosclerosis (9.8.1, 8.2) may occur in the same individual. The clinical manifestations are those produced by atherosclerosis obliterans.

9. Thromboangiitis Obliterans (Buerger's Disease)

A chronic inflammatory disease of the arteries, veins, and secondarily of the nerves, which occurs almost exclusively in men between the ages of 17 and 45. It affects all races. Almost all authentic cases occur in smokers. The extremities, particularly the lower ones, are most commonly involved but any blood vessels may be affected, and in about half of the cases the arteries and veins of the upper extremities are involved.

Pain is usually the earliest and most prominent symptom. It may appear first as intermittent claudication, and is frequently accompanied by paresthesias of pins and needles, formication, and cold or burning sensations. These symptoms are followed by rest pain, which precedes ulceration or gangrene. This is a burning, gnawing type of pain which is worse at night and which may be relieved by walking or by hanging the feet off the side of the bed.

Phlebitis occurs in about 50 percent of the cases. It is usually superficial though it may be deep, and is most commonly below the knees. It is sometimes the earliest manifestation of the disease, and is frequently migratory.

Temperature and color changes occur in the skin as with advanced atherosclerosis obliterans, and pulsations in one or more arteries are diminished or absent. When cellulitis occurs, the skin of the affected area may remain red during elevation. Localized edema due to phlebitis, inactivity, cellulitis, or a combination of these factors is common.

Trophic changes in the skin and nails frequently ensue, the skin becoming shiny, scaly, and pigmented, and the nails thick, discolored, rigid, and slow-growing. Complicating bacterial or fungal infections frequently lead to deep fissures between the toes. Gangrene may follow, with loss of the part involved. Sudden arterial occlusion may occur, with more or less extensive gangrene distal to the site of the occlusion. Ischemic neuropathy, with severe pain described as sharp, dull, shooting, pulling, or tearing, may develop.

Oscillometric readings, arteriographic studies, and reflex vasodilatation tests may be of diagnostic use as in atherosclerosis obliterans (**9.8.1**).

10. Polyarteritis Nodosa (Essential Polyangiitis, Periarteritis Nodosa, Panarteritis Nodosa, Essential Periarteritis)

This disease is more common in men and may occur at any age. The medium-sized and small arteries as well as arterioles are affected so that occlusion or hemorrhage occurs in various parts of the body. The veins are not affected. The clinical course may resemble an acute or subacute chronic infectious disease lasting from days to years, with varied and bizarre local manifestations depending upon the size and location of the blood vessels affected, usually ending in death. There may be cutaneous, muscular, neuritic, and visceral effects. In the skin and subcutaneous tissues, rashes (petechial, necrotic, erythematous), edema, and nodules (due to aneurysms or thickening of the arterial walls) may occur. Arthritis, polymyositis, and polyneuritis are common. Gastrointestinal disturbances, pulmonary involvement, coronary arterial lesions, pancreatic and hepatic dysfunction, renal involvement with hypertension (in about 30 percent of the cases) and renal insufficiency, and cerebrovascular complications have all been observed.

The usual picture is that of successive exacerbations involving one area of the body after another, with malaise, weakness, emaciation, anorexia, insomnia, and headaches. Periods of pyrexia may alternate with long afebrile intervals. Moderate or severe leukocytosis may be present, and eosinophilia frequently occurs. The sedimentation rate is almost always elevated. Anemia may be severe. Often the diagnosis is made by exclusion, but biopsy of an arterial lesion is the best though not too frequent criterion. Even with biopsy, however, the changes may not be specific for polyarteritis.

11. Cranial Arteritis (Temporal Arteritis)

A rather rare, febrile, self-limiting disease of variable duration and unknown etiology which involves the temporal and other cranial arteries. Older persons are affected. The symptoms are systemic and local. The former include fever, malaise, sweating, weakness, anorexia, and weight loss. Locally there are pain and tenderness of one or both temporal arteries, which are reddened, indurated, or nodular. The pulsations may disappear because of thrombosis. Partial or complete loss of vision often occurs. Delirium, transient coma, abnormal neurologic signs, and deafness have been observed. Anemia and slight leukocytosis (but not eosinophilia) may occur. Biopsy of an involved artery confirms the diagnosis.

12. Ergotism

In America ergotism usually results from the improper use of drugs derived from ergot, which may produce severe sympathetic stimulation with initial vasospasm. In other parts of the world, notably Europe, it occurs following the use of rye bread infected with the ergot fungus.

The effects are symmetric and most pronounced in the lower extremities. The nose and ears may be involved. The early stages characterized by coldness, numbness, and rubor or cyanosis of the limbs are reversible. With continued use of the drug, thrombosis of the blood vessels and dry gangrene develop and progress to black mummification. General symptoms of nausea, vomiting, colic, diarrhea, and even convulsions may occur.

13. Arteritis, Secondary

13.1. INFECTIOUS DISEASES. Inflammatory and proliferative alterations of small arteries and arterioles occur in many infectious diseases as a secondary feature. In the rickettsial diseases, for instance, there is widespread endothelial proliferation, degeneration, and necrosis of arterioles, capillaries, and venules with perivascular changes. Thrombosis of the larger arteries may occur. Erythema nodosum and erythema induratum are examples of inflammatory vasculitis caused by a systemic condition.

13.2. LOCAL INFLAMMATORY PROCESSES. In local inflammatory processes, both acute and chronic, the local arteries, capillaries, and venules are involved in the tissues affected. Erythema, edema, ulceration, and necrosis are the main manifestations and are produced by dilatation, increased permeability, and thrombosis of the small blood vessels as a result of infection.

14. Hypertensive Vascular Disease

Hypertensive vascular disease, although characteristically manifested by arteriolar vasoconstriction terminating in organic changes in the arterioles, occasionally produces discrete trophic, ulcerative, or gangrenous lesions of the peripheral parts of the body. An area of bluish discoloration, usually above a malleolus, becomes a hemorrhagic bleb which breaks down and forms a superficial ulcer. This slowly enlarges to a diameter of from 1 to 7 cm. There is little granulation or exudation, and healing is slow. There is moderate to severe pain.

15. Arteriolitis, Secondary

15.1. INFECTIOUS DISEASES.   As in Section 9.13.1.

15.2. LOCAL INFLAMMATORY PROCESSES, ACUTE OR CHRONIC. The manifestations are similar to those seen with arteritis (9.13.2) but are less extensive.

15.3. LUPUS ERYTHEMATOSUS DISSEMINATUS, INCLUDING ATYPICAL VERRUCOUS ENDOCARDITIS.   These conditions of widespread involvement of the small arteries and arterioles (2.14) are of unknown cause. Young women are most often affected.

Disseminated lupus erythematosus may run an acute, a subacute, or a chronic course with fever, malaise, weakness, prostration, and loss of weight. Cutaneous lesions may occur anywhere but are most common on the face and fingers. They vary from bluish to red, edematous, slightly indurated plaques. On the face they usually cover the cheeks and bridge of the nose in a butterfly configuration. Exposure to sunlight aggravates the condition. Purpura, arthralgia, and arthritis are common. Pleural, pericardial, and peritoneal effusions may occur. The lymph nodes and spleen may be enlarged. Cardiac murmurs are often observed. Azotemia and hypertension may develop but are not common. Anemia, leukopenia, thrombocytopenia, albuminuria, cylindruria, and microscopic hematuria are frequent laboratory findings. In chronic cases there are remissions and exacerbations.

The diagnosis of atypical verrucous endocarditis should be suspected when there are signs of progressive endocarditis with prolonged fever, renal damage, and negative blood cultures, but the diagnosis can be made with certainty only at necropsy (3.25).

15.4.   IDIOPATHIC ARTERIOLITIS.   Arteriolitis not associated with recognizable disease entities is sometimes observed. Some are rare cases of progressive disseminated lupus but with more vascular manifestations without cutaneous lesions or endocarditis. Gangrene of the digits and local necroses of the skin may occur.

16. Arterial Thrombosis

Thrombosis may occur in a normal or diseased artery. The occurrence in diseased vessels is considered under appropriate headings elsewhere. Thrombosis in a normal or diseased artery may be secondary to one of the following diseases.

16.1.   INFECTIOUS DISEASES.   These may cause acute arterial occlusion in two ways: (1) by direct invasion of the artery, or (2) by producing enough local inflammation, edema, and venous stasis to shut off the supplying artery. Typhoid fever, influenza, and pneumonia, as well as acute septic infections and ulcerative colitis, may have such effects.

16.2.   BLOOD DYSCRASIA.   Polycythemia vera, anemia, and leukemia.

16.3.   TRAUMA.   Trauma may cause a local thrombosis, or the systemic effects of severe injury may cause a thrombosis that is remote from the site of injury.

16.4. PARTURITION.   Thrombosis due to pressure or to reflex arterial spasm during parturition may occur.

16.5. CARDIAC INSUFFICIENCY.   Thrombosis caused by cardiac insufficiency must be distinguished from embolism, and is most common in the lungs.

16.6. DECREASED VELOCITY OF BLOOD FLOW.   The following conditions may cause sufficient slowing to result in arterial thrombosis: shock, compression, hypotension of hemorrhage, overdosage with narcotics, prolonged bed rest, and the inactivity produced by casts and orthopedic appliances.

16.7. EXPOSURE TO RADIATION.   Scarring and retraction due to x-ray, radium, or radioactive isotopes are probably responsible for some instances of thrombosis. When injected into arteries as a contrast medium, a radiopaque substance sometimes produces arteritis and occlusion.

16.8. IDIOPATHIC.   There is no apparent cause for the thrombosis. Venous thrombosis is frequently associated.

17. Abscess of Wall of Artery

Abscess may occur in any of the coats of the arterial wall. It may result from local spread of infection or may be embolic or metastatic from another focus.

18. Frostbite

Frostbite may result from momentary exposure to subfreezing temperatures or from exposure to low but above-freezing temperatures for a longer time. It occurs more readily if the blood vessels are diseased. Severe degrees of frostbite characteristically produce thrombosis of the arteries and arterioles and also involve the venous and lymphatic channels.

Frostbite has been classified into four degrees of severity, similar to the common classification of burns. Manifestations vary from a mild stage of erythema to gangrene.

19. Pernio (Chilblain)

Pernio is caused by exposure to cold and wet weather, without frostbite. It may be acute or chronic. Occlusive vascular lesions with ulceration occur only in the chronic stages of the disease. Immediately after exposure the skin becomes cool or cold and cyanotic, with edema or blebs. In the early stages there is a dermatitis accompanied by a cyanotic, reddish color and slight edema. The symptoms of itching and burning are aggravated by exposure to heat. In serious cases a hemorrhagic reaction may appear in the affected part. After susceptible patients are repeatedly exposed to the same cold stimulus, painful ulcers develop, leaving permanent scars with atrophy and fibrous changes. This type of lesion has been known as leukopernio, erythrocyanosis, and by other descriptive terms. It has been confused with erythema induratum.

20. Idiopathic Livedo Reticularis

Blotchy discoloration of the skin of the extremities, aggravated by cold and associated with increased vasomotor tone. The lesion may involve the skin of the hands and arms, but the legs and feet are most often affected. Rarely, ulceration and even gangrene may develop. (See Section 9.4.)

21. Arterial Embolism

Any foreign or abnormal particle circulating in the blood may be an embolus and cause an occlusion when it lodges in a vessel too small to permit its further passage. The most frequent source of arterial emboli are the mural thrombi or vegetations that form in the left side of the heart. Atrial fibrillation is often present. Other common origins of embolism are the shock of an operation, parturition, or myocardial infarction. An embolus may arise from a plaque or calcified area in a proximal artery such as the aorta. A patent foramen ovale or other communication between the right and left heart permits paradoxical arterial embolism to arise from thrombi in the systemic venous system. The following objects may cause embolism.

21.1. THROMBUS

21.2. FAT. Fat emboli should be suspected after trauma, particularly following fractures of major bones. Major operations may release fat by indirect introduction into the vessel or by indirect compression. Contusions to soft tissues may liberate fat particles or cause necrosis with secondary fat emboli.

21.3. AIR. Air emboli should be suspected after major trauma. In addition, they may be produced by the opening of a large vein through injury or during vascular surgery, especially in the neck; cardiac and thoracic surgery; the introduction of air into a major vessel during a therapeutic injection; transfusions or catheterization techniques; or the use of a pump oxygenator.

21.4. BACTERIA. Sepsis from local infections, blood stream infections such as occur in pneumonia, typhoid fever, meningitis, or scarlet fever may produce microbial emboli. Chronic diseases may suddenly become responsible for emboli; tuberculosis in its miliary form is an example.

21.5. NEOPLASM. The tendency of a neoplasm to invade both the vascular and lymphatic systems is inherent.

21.6. FUNGI.

21.7. INORGANIC SUBSTANCES. If injected into or near a blood vessel, inorganic substances may become embolic.

21.8. ATHEROMATOUS MATERIAL. Parts of atheromatous plaques have been found as or in emboli.

NONOCCLUSIVE

22. Aneurysm

An arterial aneurysm is a sac-like or sharply demarcated fusiform dilatation. In a "true" aneurysm the sac consists of the vessel's wall. In a "false" aneurysm the arterial wall is partially or completely destroyed and the contiguous structures form a sac-like enclosure through which the blood circulates; it usually develops as a result of a fracture of a calcific plaque. The inner wall of an aneurysm may be lined with laminated blood clots, thereby causing a reduction of pulsations. Aneurysms may be classified according to the causes given below.

22.1. CONGENITAL. The medial coat may be undeveloped or absent; dilatation may occur early in life. These aneurysms are often found intracranially in the internal carotid artery or in the circle of Willis. Rupture usually causes fatal cerebral hemorrhage.

22.2. SYPHILITIC. See Section 3.1.

22.3. ARTERIOSCLEROTIC. The medial coats of arteries affected by arteriosclerosis may rupture. This may occur at an area of calcific deposit or plaque. Common examples are saccular aneurysms occurring in the abdominal aorta and in the popliteal artery.

Arteriosclerosis with medial necrosis is the most common

cause of dissecting aneurysms (3.6; 9.23). Thrombosis of the artery is a frequent complication and at times may produce complete occlusion. Early diagnostic criteria are the physical findings of a pulsating mass or the x-ray appearance of an enlarged blood vessel, often with calcified walls.

22.4.   MYCOTIC.   The wall of the aorta or of any artery may be weakened by a suppurative process secondary to actinomycosis, tuberculosis, brucellosis, subacute bacterial endocarditis, or septicemia as in pneumonia, typhoid fever, or other infectious diseases. Local infection around a major artery may weaken it sufficiently to lead to an aneurysm or to rupture. Aneurysms occur most often where there is stress and strain on the arterial wall, e.g., near joints in the extremities.

22.5.   TRAUMATIC.   May be of the "true" or "false" variety. After injury to an artery its dilatation may be delayed.

22.6.   EMBOLIC.   An embolus may lodge in an artery and cause a weakening of the intimal and medial layers with secondary aneurysm formation.

22.7.   IDIOPATHIC.   In certain instances the true cause of an aneurysm cannot be ascertained.

23. Dissecting Hematoma (Dissecting Aneurysm)

See Sections 3.6 and 9.22.

24. Arteriovenous Anastomosis (Arteriovenous Fistula)

An abnormal communication between an artery and a vein which may be (1) direct, such as following a stab or bullet wound; (2) through a saccular aneurysm involving primarily one vessel; (3) by an abnormal dilatation of and communication through the walls of the several vessels involved; or (4) by arteries and veins opening into contiguous structures.

Arteriographic studies may show the abnormal communication. Birthmarks, hemangiomas, and related vascular lesions may be associated.

The following signs and symptoms may indicate the presence of an arteriovenous anastomosis:

Enlargement of a limb or area of body surface.

Increased local temperature.

Rubor of the affected area.

Unusual prominence of veins.

Audible bruit over the affected area; occasionally a thrill may be felt.

Increased oxygenation of venous blood from the area.

Cardiac insufficiency with enlargement of the heart and insufficiency of the aortic valve.

A pulse slowed by occlusion of the anastomosis by external pressure.

As a result of an arteriovenous fistula, short-circuiting channels are set up in which part of the blood returns to the heart before it has accomplished its function. If these channels are of large size, so much blood may be returned by these short circuits that cardiac output is increased while nutrition to the distal part fails. This may result in cardiac hypertrophy and eventually in heart failure. Arteriovenous anastomoses may be classified according to the causes given below.

24.1. CONGENITAL. The possibility of arteriovenous connections should be considered when there are congenital vascular anomalies such as cavernous hemangiomas, suddenly appearing "varicose veins," and some of the port-wine and other vascular dermal anomalies. Some congenital arteriovenous connections are locally malignant in that, after excision, new anastomoses develop with extension of the process, usually proximal. Although pathologically they do not have the appearance of a malignancy, they may result in the loss of the part and, in some cases, in the loss of life.

143

24.2. TRAUMATIC. Bullet or stab wounds are common causes of arteriovenous fistulas.

24.3. MALIGNANT. Malignancy may weaken the walls of a blood vessel by direct invasion resulting in an arteriovenous fistula.

24.4. BACTERIAL. Infection of the surrounding tissues may invade the walls of an artery and vein, thereby producing an arteriovenous fistula.

24.5. FUNGAL. Fungi may invade the walls of an artery and vein in the same manner as bacteria (above).

25. Congenital Anomalies of Artery (Other Than Aneurysm or Fistula)

The various anomalies include congenital absence of vessels, sometimes major vessels, for which collateral circulation is developed in unusually placed channels. These anomalies are classified as nonocclusive arterial diseases because the circulation to the periphery remains intact and sufficient.

26. Trauma to Artery

In addition to vascular spasm (**9.5.6**), trauma may also produce a nonocclusive organic response. A slight injury to an artery may produce a clot, which may quickly canalize and endothelialize.

27. Scalenus Anticus Syndrome

See Section **9.2.26**. This neurovascular syndrome may also produce a nonocclusive organic vascular response similar to trauma (**9.26**).

28. *Rupture of Artery*

A rupture of a major artery may be due to trauma, direct or indirect, to an accident, or to surgery. With arteriosclerosis, syphilis, or arteritis, a mild trauma may initiate rupture (3.12).

29. *Exposure to Radiation*

X-ray, radium, and radioactive isotopes have profound effects upon the vascular system (9.16.7). These are primarily due to reaction and secondarily to scarring with retraction. There may be telangiectatic changes, thrombosis, ulceration, and vascular occlusion due to contraction of scars. These changes may be progressive over a period of many years. At times they are associated with the development of malignancy.

10 / Diseases of the Veins

Functional

1. Venospasm

Venospasm, a transient, excessive contraction of the circular muscular fibers of the venous wall, may occur after direct mechanical injury of a vein or when neighboring arteries or nerves are involved in a disease process. Cutaneous venospasm may be a compensatory response to a reduction in circulating blood volume, as in shock, or it may follow severe pain or fright. It is dependent upon the integrity of the sympathetic nervous system, although an intrinsic response to local trauma may occur even when the vessel is denervated.

2. Venoparalysis

Sudden loss of normal venous tone may be observed in shock and may, in fact, be one of the etiologic factors in this state. In postural hypotension the usual physiologic increase in venous tone which occurs in the lower extremities on the assumption of the upright position is either pathologically absent or reduced. This causes a decrease in venous return and of cardiac output, leading to eventual fainting. A similar type of response is noted as a temporary phase in the individual who assumes the upright position after a prolonged period of "deconditioning." Nitrites in large doses will also produce pooling in the vessels of the lower extremities on the assumption of the upright position ("nitrite shock"). This is due to the direct vasodilating action of the drugs on the muscular coat of the veins.

Organic

OCCLUSIVE

3. Superficial and Deep Thrombophlebitis and Venous Thrombosis (Phlebothrombosis)

The pathologic change consists of two processes: thrombosis in the lumen and a variable amount of inflammation in the wall.

In superficial thrombophlebitis the process is located in the superficial vessels (long and short saphenous, cephalic, basilic, external jugular). Palpation reveals the presence of a hard linear mass in the subcutaneous tissue, associated with rubor, heat, and tenderness of the skin. Systemic symptoms are generally not present.

When large deep venous trunks are involved (axillary, subclavian, popliteal, iliofemoral), there almost invariably is enlargement of the involved limb, abnormally prominent superficial veins (unless masked by edema), and tenderness along the course of the involved vein. In most instances there are systemic signs such as fever, leukocytosis, and tachycardia.

Phlebothrombosis (venous thrombosis) involving the deep venous plexuses in the calf and plantar portion of the foot is a difficult diagnosis to make. There may be a slight increase in circumference of the calf, as determined by measurement, tenderness to deep palpation in this site, presence of an indefinite mass in the muscle, and pain on dorsiflexion of the foot. Systemic symptoms are usually minimal. No local signs of increased venous pressure occur.

In the case of *superficial* thrombophlebitis resolution generally takes place in a few weeks, leaving either no trace of the process, except for possibly a brown line of pigment in the overlying skin, or a fibrous, nontender, palpable subcutaneous cord. With popliteal and iliofemoral *deep* thrombophlebitis, the frequent residual thickening of the wall, obstruction of the lumen, and destruction of the valves may make the deep venous system incompetent. This may result in the production of the postphlebitic syndrome: persistent pitting or nonpitting edema, secondary varicosities, pigmentation, night cramps, stasis dermatitis, and stasis ulceration.

The sequelae in axillary or subclavian venous thrombosis are usually not as serious. However, swelling may persist for years, there may be a sense of heaviness or dull aching whenever the arm is exercised, or at times the pain and discomfort may be continuous.

With phlebothrombosis, sequelae generally do not occur, the only danger associated with the condition being the relatively frequent occurrence of pulmonary embolism.

3.1.   THROMBOSIS DUE TO INTIMAL DAMAGE

a. Direct trauma may result from crushing injuries, dislocations, fractures, and operative procedures in the pelvis. Prolonged pressure on the calf muscles (as during an operation or in the immediate postoperative period), intermittent compression (as in the various neurovascular syndromes of the upper extremity), and sitting in one position on long trips are traumas in which stasis also contributes to the formation of a clot (see below).

b. Indirect injury may result from sudden and severe or moderate but repeated contractions of large muscle groups which produce a bursting force of considerable magnitude in the regional venous system. Venous angulation in the popliteal space, as produced by kneeling, squatting, or tendinous pressure on the popliteal veins, may contribute to injury of the intima.

c. Intravenous administration of irritants, such as sclerosing or hypertonic solutions, may injure the intima.

d. Inflammatory suppurative lesions may cause phlebitis in contiguous veins.

e. Superficial migratory thrombophlebitis, a specific type, is found in about 40 percent of cases of thromboangiitis obliterans (**9.9**). It is characterized by the presence of small, red, discrete and tender nodules located on the extremities in the course of superficial veins. Together with the overlying and surrounding area of inflammation, the lesions eventually assume a linear shape, with the affected vessel felt as a firm, indurated cord. The process appears in crops, hence the designation "migratory."

Thrombophlebitis migrans is a similar entity except that there are no associated signs of arterial involvement. Furthermore, the condition may involve the intracranial sinuses, as well as the mesenteric, renal, portal, and possibly pulmonary veins, and the deep veins in the extremities.

f. Thrombosis of the vein generally occurs when the adventitia is involved in direct malignant invasion, although in some instances it may be delayed until the tumor has reached the lumen of the vessel.

g. Superficial varicophlebitis is a relatively frequent complication of varicosities.

h. Severe local ischemia following acute embolic or thrombotic arterial occlusion or extensive chronic occlusive arterial disease may cause sufficient change in the intima of veins to lead to thrombosis.

3.2. THROMBOSIS DUE TO CHANGES IN THE CLOTTING MECHANISM OF THE BLOOD

a. Increased coagulability of the blood occurs in visceral carcinoma of an advanced degree, particularly of the head and tail of the pancreas and, less often, of the stomach, lung, and gallbladder.

b. Infectious diseases of bacterial or viral origin may be associated with venous thrombosis. Common among these are typhoid fever, actinomycosis, influenza, rheumatic fever, and pneumonia.

c. Certain hematologic conditions predispose to blood coagulation. Among these are the primary and secondary types of polycythemia. Severe anemia is associated with changes which favor blood coagulation. Other blood dyscrasias in which venous thrombosis may occur are lymphatic and myelogenous leukemia.

3.3. THROMBOSIS DUE TO VENOUS STASIS

a. Among the large number of factors which predispose to venous stasis in the lower extremities are prolonged bed rest, immobilization of a limb, Fowler's position, use of pillows placed under the knees, and sitting for many hours with tight garments around the lower extremities. In patients suffering from congestive heart failure, venous stasis may result from or be aggravated by the increased central venous pressure.

b. Elevated intra-abdominal pressure also raises venous pressure in the lower limbs, thereby producing venous stasis. Such a condition may result from the presence of abdominal neoplasms and aneurysms, ascites, a gravid uterus, and the use of tight abdominal binders.

3.4. THROMBOSIS DUE TO MULTIPLE FACTORS.

With surgical procedures venous thrombosis may result from a number of factors. Venous stasis is present because of immobilization during the early postoperative period. Because of the weight of the legs, there is a tendency for the deep veins in the calf to become collapsed and remain so for relatively long periods of time. As a result, the intimal folds are in contact with each other, an occurrence which leads to irritation and a tendency to clot formation. Finally, the tissue destruction associated with the operative procedure may produce alterations in the plasma in the form of greater viscosity and an elevation of the fibrinogen content, changes which predispose to intravascular clotting.

NONOCCLUSIVE

4. Varicosities

4.1. PRIMARY VARICOSITIES. Although the cause is uncertain, the process responsible for varicosities is incompetency of the venous valves with regurgitation of blood into the superficial venous system distally.

4.2. SECONDARY VARICOSITIES

a. Secondary varicosities follow deep vein thrombophlebitis of the lower extremities. The underlying mechanism is either phlebitic destruction of a critical valve at the site of occlusion or a permanent block in this region. In either case a great load is placed upon the poorly supported regional superficial venous system with the result that the valves in the markedly distended vessels become incompetent, producing regurgitation of blood.

b. Any mechanism which increases local venous pressure in the lower extremities may lead to varicosities, e.g., congenital or acquired arteriovenous fistula, intra-abdominal neoplasms, ascites, and a gravid uterus. In "arterial varices," an entity which is considered to be a modification of a congenital arteriovenous fistula, communication is present between the arterial and venous systems. The venous pressure is high and the venous valves may become incompetent.

5. Phlebectasia (Venous Anomalies)

Phlebectasia may be congenital, secondary, or acquired. As a congenital vascular anomaly, there is significant enlargement and fusiform dilatation of the venous channels in the skin of an extremity without demonstrable evidence of abnormal arteriovenous communication. The condition may result secondarily from primary atrophic diseases of the skin. It may be produced by overexposure to roentgen rays, radium, ultra-violet light, or sunlight, or by a persistently increased venous pressure. Of diagnostic importance are the following signs and symptoms.

Presence of numerous superficial thin-walled vascular structures, giving the extremity a cyanotic appearance.

Complaints of sensations of heaviness, aching, tenseness, and fatigue in the involved limb, produced by physical effort.

Absence of abnormal pulsations, thrills, or bruits, ruling out arterial connections.

Absence of increased pressure in the involved vessels.

Venographic demonstration of the venous sinusoidal character of the vessels.

6. Phlebosclerosis

The superficial and deep veins of the lower extremities are prominent, not because of distention by blood, but because the walls of the vessels have lost their normal elasticity and collapsibility. The vessels may be felt as hard subcutaneous cords which may be mistaken for tendons. Pathologically, there is thickening of the walls, with an increase of connective tissue in the media, atrophy of muscle fibers, and fibrosis of the intima. Although some narrowing of the lumen occurs as a result of these changes, there is no particular tendency to thrombosis.

7. Periphlebitis and Phlebitis Without Thrombosis

These conditions may occur in association with a number of different abnormalities, such as tuberculids, syphilids, erythema nodosum, nontuberculous erythema induratum, and chronic indurated cellulitis. They may also be noted in the vicinity of such pyogenic infections as furuncles, abscesses, and osteomyelitis. Pathologically, it is part of a more widespread inflammatory process involving capillaries, lymph vessels, and small arteries.

A specific type of periphlebitis and phlebitis consists of involvement of a superficial vein of the chest wall, particularly below the nipple extending from the anterior axillary fold toward the epigastrium. The vessel is tender and painful at first and later is felt as a firm cord attached to the skin. The process slowly resolves and after six to eight weeks disappears.

8. Rupture of Vein

Rupture of a vein is followed either by a hemorrhage into the surrounding tissues to form an ecchymosis or a hematoma, or by free external bleeding if the vessel is superficial and erosion through the skin has occurred. The condition may result from severe contusion of the wall of a normal vein or from even slight trauma to a diseased vessel, such as a thinned-out, dilated varix. If the overlying skin is intact, the hemorrhage is usually limited by the increase in tissue pressure which follows the development of the hematoma. On the other hand, external bleeding may result in shock and even exsanguination if it is not quickly controlled.

9. Congenital Hypoplasia of Veins

The superficial veins are small and undeveloped as compared to other structures in the limb. This condition occurs particularly among women, and on occasion it may lead to venous insufficiency and orthostatic edema of the lower extremities.

11 / Diseases of
the Lymphatics

Relative to multiple diagnostic criteria, the etiology of diseases of the lymphatic system is still obscure, although factors which cause impaired lymphatic drainage are often recognizable. The morbid anatomy of lymphatic disease can frequently be identified with the use of new diagnostic tools and, in some instances, by biopsy. The site and the extent of obstruction may be identified with the aid of lymphangiography. The physiologic diagnosis will be more readily accomplished with increased understanding of the different types of edema. The functional and therapeutic diagnosis of lymphatic disease can be derived from a consideration of the other parts of the diagnosis, which indicate the physical disability which the abnormality of the lymphatic system causes the individual patient and the limitations which, in the opinion of the examiner, should be imposed (1, 8).

Functional

Functional diseases of the lymphatic system differ from comparable arterial and venous dysfunctions in that they do not appear to be significantly related to vasomotor derangements. They are most commonly due to disturbed function of the lymphatic vessels and to local factors which influence the distribution of body fluids. The latter include temperature and other effects of environment upon the local part, the composition of body fluids, and the hydrostatic pressure in the veins and capillaries. Flow through the lymphatic system is also influenced by the presence of local metabolites and by variations in osmotic pressure. Important factors in lymphatic return are gravity and movement of the extremities. It is well recognized that prolonged dependency of extremities predisposes to lymphedema in the dependent parts. This edema is augmented by immobilization and by environmental factors. Some conditions which are considered to be diseases of the lymphatic system may in fact be due chiefly to functional factors which have not as yet been adequately identified. This may be true for many instances of so-called lymphedema praecox. Edema of the lower extremities, which occurs commonly in women, particularly in warm weather, and is referred to as "simple" lymphedema, is usually on a functional basis. It is very possible that some forms of congenital lymphedema are, at least in part, due to functional abnormalities.

Organic

Organic diseases of the lymphatic system may be due to obstruction of the lymphatic channels, to lymphangiectasia, or to congenital underdevelopment. It is frequently difficult or impossible to identify clearly the anatomic cause of lymphedema. This applies to noninflammatory "primary" lymphedema and to lymphedema due to any persistent cause. Prolonged lymphatic stasis causes an increase in the protein content of the lymph and proliferation of fibroblasts. Increased fibrosis in turn contributes to further stasis. Inadequate lymphatic drainage predisposes to infection in the involved tissue, which results in thrombosis within the lymph vessels. Thus a vicious cycle is established which tends to perpetuate and increase lymphedema, occasionally with the development of massive enlargement of the involved extremity, a condition to which the term *elephantiasis* is frequently applied. The present classification, although often inadequate, will be useful until further physiologic data on the lymphatics are acquired.

OBSTRUCTIVE

1. Noninflammatory Lymphedema

1.1. PRIMARY LYMPHEDEMA. This term indicates incomplete knowledge of the cause and mechanism of the edema.
a. *Lymphedema praecox.* A clinical syndrome involving the lower extremities, most commonly in young women. One or both limbs may be involved.
b. *Congenital lymphedema.* Involvement of the upper or lower extremities and sometimes of portions of the face or trunk. Edema may be noted at birth or may only become evident during adolescence. The term *Milroy's disease* is usually applied only to lymphedema which is both congenital and hereditary. Congenital lymphedema, unlike obstructive types, consists of widely dilated lymph channels with lymphatic thromboses or evidence of inflammation.

1.2. SECONDARY LYMPHEDEMA
a. Surgical removal of lymphatics and lymph nodes.
b. Obstruction of the involved lymphatics from fibrosis and scarring due to the effects of radiation.
c. Invasion of the lymph nodes by either primary or metastatic neoplasm.

2. Inflammatory Lymphedema

2.1. PRIMARY LYMPHANGITIS. This category includes inflammation involving lymphatic structures where no causal agent can be identified. The etiology of this type of lymphatic disease should be designated as "unknown."
2.2. SECONDARY LYMPHANGITIS. There are numerous known

causes for inflammation of the lymphatics, e.g., invasion by parasites (especially filariasis) and local tissue injury or infection as with ulcerations, insect bites, burns, or furuncles. Cellulitis and lymphangitis are commonly recurrent. The streptococcus is considered to be the most frequent infecting organism. The terms *erysipelas* and *erysipeloid* are then commonly employed to describe the disease.

NONOBSTRUCTIVE

3. Lymphatic Fistulas Causing Lymphedema

4. Other Conditions Causing Lymphedema (Specify Condition)

LYMPHATIC TUMORS

5. Lymphangioma

A benign growth consisting of anastomosing, endothelium-lined channels that contain lymph.

5.1. SIMPLEX. A lymphangioma containing lymph vessels of small caliber. It is usually a sharply circumscribed pale swelling and is often compressible.

5.2. CYSTICUM (HYGROMA OR CYSTIC LYMPHANGIOMA). This is a lymphangioma containing multilocular cysts which can rarely be recognized clinically. It is often congenital and usually occurs in the neck or sacral region.

6. Lymphangiosarcoma

A malignant growth consisting of solid nests of anaplastic endothelial cells and poorly formed channels lacking red blood cells. Microscopically, the separation of this neoplasm from malignant hemangioendothelioma is not obvious, since in both lesions the crudely formed channels are often devoid of red blood cells. It is frequently a deep-seated, pale, firm mass.

12 / Diseases of the Minute Vessels

Not only the capillaries but also the finest arterioles and venules are included under the term *minute vessels.*

In conditions leading to increased pressure within the lumen or to damage to the capillary walls, excessive serum and formed elements may escape. When there is an extravasation of cells into the skin or mucous membranes, the term *petechiae* is used for minute, often multiple hemorrhages 2 mm in diameter or less, and the term *purpura* is used for larger hemorrhages.

Increased Fragility of Vessels

1. Infectious (Bacterial) Purpura

Petechiae are characteristic of bacteremias and septicemias, notably as occurring in subacute bacterial endocarditis.

2. Toxic Purpura

2.1. ARSENIC. Contained in arsphenamine derivatives and in Fowler's solution.

2.2. PHOSPHORUS

2.3. PHENOLPHTHALEIN

2.4. COUMARIN DERIVATIVES AND VITAMIN-K BLOCKING AGENTS. These drugs have an effect on the capillaries which is distinct from their hypothrombinemic effect.

2.5. SNAKE AND INSECT VENOM

2.6. OTHER AGENTS

3. Allergic Purpura

A condition which may be recognized by a history compatible with an allergic diathesis together with the findings of urticaria, eosinophilia, or erythema. In *Schönlein's purpura* the manifestations are primarily articular. In *Henoch's purpura* visceral phenomena predominate. Microscopic examination may show perivascular inflammation around the small vessels. These purpuras are to be distinguished from thrombocytopenic purpura in which platelet antibodies are present.

4. Purpura Due to Avitaminosis

4.1. VITAMIN C. A deficiency of vitamin C results in scurvy, which is characterized by easy bruising, bleeding gums, and depletion of the body stores of ascorbic acid. Failure of the intercellular cement substance to form results in both fragility and permeability of the capillaries.

4.2. VITAMIN K. A deficiency of vitamin K results in a reduction in the levels of a variety of factors necessary for blood coagulation.

5. Von Willebrand's Disease

A constitutional, inherited abnormality of the capillaries with prolonged bleeding time.

6. Idiopathic Purpura

Purpuras of unknown causation include such conditions as senile and menstrual purpura.

Increased Permeability of Vessels

Normally the capillary walls retain the solids of the blood and certain dissolved and suspended material of high molecular weight. The capillary wall acts as an osmotic membrane, allowing fluids and electrolytes to flow freely in accordance with physical laws. Under certain conditions the capillary wall may be changed so as to allow protein and other constituents to flow through.

7. Sensitivity to Physical Agents

Such sensitivity results in local swelling due to extravasation of fluid into the tissue spaces of the skin. The swelling may be pale or red and may be due to one of the following causes.

7.1. MECHANICAL IRRITATION. Scratching, pressure, friction are examples.

7.2. COLD. Allergic release of histamine.

7.3. HEAT. Thermal damage to the capillary walls.

8. Purpura Secondary to Increased Venous Pressure

Increased venous pressure leads to an increase in pressure in the capillaries. Small hemorrhages may result from rupture of these vessels. Such purpuric spots are usually located about the ankles, feet, and hips.

9. Hematogenic Purpura

In contrast to those blood dyscrasias in which purpura is a secondary manifestation of a primary deficiency of a formed element or clotting factor, there are instances in which the blood dyscrasia is believed to have a direct effect on the wall of the capillary. Secondary factors may operate simultaneously. Myeloid and lymphocytic leukemia, aplastic anemia, and macroglobulinemias may appear in this group.

10. Frostbite

See Section 9.18.

Purpura Secondary to Deficiencies in the Circulating Blood

11. Platelet Deficiencies

11.1.   IDIOPATHIC THROMBOCYTOPENIC PURPURA.   This type may include an element of increased capillary fragility.

11.2.   CHEMICAL.   This type includes the effects of myelosuppressive agents and drugs acting through individual sensitivities (platelet agglutinins).

11.3.   BLOOD DYSCRASIAS

11.4.   HYPERSPLENIC STATES

11.5.   INFECTIONS

11.6.   THROMBOTIC THROMBOCYTOPENIC PURPURA

12. Disturbances in the Clotting Mechanism

13 / Neoplasms of the Blood Vessels

1. Capillary Hemangioma

Capillary hemangiomas are benign growths composed of capillary vessels and varying in size from minute tumors to large port-wine marks. The nevus flammeus nuchae is a common inconsequential hemangioma which appears in infants as a superficial light red or pinkish growth in the occipital region. It gradually disappears in the majority of cases.

The spider angioma (nevus araneus) consists of a central red cutaneous punctum with many fine capillary strands radiating like spokes of a wheel for a few millimeters to several centimeters. It may be associated with hepatic disease or pregnancy, or it may occur independently.

The sclerosing hemangioma is a capillary hemangioma with profuse connective tissue proliferation. Just beneath the surface of the skin a solid mass is formed which clinically resembles a small cutaneous fibroma with a faint hue.

2. Cavernous Hemangioma

The blood vessels are more dilated than in the capillary type. There is an expanding connection between the general circulation and the channels of the fundamental capillary hemangioma so that the capillaries become distended to form pools or sinuses separated by septa.

3. Hypertrophic Hemangioma

This is the benign analogue of the malignant hemangioendo-thelioma (13.5). It is a solid, noncompressible tumor which is often locally aggressive and tends to recur after surgical re-moval. Clinically, it resembles a small fibroma of the skin, and therefore its true nature is often revealed only by patho-logic examination.

4. Racemose (Cirsoid) Hemangioma

This type of tumor may arise independently or through the transformation of a pre-existent hemangioma. The distinguish-ing feature is the size of the anteriovenous fistulas. The tumor may gradually become evident or, usually in adult life, sud-denly present itself. Dilated, tortuous, throbbing vessels of this tumor present a pulsating mass that is capable of eroding bone.

5. Hemangioendothelioma (Benign, Malignant)

The hemangioendothelioma has its origin in the vascular endothelial cell. Although the majority are of malignant form, malignant tumors that recur after surgical removal are rare. This tumor is a soft, dark red mass of 1 to 6 or 8 cm or more in diameter which tends to ulcerate and bleed and which may have satellite nodules that are usually painless. This tumor may occur at any age, although it appears more frequently after adolescence.

6. Hemangiopericytoma

This is a vascular tumor formed by endothelial tubes and sprouts derived from the contractile pericytes outside the reticulum sheath of the capillary wall. Although ordinarily benign, on occasion it may demonstrate wide infiltration with metastases. The benign glomus tumor is of this type, being a "hypertrophied caricature" of the specialized arteriovenous anastomoses (Sucquet-Hoyer canals) found in the periphery. It consists of blood vessels embedded in smooth muscle, epithelial cells, and nonmyelinated nerve fibers. These benign tumors may be situated anywhere in the skin but classically they are found on the hands and feet, frequently beneath the nails. Typically, the tumor causes paroxysms of severe radiating pain, especially on pressure. The tumor is usually small, seldom measuring more than a few millimeters in diameter, and when superficial is slate gray in color.

7. Systemic Hemangiomas

These are diffuse vascular tumors which usually occupy an entire extremity or portion of the head or trunk. As much as an entire half of the body may be involved in this congenital neoplastic process.

8. Congenital Neurocutaneous Syndromes Associated with Angiomatosis

Neuroectodermal defects, involving the central nervous system and peripheral nerves, are frequently found to be associated with hemangiomatous lesions. They may be intracranial, dermal, and visceral in distribution. The four congenital neurocutaneous syndromes listed below have been found to be associated with angiomatosis.

8.1. NEUROFIBROMATOSIS (RECKLINGHAUSEN'S DISEASE) WITH ANGIOMAS OF THE SKIN

8.2. TUBEROUS SCLEROSIS OF THE BRAIN, ADENOMA SEBACEUM (PRINGLE'S DISEASE), AND REGIONAL ANGIOMA

8.3. ENCEPHALOFACIAL ANGIOMATOSIS

8.4. HEMANGIOMATOSIS OF THE CEREBELLUM AND RETINA

9. Hemangiomas of Organs Other Than the Skin

Such hemangiomas occur in the orbit and retina, tongue, gastrointestinal tract, liver, and bone.

10. Telangiectasis*

Telangiectasis may not be a pure neoplasm. It may be a varix-like dilatation of pre-existing vascular channels (venules, capillaries, or arterioles) rather than a neoplastic proliferation of new vessels.

10.1. HEREDITARY HEMORRHAGIC TELANGIECTASIS.* This is characterized by numerous dilatations of the cutaneous and mucous membranous capillaries and venules. These anomalies seldom measure over 4 mm in diameter. Rupture of the lesions in the mucous membranes give rise to epistaxis, hematuria, melena, etc. The disease is said to be transmitted by either sex as a simple Mendelian dominant.

10.2. PAPILLARY VARICES (SENILE ANGIOMA, CAYENNE-PEPPER SPOT). Small, red, compressible, localized cutaneous swellings, consisting of a single dilated vessel and occurring with increasing frequency after middle age. They are strictly benign.

11. Angiosarcoma†

The term *angiosarcoma* is seldom used. Many pathologists reserve the term *sarcoma* for neoplasm arising from mesenchymal derivatives other than blood vessels. If many of the neoplastic cells are anaplastic but in places sufficiently differentiated to

* Standard Nomenclature uses *Hemangiomatosis.*
† Standard Nomenclature uses *Hemangiosarcoma.*

form vascular spaces, the diagnosis of malignant hemangio-endothelioma rather than angiosarcoma is made. Some sarcomas are so highly undifferentiated that the parent tissue cannot be ascertained.

12. Kaposi's Sarcoma*

The term *Kaposi's sarcoma* is applied to multiple, pigmented lesions composed of dilated capillaries, fibroblastic proliferations, inflammatory cells, and hemosiderin deposits. The hemosiderin deposition is due to extravasations of blood from ruptured capillaries. The lesions usually appear first in the skin of the extremities. There is a bluish mass of slow-growing blood vessels extending into the adjacent tissues. Males are more commonly affected than females. Visceral lesions do occur, but they are usually undetectable clinically. It is not at all certain whether this entity is really a neoplasm or an inflammation.

* Standard Nomenclature uses *Multiple Hemorrhagic Hemangioma of Kaposi.*

Part III | Nomenclature and Criteria for the Pathologic Diagnosis

14 / Nomenclature for the Pathologic Diagnosis

15. Congenital Anomalies of the Heart and Great Vessels*

THE HEART AS A WHOLE

1. Ectopia cordis
2. Dextroposition
3. Dextrocardia
4. Isolated levocardia or isolated sinistrocardia

INDIVIDUAL CHAMBERS

5. Hypoplasia of the right ventricle
6. Right ventricular infundibular stenosis
7. Cor triatriatum (accessory left atrial chamber)
8. Supravalvular stenosing ring of the left atrium
9. Subaortic stenosis

ATRIAL SEPTUM

10. Patent foramen ovale
11. Atrial septal defect

VENTRICULAR SEPTUM

12. Ventricular septal defect
13. Aneurysm of the ventricular septum
14. Absence of the ventricular septum

---

* To facilitate cross-referencing, the numbering of the sections in the chapter on nomenclature conforms to the numbering of the corresponding chapters on pathologic diagnosis.

15. Large ventricular septal defect and pulmonary stenosis (tetralogy of Fallot)
16. Small ventricular septal defect and pulmonary stenosis

ORIGIN OF THE GREAT ARTERIAL VESSELS

17. Complete transposition of the great vessels
18. Corrected transposition of the great vessels
19. Origin of both great vessels from the right ventricle
20. Persistent truncus arteriosus
21. Partial persistent truncus arteriosus (aorticopulmonary window, aorticopulmonary septal defect)

VALVES

22. Hypoplasia of the tricuspid valve
23. Tricuspid stenosis
24. Tricuspid atresia
25. Ebstein's malformation of the tricuspid valve
26. Pulmonary atresia with intact ventricular septum
27. Pulmonary valvular stenosis with intact ventricular septum
28. Bicuspid pulmonary valve; quadricuspid pulmonary valve
29. Congenital absence of the pulmonary valve
30. Congenital mitral insufficiency
31. Anomalous mural insertion of the chordae tendineae of the mitral valve
32. Double orifice of the mitral valve
33. Mitral stenosis
34. Mitral atresia
35. Coexistent mitral atresia and aortic atresia
36. Congenital aortic stenosis
37. Aortic atresia
38. Bicuspid aortic valve
39. Quadricuspid aortic valve

MYOCARDIUM

40. Idiopathic myocardial hypertrophy

41. Localized hypertrophy of the myocardium
42. Glycogen storage disease of the myocardium
43. Congenital tumor of the myocardium

ENDOCARDIUM

44. Fibroelastosis (endocardial sclerosis)
45. Anomalous endocardial cords

PERICARDIUM

46. Anomalies of the pericardium

CORONARY VESSELS

47. Atresia of the right atrial ostium of the coronary sinus
48. Unusually large communication of the coronary sinus with the left atrium
49. Enlargement of the coronary sinus
50. Absence of the coronary sinus
51. Coronary artery—coronary sinus arteriovenous fistula
52. Single coronary artery
53. Origin of the left circumflex artery from the right coronary artery
54. Origin of both coronary arteries from the same aortic sinus (Valsalva)
55. Origin of a coronary artery from the pulmonary arterial trunk
56. Congenital coronary arterial aneurysms
57. Communication of a coronary artery with a cardiac chamber

ANOMALIES OF THE ASCENDING AORTA

58. Supravalvular aortic stenosis
59. Origin of the right pulmonary artery from the ascending aorta
60. Communication of the ascending aorta with the pulmonary trunk (aorticopulmonary septal defect, aorti-

copulmonary window, partial persistent truncus arteriosus)

61. Hypoplasia of the ascending aorta

ANOMALIES OF THE AORTIC ARCH SYSTEM

62. Interruption of the aortic arch
63. Tubular hypoplasia of the aortic arch
64. Coarctation of the aorta
65. Patent ductus arteriosus
66. Absence of a ductus arteriosus
67. Vascular rings

PULMONARY VEINS

68. Anomalous connection of the pulmonary veins
69. Pulmonary venous stenosis or atresia
70. Pulmonary arteriovenous fistula

CENTRAL SYSTEMIC VEINS

71. Persistent left superior vena cava
72. Termination of the left superior vena cava in the left atrium
73. Termination of the inferior vena cava in the left atrium
74. Continuity of the inferior vena cava with the azygos system

16. Atherosclerotic Coronary Artery Disease

1. Coronary atherosclerosis
2. Infarction of the myocardium
3. Fibrosis of the myocardium
4. Rupture of the myocardium
5. Hemopericardium
6. Aneurysm of the heart

7. Rupture of the papillary muscle
8. Mural thrombosis
9. Hypertrophy of the myocardium
10. Dilatation of the myocardium

17. Hypertensive Heart Disease

1. Hypertrophy of the myocardium
1. Dilatation of the myocardium
3. Necrosis and fibrosis of the myocardium
4. Coronary arterial lesions
5. Valvular lesions

18. Pulmonary Heart Disease

1. Acute pulmonary heart disease (acute cor pulmonale)
2. Chronic pulmonary heart disease (chronic cor pulmonale)

19. Rheumatic Heart Disease

1. Rheumatic myocarditis
2. Rheumatic valvulitis and endocarditis
3. Rheumatic endocarditis of the atrium
4. Rheumatic pericarditis
5. Rheumatic vasculitis

20. Syphilis of the Heart and Aorta

1. Syphilitic aortitis
2. Syphilitic aneurysm of the aorta
3. Involvement of the aortic valve (syphilitic valvulitis)
4. Coronary artery involvement in syphilitic aortitis
5. The myocardium in syphilis
6. Congenital syphilis of the heart and great vessels

173

21. Other Diseases of the Aorta and Pulmonary Artery

1. Atherosclerosis of the aorta
2. Calcification of the aorta
3. Atherosclerosis of the pulmonary artery
4. Medial necrosis
5. Granulomatous giant cell arteritis
6. Thrombosis of the pulmonary artery
7. Embolism of the pulmonary artery

22. Other Diseases of the Coronary Arteries

1. Arteritis (endarteritis, mesarteritis, periarteritis)
2. Polyarteritis nodosa (essential polyangiitis, periarteritis nodosa, panarteritis nodosa)
3. Thromboangiitis obliterans
4. Aneurysm
5. Embolism
6. Rupture (spontaneous)

23. Other Diseases of the Endocardium and Valves

1. Bacterial endocarditis
2. Nonbacterial endocarditis (indeterminate endocarditis)
3. Tuberculosis
4. Annular sclerosis
5. Valvular atheroma
6. Valvular sclerosis (calcific nodular valvular sclerosis, calcareous valvular disease, Mönckeberg's aortic sclerosis, primary ascending sclerosis of the aortic valve)
7. Mural endocardial fibrosis (fibroelastosis, endomyocardial fibrosis)
8. Rheumatoid valvulitis
9. Mural thrombosis (endocardial thrombosis)
10. Endocardial blood cysts
11. Anatomic signs of valvular dysfunction

24. Other Diseases of the Myocardium

1. Infectious myocarditis
2. Isolated myocarditis (Fiedler's myocarditis, idiopathic myocarditis)
3. Myocarditis associated with hypersensitivity reactions
4. Metabolic heart disease
5. Myocardial disease in familial myopathies
6. Idiopathic ventricular hypertrophy
7. Atrophy of the heart

25. Other Diseases of the Pericardium

1. Acute infectious pericarditis
2. Acute nonbacterial pericarditis
3. Acute nonspecific pericarditis (benign, idiopathic, viral)
4. Granulomatous pericarditis
5. Chronic pericarditis
6. Parasitic disease of the pericardium
7. Hemopericardium
8. Hydropericardium
9. Adipose changes in the pericardium
10. Neoplasm of the pericardium

26. Diseases of the Conduction System

1. Congenital disease
2. Rheumatic disease
3. Syphilitic disease
4. Atherosclerotic disease
5. Myocarditis
6. Neoplasms
7. Other involvement of the conduction system

15 / Congenital Anomalies of the Heart and Great Vessels

Cardiovascular malformations may be classified according to the various anatomic components of the heart and great vessels involved.

The Heart as a Whole

1. Ectopia Cordis

The rare situation in which the heart lies outside the thoracic cage. It may protrude through a congenital defect in the anterior thoracic wall, or it may lie in the abdominal cavity.

2. Dextroposition

All or part of the heart lies in the right hemithorax. There need not be any associated cardiac malformation and the anomaly may simply represent accommodation of the heart to peculiarities of other thoracic organs.

3. Dextrocardia

The apex of the heart lies in the right hemithorax (4.19). This phenomenon may appear in one of two situations:

3.1. DEXTROCARDIA WITH SITUS INVERSUS. Here the heart is essentially a mirror image of the heart in situs solitus. The arterial chambers lie on the right side and the venous chambers on the left. Although intracardiac malformations are commonly associated with situs inversus, they are not universal and the heart may be normal except for its mirror image arrangement. The mirror image refers to left and right relationships; the anteroposterior arrangements are like those in situs solitus.

3.2. DEXTROCARDIA WITHOUT SITUS INVERSUS (ISOLATED DEXTROCARDIA). In the first form the heart is as in situs inversus with the right chambers being arterial and the left chambers venous. In the second form the normal left and right relationships are preserved so that the arterial chambers lie on the left and the venous chambers on the right. Because isolated dextrocardia is commonly associated with major intracardiac malformations, the diagnosis requires further qualification if the entire abnormality is to be identified. Among the associated malformations are common ventricle, ventricular septal defect with pulmonary stenosis, and corrected transposition of the great vessels.

4. Isolated Levocardia or Isolated Sinistrocardia

These terms may be applied when the cardiac apex points to the left in a patient with situs inversus of other organs (4.20). Isolated levocardia is essentially the mirror image of isolated dextrocardia occurring in situs solitus of other organs, and has a high degree of association with intracardiac malformations.

Individual Chambers

The primary malformations of individual chambers are abnormal size and localized obstructions. Dilatation of chambers is usually secondary to the functional effect of a disturbance at another site, particularly at the valves.

5. Hypoplasia of the Right Ventricle

This usually takes the form of preservation of the outflow part of the chamber and deficiency of the inflow portion. At times this deficiency may be complete, with little or no element of the inflow part being identifiable, particularly in certain cases of tricuspid atresia.

In other instances the condition is an isolated malformation. The right ventricular chamber is generally small, with the major deficiency being in the inflow portion. The restricted size of the chamber is, in effect, an obstructive lesion during ventricular diastole and may be associated with a right-to-left shunt at the level of the foramen ovale.

In instances of pulmonary atresia with intact ventricular septum, the right ventricular chamber may be diminutive in size. Here the inflow and outflow elements are identifiable and the size of the chamber is considered secondary to the altered dynamics of the valvular obstruction (15.26).

6. Right Ventricular Infundibular Stenosis

This may be represented by one of four anatomic situations. The first is secondary to congenital pulmonary valvular stenosis, and is characterized by pronounced hypertrophy of the right ventricle, particularly of the muscle bundles in the infundibulum (4.13).

The second and third types of infundibular stenosis are

178

primary. In the second type the stenosis, of muscular form, simulates that seen in association with pulmonary valvular stenosis. The third type is similar to the membranous type of subaortic stenosis. A fibrous collar encircles the junction of the inflow and outflow portions of the right ventricle, thereby producing a narrowing that is sometimes referred to as the lower ostium of the infundibulum. Either of these primary types of infundibular stenosis of the right ventricle may be associated with a ventricular septal defect lying proximal to the zone of obstruction.

The fourth type of infundibular stenosis is part of the tetralogy of Fallot. A hypertrophied crista supraventricularis participates with the septal and anterior walls of the right ventricle in forming a narrow tract beneath the pulmonary valve.

7. Cor Triatriatum (Accessory Left Atrial Chamber)

This is a condition considered to be primarily a malformation of the pulmonary veins wherein there is failure of the incorporation of the major pulmonary venous stems into the definitive left atrium (4.12). It results in an accessory left atrial chamber. This cor triatriatum or triatrial heart is characterized by the junction of the pulmonary veins with an atrium-like chamber which is above and separate from the left atrium. The two chambers communicate through a narrow opening. If the opening is sufficiently narrow, an obstructive phenomenon occurs and the altered dynamics simulate those of mitral stenosis.

8. Supravalvular Stenosing Ring of the Left Atrium

This is a rare condition in which a fibrous ring lies in the lower aspect of the left atrium just above the mitral valve. The restricted diameter of this area causes obstruction to blood flow.

179

9. Subaortic Stenosis

This is represented by a restricted caliber of the outflow portion of the left ventricle (4.7). Muscular and membranous types occur.

9.1. MUSCULAR TYPE. This type is characterized by pronounced hypertrophy of that portion of the ventricular septum which forms the outflow tract of the left ventricle. Secondary endocardial thickening may occur over the area of muscular thickening and on the opposite wall of the outflow tract on the ventricular aspect of the anterior leaflet of the mitral valve.

9.2. MEMBRANOUS TYPE. This type is characterized by an essentially normal ventricular septum. The obstruction is caused by a fibrous ring encircling the outflow tract, usually about 1 cm below the aortic valve. The fibrous stenosing ring involves not only the endocardium over the septal wall of the outflow tract, but also that part of the wall of the outflow tract which is formed by the anterior leaflet of the mitral valve.

Atrial Septum

10. Patent Foramen Ovale

Patent foramen ovale is a term used in one of two ways: (1) to designate the type of patent foramen ovale characteristic of the normal interatrial passage in the fetal heart, or (2) to designate a permanent interatrial communication at the fossa ovalis. It is recommended that the term *atrial septal defect* be applied to the latter type of condition. In this way *patent foramen ovale* would be synonymous with the terms *probe patent foramen ovale* and *valvular competent patent foramen ovale.* The latter of the two terms is preferable in that it indicates specifically that a potential channel exists through which blood may flow from the right atrium into the left but because of a valve flap is prevented from flowing in the reverse direction when the pressure in the left atrium is higher (4.28).

11. Atrial Septal Defect

This is a permanent opening in the atrial septum. Several types may be recognized according to the position of the defect relative to the fossa ovalis.

11.1. ATRIAL SEPTAL DEFECT AT THE FOSSA OVALIS. This is commonly called *ostium secundum defect.* It lies anterior to the coronary sinus and, regardless of size, is separated from the atrioventricular valves by some septal tissue. The defect at the fossa ovalis is usually represented by a single opening. Less commonly, one or several bands of septal tissue may convert the defect into several openings. Sometimes a lacework of delicate fibers crosses the defect.

The valve of the inferior vena cava (eustachian) lies posterior and slightly to the right of the atrial septum. When the atrial septal defect is large and extends to the posterior atrial wall, the valve of the inferior vena cava is large. Under these circumstances the anterior edge of the valve of the inferior vena cava may be regarded erroneously as the posterior edge of the septal defect.

11.2. ATRIAL SEPTAL DEFECT INFERIOR TO THE FOSSA OVALIS. This is usually part of a developmental complex, including malformation of the atrioventricular valves, often called a *persistent ostium primum* type of atrial septal defect. Atrioventricular valvular tissue rather than septal tissue lies at the lower edge. The valvular malformation is characterized by clefts in one or both atrioventricular valves. When present in both the tricuspid and mitral valves, the clefts involve the

181

septal and anterior leaflets respectively. One of two possible formations exists: (1) The two clefts are continuous so that instead of both the mitral and tricuspid valves being present in the usual sense, there is one valve common to both sides of the heart; in this circumstance the *complete* variety of persistent common atrioventricular canal is present. (2) A bridge of valvular tissue separates the clefts in each of the two valves; this malformation may be termed the *transitional* or *intermediate* type of persistent common atrioventricular canal. If a cleft is present in only one of the two atrioventricular valves (usually the mitral) and if the ostium primum type of atrial septal defect is associated, the complex may be termed the *partial* type of persistent common atrioventricular canal. A synonym for this variety is *persistent ostium primum with cleft mitral valve.*

For the varieties of persistent common atrioventricular canal here defined, the term *endocardial cushion defect* has been applied by some authors. In each variety of persistent common atrioventricular canal, there is a deficiency in the membranous portion of the ventricular septum and in that part of the muscular septum which lies inferior to this area. In the partial variety the potential interventricular communication is usually closed by adhesions of valvular tissue and chordae tendineae to the upper aspect of the deficient ventricular septum. In the other varieties, particularly in the complete variety, spaces between the chordae allow interventricular communication.

11.3. ATRIAL SEPTAL DEFECT SUPERIOR TO THE FOSSA OVALIS. This is a specific type of atrial septal defect which lies above the fossa ovalis and so near the superior vena cava that the vein appears to override the defect. Although these have been classed as *ostium secundum* defects, this is not correct, as the region of the fossa ovalis is readily identified as occupying a position beneath the communication. Other designations used are *superior vena caval* or *sinus venosus* type of atrial septal defect. This type is probably always associated with anomalous connection of all or some of the right pulmonary veins to the superior vena cava or to the right atrium near the entrance of the superior vena cava.

11.4. ATRIAL SEPTAL DEFECT POSTERIOR TO THE FOSSA OVALIS. Although some defects of the fossa ovalis type may involve all of the septal tissue posterior to the fossa ovalis, there is a rare instance wherein the fossa ovalis is normal and a defect lies posterior to it. This rare type of defect is associated with anomalous connection of the right pulmonary veins to the right atrium entering near the defect.

Ventricular Septum

The major anomaly of the ventricular septum is the ventricular septal defect. A basis for subdivision of ventricular septal defects is the identification of their relationship to certain structures in the normal ventricular septum. From the right ventricular aspect, four anatomic landmarks may be identified, starting superoanteriorly and proceeding posteroinferiorly. These are (1) the pulmonary valve, (2) the parietal limb (or band) of the crista supraventricularis, (3) the so-called papillary muscle of the conus, and (4) the membranous septum.

The crista supraventricularis is recognized as having two limbs, the parietal and septal. The parietal limb of the crista lies in the anterior wall of the right ventricular outflow tract and extends from near the basal aspect of the anterior tricuspid leaflet to the pulmonary valve at the junction of its left and right cusps. The septal limb begins at the pulmonary valve and extends downward obliquely along the ventricular septum.

The so-called papillary muscle of the conus represents the site of myocardial attachment of the chordae tendineae from the adjacent portions of the anterior and septal tricuspid leaflets. In some hearts this area is represented as a distinct papillary muscle, whereas in others no specialized muscular formation is present. The membranous septum lies posteroinferiorly to the papillary muscle of the conus and is overhung by the anterior portion of the septal leaflet of the tricuspid valve.

Regions in the septal wall of the outflow tract of the left ventricle may be identified as counterparts of the landmarks on the right side. The long axis of the left ventricular outflow tract is oblique to the outflow tract of the right ventricle. For this reason landmarks which run from a given point posteroinferiorly on the right will run almost directly posteriorly on the left.

The junction of the crista supraventricularis with the pulmonary valve on the right side corresponds with the junction of the right and left aortic cusps on the left side. The body of the parietal limb of the crista supraventricularis on the right lies against the right aortic sinus, and the region just inferior to the parietal limb of the crista lies below the right aortic cusp on the left. The septal branch of the crista supraventricularis corresponds in the left ventricular aspect to muscle inferior to but not continuous with the aortic valve.

Whereas the membranous portion of the ventricular septum is overhung on the right side by the septal leaflet of the tricuspid valve, this membrane on the left lies beneath the adjacent parts of the right and posterior aortic cusps. In some hearts none of the membranous septum extends far enough forward to lie beneath the right aortic cusp, lying immediately adjacent only to the posterior cusp. Posteriorly, on the left, the membranous septum joins the ventricular aspect of the anterior (aortic) leaflet of the mitral valve.

The majority of ventricular septal defects lie in close relationship to elements of the crista supraventricularis.

12. Ventricular Septal Defect

This fundamentally simple anatomic deficiency has a number of possible sites of occurrence that are of considerable importance in terms of surgical correction (4.25).

12.1. VENTRICULAR SEPTAL DEFECT SUPERIOR TO THE CRISTA SUPRAVENTRICULARIS. This is an uncommon type which lies superior to the junction of the parietal and septal limbs of the crista supraventricularis and is therefore bordered on the right by the pulmonary valve. When viewed from the left side, the defect lies in the anterior portion of the outflow part of the ventricular septum, immediately beneath the adjacent portions of the left and right aortic leaflets.

12.2. VENTRICULAR SEPTAL DEFECT INFERIOR TO THE CRISTA SUPRAVENTRICULARIS AND SUPERIOR TO THE PAPILLARY MUSCLE OF THE CONUS. Defects of this type lie in a confined position between the crista supraventricularis and the papillary muscle of the conus. On the left side the defects lie inferior to the right aortic cusp (the right aortic sinus is walled by the crista supraventricularis). The membranous septum is intact.

12.3. VENTRICULAR SEPTAL DEFECT INFERIOR TO THE CRISTA SUPRAVENTRICULARIS AND TO THE PAPILLARY MUSCLE OF THE CONUS. This common type of defect is frequently referred to as the *membranous type of ventricular septal defect,* even though it usually involves more than the membranous portion. The most posterior extremity of the defect (posterior to the papillary muscle of the conus) does involve the membranous portion, and that part which lies superior to the papillary muscle of the conus involves muscle of the outflow tract of both the right and left ventricles.

On the right this defect is in part overhung by the septal leaflet of the tricuspid valve. On the left it lies below varying extents of the right and posterior aortic cusps.

12.4. VENTRICULAR SEPTAL DEFECT OF THE "A–V COMMUNE" TYPE. Isolated ventricular septal defects which have been categorized as being of the A–V commune type are defects of the ventricular septum which bear similarity to the ventricular part of the complex of malformations known as persistent common atrioventricular canal.

185

Two varieties of this defect, the *posterior* and the *anterior,* may be identified. The posterior, which is less common, may involve all of the membranous part of the ventricular septum and then extend posteriorly under the septal leaflet of the tricuspid valve. The upper wall of the defect is formed by atrioventricular valvular tissue representing confluence of septal tricuspid and anterior mitral leaflets. From the left side, therefore, the defect lies under the anterior leaflet of the mitral valve.

The anterior variety occurs more often than the posterior. On the right side it is posterior to the parietal limb of the crista supraventricularis and extends forward against the septal limb. From the left the defect lies in front of the membranous portion of the septum and extends obliquely downward into and along the long axis of the outflow tract of the left ventricle. This is in contrast to the usual variety which lies inferior to the crista supraventricularis and in which the long axis is horizontal and at right angles to the long axis of the outflow tract of the left ventricle.

It is evident that there is some overlap in the positions of the usual variety of ventricular septal defect and in that of the type of defect being discussed here. In addition to the distinctions outlined, one difference revolves around the relationship of the defect to the septal limb of the crista supraventricularis. The usual defect does not extend along this muscle bundle, whereas the anterior variety of the A–V commune type of defect has a distinct relationship to the lower edge of this muscle bundle.

12.5. MUSCULAR VENTRICULAR SEPTAL DEFECT. This type of defect may occur in any portion of the muscular part of the ventricular septum and is often multiple. Characteristically, the ventricular septum which harbors such defects is a highly trabeculated structure not only on the right but on the left side as well. Rather than being perforations of the ventricular septum, defects of this type are often tortuous channels between muscular bundles.

12.6. LEFT VENTRICULAR–RIGHT ATRIAL COMMUNICATION. Special forms of ventricular septal defects, either alone or in combination with malformations of the tricuspid valve, may cause communication between the left ventricle and the right atrium. The pure form of this malformation is a true defect of that part of the membranous portion of the ventricular septum which enters into the formation of the floor of the right atrium. An isolated defect in this location causes an absolute communication between the left ventricle and the right atrium.

In other forms a ventricular septal defect posterior to the crista supraventricularis may be associated with a cleft or a double orifice of the tricuspid valve. With such a combination, streamline flow through the ventricular septal defect may, by chance, coincide with the position of the cleft or double orifice in the tricuspid valve, thereby allowing left ventricular blood to be carried through the right ventricle into the right atrium. Under other circumstances, coexistence of a ventricular septal defect in this position and of a cleft or double orifice of the tricuspid valve shows adhesions between the edges of the ventricular septal defect and those of the cleft, or an extra opening of the tricuspid valve. Here again, a direct channel exists between the left ventricle and the right atrium.

13. Aneurysm of the Ventricular Septum

An aneurysm involves the membranous portion of the ventricular septum. Because of the anatomic location of this structure, the aneurysm bulges into the right ventricle inferior to the junction of the septal and anterior leaflets of the tricuspid valve. As a rule, these aneurysms are imperforate and represent incidental findings.

14. Absence of the Ventricular Septum

This absence is associated either with an intact or with an almost totally absent atrial septum. With the latter the atrioventricular valvular structure is usually of the common variety, without separation into tricuspid and mitral valves. This form of heart may be termed *cor biloculare*. In cor biloculare the arterial origin from the single ventricle is abnormal in that the aorta is transposed and lies anteriorly while the usually hypoplastic or atresic pulmonary trunk lies posteriorly. When the pulmonary trunk is hypoplastic, there is usually a stenotic muscular channel which extends through the wall of the single ventricle upward to the level of the pulmonary valve.

When two atria are present in association with one ventricle, the term *cor triloculare biatriatum* is applicable. The single ventricle is usually one of two forms. The most common is that in which the internal structure of the ventricle bears considerable similarity to that of the two ventricles in corrected transposition of the great vessels. The right and left atrioventricular valves enter the common ventricle. The crista supraventricularis is directed toward the left and bears the mirror image relationship to the aorta that the crista supraventricularis bears to the pulmonary valve in a normal heart. The crista may be said to divide the outflow tract of the common ventricle into an anterior subaortic pocket and a posterior subpulmonary channel. The subaortic pocket extends more superiorly than does the subpulmonary pocket because the valve of the transposed aorta lies at a body level higher than that of the pulmonary valve.

The second variety of cor triloculare biatriatum is one in which obstruction to pulmonary blood flow occurs. The single ventricle may be compared to the two ventricles in the tetralogy of Fallot. The aorta arises to the right of the pulmonary valve and an infundibular channel runs through the anterior wall of the muscle of the common ventricle to lead to a stenotic, or at least narrow, pulmonary trunk. The two semilunar valves lie at about the same body plane with the aortic valve to the right of the pulmonic.

Only under rare circumstances is a single ventricle not associated with an abnormal position of the great arteries.

15. Large Ventricular Septal Defect and Pulmonary Stenosis (Tetralogy of Fallot)

The association of a large ventricular septal defect with free interventricular communication and with obstruction in the pathway between the right ventricle and the pulmonary arteries usually takes a fairly specific anatomic form called the *tetralogy of Fallot* (4.35). The defect lies at the crest of the ventricular septum just in front of the membranous portion. The parietal limb of the crista supraventricularis has an abnormal shape, being vertically rather than obliquely oriented. The defect lies behind the crista supraventricularis. The aorta arises from both ventricles above the defect. The degree of so-called overriding of the aorta varies. In some instances of the tetralogy of Fallot approximately two-thirds of the aorta originates from the left ventricle and one-third from the right; in other instances the aorta may arise entirely over the right ventricle. Even in the latter case the aortic valve maintains normal continuity with the anterior leaflet of the mitral valve. This condition must be distinguished from the condition known as *origin of both great vessels from the right ventricle.*

In the tetralogy of Fallot the obstruction to pulmonary flow may lie in one of several areas, singly or in combination. The abnormally placed crista supraventricularis together with the anterior septal wall of the outflow tract of the right ventricle form an infundibular chamber which usually is stenotic. The pulmonary valve usually is bicuspid and contributes to the stenosis. The pulmonary trunk commonly is narrower than normal but seldom contributes significant obstruction.

Hypertrophy of the right ventricular wall is a universal phenomenon since the right ventricle shares with the left the function of developing systemic pressure during systole.

Malformations of the aortic arch system are commonly associated with the tetralogy of Fallot, being observed in approximately 20 percent of the cases. The most common variety is represented by a right aortic arch from which the branches arise in mirror image fashion of the normal; that is, the first branch is a left innominate artery, the second branch the right common carotid, and the third branch the right subclavian artery. Less common forms of aortic arch malformations in association with the tetralogy of Fallot include a right aortic arch and origin of the left subclavian artery as the fourth branch of the aorta, a condition which represents the mirror image of the more commonly observed anomalous right subclavian artery.

The ductus arteriosus not infrequently shows alterations from the normal. In those cases where a right aortic arch and left innominate artery exist, the ductus arteriosus may extend from the base of the innominate or left subclavian artery, on one hand, to the left pulmonary artery, on the other. When a right aortic arch is present, the ductus arteriosus may be on the right side extending from the aortic arch above to the right pulmonary artery below. The ductus arteriosus is absent in some instances of the tetralogy of Fallot.

Anomalies of the coronary arteries may also coexist with the tetralogy of Fallot. A major variety of anomaly consists of a large coronary artery crossing the outflow tract of the right ventricle. In some instances this may be the anterior descending coronary artery arising from the right coronary artery, or it may, in other instances, represent large collaterals from the anterior descending coronary artery to the bed of the right coronary artery.

16. Small Ventricular Septal Defect and Pulmonary Stenosis

An uncommon combination of defects is pulmonary stenosis in association with a small ventricular septal defect. In such a combination the pulmonary stenosis is of the type usually observed in isolated stenosis of the pulmonary valve. The defect of the ventricular septum may be in the muscular portion.

Origin of the Great Arterial Vessels

When the term *transposition of the great vessels* is used without further qualification, it should be taken to indicate some abnormal relationship between the two great vessels. It is a general term that is at times erroneously used to refer to the specific condition correctly called *complete transposition of the great vessels.*

There is a large variety of anatomic situations in which the great vessels arise abnormally. The most common single variety is the complete transposition.

17. Complete Transposition of the Great Vessels

This is a condition in which the aorta arises exclusively from the right ventricle and the pulmonary trunk arises from the left ventricle (4.29). Under these circumstances the transport of systemic venous blood to the lesser circulation and of pulmonary venous blood to the greater circulation depends on the existence of some communication between the two sides of the circulation. Among the common communications are patent ductus arteriosus and atrial septal defect. Ventricular septal defect represents the third most common communication, occurring in approximately half of the cases. Enlarged bronchial arteries constitute another form of communication between the two circulations. Only rarely does a pulmonary vein connect anomalously to the right side of the circulation, a desirable situation since the abnormal communication allows delivery of oxygenated blood to the right side of the heart and ultimately to the aorta.

The coronary arteries arise from the aorta. Because the infundibular portion of the right ventricle is poorly developed, the aortic and pulmonary valves lie at the same body

191

plane. The atrioventricular valves are normally developed. The anterior leaflet of the mitral valve makes continuity with the pulmonary valve in a way similar to the continuity of the mitral valve with the aortic valve of a normal heart.

18. Corrected Transposition of the Great Vessels

This is a condition in which the great vessels are related to each other as they are in complete transposition of the great vessels, but in spite of this abnormal relationship the route of blood flow is normal (4.18). In its purest form this condition reveals four cardiac chambers, the two atria being normal and the atrial septum being normally oriented. Beyond the atria the atrioventricular valves and the ventricles represent in their structure mirror images of the normal. Thus the right atrioventricular valve has similarity in structure, but in mirror image, to that of a normal mitral valve and, further, the anterior leaflet of the right atrioventricular valve is continuous with elements of the posteriorly lying pulmonary valve. This represents a mirror image arrangement of the normal connection of the mitral valve with the aortic valve. On the left side the atrioventricular valve is basically constructed as a tricuspid valve, although further malformation is characterized by variations of the fully developed picture of Ebstein's anomaly usually seen in the tricuspid valve. Abnormal attachments of the valvular tissues and associated short chordae frequently are responsible for incompetence of the left atrioventricular valve.

The interior of the right-sided ventricle bears similarity in its general structure to the normal left ventricle, and the left-sided ventricle in corrected transposition of the great vessels bears similarity, but in mirror image, to the normal right ventricle. The outflow portion of the left-sided ventricle rises above the level of the right-sided ventricle. Because of this peculiarity, the aortic valve in corrected transposition lies at a considerably higher plane than does the pulmonary valve. Just as the pulmonary valve of the normal heart has no connection with atrioventricular valvular tissue, so the aortic valve in corrected transposition of the great vessels has no continuity with atrioventricular valvular tissue.

The right-sided (venous) ventricle of corrected transposition lies in a more posterior position than does the left-sided (arterial) ventricle. This is in contrast to the arrangement of the normal heart.

A ventricular septal defect is commonly associated (in approximately 50 percent of cases) with corrected transposition of the great vessels. Stenosis of the pulmonary valve or subpulmonary stenosis of the outflow tract of the transposed right-sided ventricle occurs occasionally. The latter lesion is similar to subaortic stenosis occuring in the left ventricle of normally oriented hearts. Isolated dextrocardia may be associated.

Exceptionally, the ventricular septum is absent. In some of these cases both atrioventricular valves are present, and in other cases either the right or left valve is atresic. It becomes a matter of semantics whether or not hearts with this general pattern should be classified as corrected transposition of the great vessels. It seems more appropriate to define the ventricular and great vascular arrangement simply as *single ventricle with transposition* rather than to apply the term *corrected transposition of the great vessels* when the ventricular septum is absent.

19. Origin of Both Great Vessels from the Right Ventricle

A peculiar form of malposition of the great vessels is seen in the circumstance where both great vessels arise from the right ventricle and where the only outlet for the left ventricle is a ventricular septal defect. The abnormal position between the great arteries occurs only at the cardiac level, whereas above the cardiac level the general relationship between the aorta and the pulmonary artery is essentially normal, or nearly so. Two major divisions of origin of both great vessels from the right ventricle may be identified according to the position of the ventricular septal defect relative to the semilunar valves. In the first subgroup, the larger, the ventricular septal defect lies inferior to the crista supraventricularis. The defect is therefore entirely surrounded by muscle or by muscle and atrioventricular valvular tissue. In any circumstance the defect is separated from the semilunar valves by muscular tissue. The remoteness in relationship between the semilunar valves and the ventricular septal defect, which is characteristic of this subgroup, is in contrast to the second subgroup. In this subgroup both great vessels arise from the right ventricle, the ventricular septal defect lies above the crista supraventricularis, and the defect is in direct continuity only with the pulmonary valve (Taussig-Bing complex) or with the pulmonary and the aortic valves together.

One of the major peculiarities in origin of both great vessels from the right ventricle is that the ascending aorta in the supracardiac position has a normal relationship to the pulmonary trunk. At the cardiac level, however, the aorta fails to continue downward and to the left to join the left ventricle; instead the aorta ends at the base of the right ventricle. The two semilunar valves lie at about the same body plane. The ventricular septal defect usually is of the functionally large variety, although in a rare instance it may be small and represent an obstruction to the left ventricular outflow.

Malformations of the aortic arch in the form of tubular hypoplasia, coarctation, and patent ductus arteriosus have a tendency to be associated with origin of both great vessels from the right ventricle.

20. Persistent Truncus Arteriosus

In this condition a single arterial vessel leaves the heart, and from this vessel arise the pulmonary, aortic, and coronary branches (4.23). The single vessel usually lies above the associated ventricular septal defect and then takes origin from both ventricles. Four subdivisions of persistent truncus arteriosus may be made according to the manner of origin of the pulmonary arteries from it.

20.1. A distinct pulmonary trunk and ascending aorta arise from the *common trunk*.

20.2. The pulmonary arteries, with their ostia close together, arise from the *back of the truncus arteriosus*.

20.3. The pulmonary arteries arise from the *lateral aspects of the truncus arteriosus*.

20.4. No pulmonary arteries are identifiable, the blood supply to the lungs being derived by way of the bronchial arteries.

21. Partial Persistent Truncus Arteriosus (Aorticopulmonary Window, Aorticopulmonary Septal Defect)

See Section 15.60.

Valves

Malformations of the valves include such conditions as hypoplasia, stenosis, and atresia. There is a tendency toward synonymous use of these terms, but greater specificity of understanding results when each of these terms is used to denote a specific entity, each different from the other.

Hypoplasia refers to a diminutive state of a valve wherein the basic structure and interrelationships of its components are normal. *Stenosis* refers to an abnormal structure of the valvular elements which results in obstruction to the flow of blood through the valve. The term implies that some opening is present. Therefore the expression *complete stenosis* is meaningless. *Atresia* refers to the absence of any opening. Because this is an absolute condition, such expressions as *slight atresia, partial atresia,* or *severe atresia* are also meaningless.

TRICUSPID VALVE

22. Hypoplasia of the Tricuspid Valve

This is perhaps always a secondary phenomenon resulting from a right ventricular malformation (such as hypoplasia of the right ventricle) or from atresia of the pulmonary valve associated with intact ventricular septum.

The elements of the tricuspid valve are identifiable but smaller than normal and often diminutive. Although this condition may result from a malformation upstream in the circulation, it might constitute an obstructive lesion if the basic malformation were corrected.

23. Tricuspid Stenosis

This is a rare malformation resulting from congenital interadhesion (or lack of differentiation) of the individual leaflets. The basic gross derangement resembles tricuspid stenosis resulting from rheumatic endocarditis, and in individuals beyond the age of infancy it may be impossible to differentiate the congenital and rheumatic varieties of stenosis. In Ebstein's malformation of the tricuspid valve, a stenotic element may be identified in some cases.

24. Tricuspid Atresia

In tricuspid atresia neither valvular elements nor orifice is identifiable, and the only outlet for right atrial blood is an interatrial communication. The latter may take the form of a true atrial septal defect, but the more usual opening is a valvular competent type of patent foramen ovale. The potential size of the patent foramen ovale varies, usually being comparatively large but in some cases sufficiently narrow to constitute an obstruction to right atrial outlet.

As a result of the basic derangements in tricuspid atresia, right atrial blood is carried into the left atrium where it mixes with blood returning from the pulmonary veins. The mixture flows through the mitral valve into the left side of the ventricular portion of the heart, whence it is distributed to the pulmonary trunk and the aorta.

There are variations in the state and interrelationships of the pulmonary trunk and the aorta as well as in the structure of the ventricular portion of the heart. An anatomic classification of tricuspid atresia based on these variations is given below.

24.1. GREAT VESSELS NORMALLY INTERRELATED

a. *Coexistent tricuspid and pulmonary atresia.* The ventricular septum is intact and the right ventricular chamber is a blind structure of microscopic size hidden in the wall of the large left ventricle. The ductus arteriosus is patent.

b. *Hypoplasia of the right ventricle, stenotic ventricular septal defect.* This is the classic and most common variety of tricuspid atresia. The right ventricle is represented only by a hypoplastic infundibulum which communicates with the large left ventricle through a slit-like, narrow muscular ventricular septal defect (which constitutes a zone of subpulmonary stenosis). The pulmonary valve and trunk are more narrow than normal and the pulmonary valve may be tricuspid.

c. *Single ventricle, absence of pulmonary or subpulmonary stenosis.* The ventricular portion of the heart does not exhibit parts which may be identified specifically as right and left ventricular. Instead, a single ventricle is present from which the normally interrelated pulmonary trunk and aorta both arise. There is no pulmonary or subpulmonary stenosis.

d. *Hypoplasia of the right ventricle, wide ventricular septal defect.* The essential structural pattern is like that in Section 24.1b, but in this rare form of tricuspid atresia, the ventricular septal defect is wide. The wall of the deformed right ventricle is thick and the pulmonary trunk is tense, thick-walled, and wide.

24.2. TRANSPOSITION OF THE GREAT VESSELS. In this major type of tricuspid atresia, the ascending aorta lies anterior and parallel to the pulmonary trunk. Each arises from a single ventricle.

a. *Subpulmonary stenosis.* A stenotic muscular channel runs through the base of the heart to the transposed origin of the pulmonary trunk. Although the pulmonary trunk and valve are narrower than normal, the zone of greatest obstruction to pulmonary blood flow lies in the muscular channel.

b. *Absence of pulmonary stenosis.* The essential relationships are like those in Section 24.2a, with the important exception that no obstruction to pulmonary blood flow exists. As a consequence the pulmonary trunk is wide and thick-walled.

25. Ebstein's Malformation of the Tricuspid Valve

Classically, portions of the tricuspid valve are attached at a level lower than the annulus fibrosus (4.16). In the usual instance of the fully developed condition, the septal and posterior leaflets are attached to the right ventricular wall at varying distances between the annulus fibrosus and apex. Not only is there malinsertion of the basal parts of these leaflets, but multiple attachments of the valvular tissue to the ventricular wall often occur so that little in the way of functional tissue remains in the involved portion of the valve. The anterior leaflet is normally formed and attached.

The part of the right ventricle which lies proximal to the

malinsertion of tricuspid valvular tissue is in continuity with the right atrium, forming with the latter a large receiving chamber. The effective volume of the right ventricle is reduced. In many instances the only portion of the right ventricle that functions as such is hardly more than the outflow portion of the chamber. Classically, there is considerable atrophy of the right ventricular wall both proximal and distal to the malinsertion of the tricuspid valve. In the outflow part of the right ventricle, the thinning and dilatation of the chamber may give rise to a roentgenographically false impression of dilatation of the pulmonary artery. The pulmonary artery is of normal caliber or narrower than normal, and the pulmonary valve is normal.

In most instances of Ebstein's malformation, there is interatrial communication (4.34). This usually takes the form of a valvular competent patent foramen ovale, although in some instances, there is a true atrial septal defect. Only rarely is the atrial septum intact. Exceptionally, Ebstein's malformation of the tricuspid valve may be associated with a ventricular septal defect communicating with the outflow portion of the right ventricle.

PULMONARY VALVE

26. Pulmonary Atresia with Intact Ventricular Septum

In this condition the pulmonary valve is represented by a fibrous diaphragm which forms an absolute barrier between the right ventricular cavity and the pulmonary artery. From the upper aspect of the fibrous diaphragm, three equidistant raphe radiate to the pulmonary arterial wall.

When the tricuspid valve is present, pulmonary atresia with intact ventricular septum may present one of two patterns with regard to right ventricular size. In the first type the chamber of the right ventricle is minute, although the wall may be decidedly hypertrophied. The tricuspid valve, although normally formed, is hypoplastic. It is not uncommon for sinusoids in the right ventricular wall to be enlarged and to converge ultimately to form one or several vessels which penetrate the epicardium and make continuity with the standard branches of the coronary artery in this layer of the heart.

In the second type of pulmonary atresia with intact ventricular septum, the right ventricular chamber is either of normal size or enlarged. The tricuspid valve is wide and often gives evidence of having been incompetent. In some instances the incompetence appears to result from undue shortening of chordae and valvular tissue; in other instances minor degrees of Ebstein's malformation are apparent in the valve.

In all instances of pulmonary atresia with intact ventricular septum, there is an interatrial communication, usually a valvular competent patent foramen ovale. The left side of the heart is normal. A patent ductus arteriosus serves to carry blood to the pulmonary arterial system. The pulmonary trunk often is somewhat narrower than normal, although its two major branches are within the range of normal.

A special variety of pulmonary atresia with intact ventricular septum has been discussed under tricuspid atresia (15.24.1a). This is the type in which there is coexistent tricuspid atresia. The right ventricular chamber is a cavity of microscopic size hidden in the right upper aspect of the wall of the left ventricle. Cases of this type are sometimes erroneously referred to as examples of single ventricle.

27. Pulmonary Valvular Stenosis with Intact Ventricular Septum

A comparatively common condition is congenital stenosis of the pulmonary valve associated with intact ventricular septum (4.13). The pulmonary valve has considerable similarity from patient to patient. The valvular tissue is fused and has a central perforation. The upward prolongation of the valvular tissue coupled with its narrow central opening gives the valve the configuration of a truncated cone, referred to as a *dome-shaped stenosis*.

As a consequence of pronounced right ventricular hypertension secondary to pulmonary valvular stenosis, the right ventricular chamber shows marked concentric hypertrophy. This may be responsible for secondary obstruction in the infundibular region.

The tricuspid valve often shows fibrous thickening.

In some instances the atrial septum is intact, and in other cases there is a valvular competent patent foramen ovale.

28. *Bicuspid Pulmonary Valve; Quadricuspid Pulmonary Valve*

Bicuspid pulmonary valve is commonly associated with the tetralogy of Fallot and here it is probably always stenotic. When the bicuspid pulmonary valve occurs in isolated form, the pulmonary trunk is of normal width and the two leaflets are flexible and of considerable length, probably not being responsible for any significant degree of obstruction.

The quadricuspid pulmonary valve is usually represented by three leaflets of nearly equal size, and the fourth, or extra, leaflet is hypoplastic. This malformation does not appear to be associated with any significant functional valvular derangement.

29. *Congenital Absence of the Pulmonary Valve*

Absence of the pulmonary valve or pronounced hypoplasia to a point of functional incompetence are uncommon conditions. They may occur as independent malformations, but more frequently they are associated with some other malformation, particularly the tetralogy of Fallot.

MITRAL VALVE

Malformations of the mitral valve as isolated conditions are comparatively uncommon. More often they are associated with other conditions. An example is the cleft associated with persistent common atrioventricular canal. Another is the Ebstein-like deformity, which may accompany corrected transposition of the great vessels and endocardial sclerosis of the left ventricle. Sections 15.30–34 describe isolated congenital lesions of the mitral valve.

30. Congenital Mitral Insufficiency

Of the several varieties that occur, one is manifested by a cleft in the anterior leaflet of the valve in the same location that is ordinarily encountered in persistent common atrioventricular canal. The cleft extends from the free edge of the leaflet for varying distances toward its base. Often accessory chordae extend from the edges of the cleft to the nearby ventricular septum.

31. Anomalous Mural Insertion of the Chordae Tendineae of the Mitral Valve

This ectopic insertion may be responsible for abnormal apposition of the valvular tissue during ventricular systole, thereby causing mitral insufficiency.

32. Double Orifice of the Mitral Valve

The accessory orifice in one of the leaflets usually has a circular shape, and chordae extend in a parachute-like fashion to an underlying apical portion of an accessory papillary muscle. It is probable that the accessory orifice allows incompetence of the mitral valve to occur.

33. Mitral Stenosis

Congenital mitral stenosis represents one of the most uncommon malformations (4.11). It is often difficult to distinguish this type from acquired rheumatic mitral stenosis, since the basic deformities show considerable similarity. There is fusion of the two leaflets at the commissures and shortening of the chordae, creating a funnel type of mitral valve. In young infants valves of this type are justifiably considered congenital, whereas in children the possibility of rare occurrence of early rheumatic endocarditis makes distinction between a congenital and an acquired variety of mitral stenosis difficult or impossible.

34. Mitral Atresia

In mitral atresia there is no valvular tissue or orifice at the expected location of the mitral valve. Herniation of the anterior edge of the valve of the foramen ovale into the right atrium is the result of flow from the left atrium. The opening between the atria is usually confined so that considerable obstruction to pulmonary venous flow represents an essential functional phenomenon.

The right atrium, which functions as a common atrium, is large. The ventricular portion of the heart varies from patient to patient. Most commonly there is a single ventricle and transposition of the great vessels. Pulmonary stenosis is absent. Less commonly the great vessels are normally oriented and both ventricles are present. In the latter circumstance the left ventricle receives blood through an interventricular communication, which may be a septal defect or, more commonly, multiple muscular septal defects.

In a rare instance of mitral atresia, the interatrial communication that is usually present is either closed by virtue of premature closure of the foramen ovale or is so small an opening that it is ineffective. When this happens, a collateral venous channel may extend from either one of the pulmonary veins or from the left atrium, on one hand, to a systemic vein such as the superior vena cava or the left innominate vein, on the other. This anomalous channel has been referred to as the *levoatriocardinal vein*.

35. Coexistent Mitral Atresia and Aortic Atresia

When mitral atresia is present, usually the aortic valve is normally formed, although the aorta may be transposed. In uncommon circumstances the aortic valve is also atresic (4.38). The entire picture somewhat resembles, in mirror image, the arrangement wherein tricuspid and pulmonary atresia coexist in association with an intact ventricular septum. In this combination on the left side of the heart, the arrangement at the foramen ovale is the same as in isolated mitral atresia. There is, in addition, significant hypoplasia of the ascending aorta similar to that which occurs in aortic atresia. The functional derangements in coexistent mitral and aortic atresia are similar to those in aortic atresia alone (15.37).

AORTIC VALVE

Significant malformations of the aortic valve are more often obstructive than insufficient in nature.

36. Congenital Aortic Stenosis

In each of two recognized forms the aortic valve is somewhat similar to the dome-shaped malformation of the pulmonary valve in isolated pulmonary stenosis. In the less common variety of aortic stenosis, the valvular tissue is represented by a dome-shaped structure with a central perforation. In the more common variety, the aortic valve is represented by one leaflet which forms only one valvular commissure. Opposite the single commissure the valve may show a raphe which extends from the aortic aspect of the valve to the adjacent aortic wall. In some instances this raphe is shallow and offers little support to the valvular tissue; in other instances, it has considerable height and thus offers more support (4.7).

37. Aortic Atresia

The valve is represented by a fibrous membrane. From the central portion of its aortic aspect three equidistant raphe radiate to the aortic wall. The ventricular septum is intact. Classically, the left ventricular chamber is minute, and the mitral valve, though essentially normal, is diminutive in size. The left ventricular wall is greatly hypertrophied. As in pulmonary atresia with intact ventricular septum and small right ventricular chamber, converging sinusoids may carry blood from the obstructed ventricle into the epicardial ramifications of the coronary arteries.

In aortic atresia there is an interatrial communication similar to that occurring in mitral atresia. Because all of the blood from the left side of the circulation is diverted into the two right-sided chambers, there is enlargement of the right atrium and the right ventricle. A patent ductus arteriosus serves as the channel for delivery of blood from the pulmonary arterial system into the aorta. The aortic arch and descending portion of the aorta are of normal caliber, but the ascending aorta, classically, is hypoplastic. Functionally, the ascending aorta simply represents a channel for retrograde delivery of blood to the coronary arteries, the latter arising from the aorta above the level of the atresic valve.

38. Bicuspid Aortic Valve

The bicuspid aortic valve may occur as an isolated malformation. It accompanies approximately 85 percent of the cases of coarctation of the aorta and is found in an occasional instance of congenital polycystic kidneys.

Although hypothetically the bicuspid aortic valve may function normally, there is probably always a minor degree of stenosis or an element of insufficiency. Valves of this type are particularly subject to acquired disease such as calcific stenosis or bacterial endocarditis.

39. Quadricuspid Aortic Valve

As in the case of the quadricuspid pulmonary valve, the aortic valve may be composed of four leaflets. Often one of the four leaflets is rudimentary with the other three tending to approach normal size.

Myocardium

Primary malformations of the myocardium are rather uncommon. Included among these malformations are several types of hypertrophies, glycogen infiltration, and tumors.

40. Idiopathic Myocardial Hypertrophy

As a congenital disease idiopathic myocardial hypertrophy has lost favor and the term is rarely used today. Aside from patients with malformations that are readily recognized as causes of myocardial hypertrophy, there remains a group of patients in which left ventricular endocardial sclerosis (fibroelastosis) and myocardial hypertrophy coexist (15.44).

41. Localized Hypertrophy of the Myocardium

This type of hypertrophy may involve the ventricular septum and the right ventricular infundibulum. Such changes cause either subaortic stenosis or right ventricular infundibular stenosis (15.5–9).

42. Glycogen Storage Disease of the Myocardium

This may be part of the systemic alteration in metabolism of glycogen known as von Gierke's disease, or it may be part of a condition in which glycogen is stored abnormally in cardiac and skeletal muscles without the hepatic involvement characteristic of von Gierke's disease (4.10).

43. Congenital Tumor of the Myocardium

This usually takes the form of a rhabdomyoma. Usually the tumors are multiple. A close association with tuberous sclerosis exists. The nature of the condition is disputed, with opinions variously held that it is a true tumor, a congenital malformation (hamartoma), or a localized form of glycogen storage disease of the myocardium.

Endocardium

44. Fibroelastosis (Endocardial Sclerosis)

Fibroelastosis is the most common of the few endocardial anomalies (4.9). The characteristic abnormality is a heavy, fibrous thickening of the endocardium of the left ventricle in which an obvious gross layer may be identified. Histologically, this is composed of laminations of the elastic tissue and of collagen. Two general types are recognized. In the first the left ventricle is dilated, and the disease may be referred to as *endocardial sclerosis of the dilated type;* in the second and less common type the left ventricular chamber is smaller than normal, and may be termed the *contracted type of endocardial sclerosis.*

Any condition in which the left ventricular chamber is enlarged may display secondary endocardial thickening. Differentiation is made by the degree of involvement, which is considerably less than in the primary type.

At times there is seen in this condition associated fibrous thickening of the mitral or of the aortic valve which causes stenosis or incompetence of the involved valve. At other times the mitral valve is essentially uninvolved but, because of abnormal papillary muscle orientation, the valve is incompetent.

The left atrium commonly is enlarged and its endocardium thickened. In all probability these changes are secondary to the functional alteration of the left ventricle caused by the primary disease of that chamber.

45. Anomalous Endocardial Cords

In the left ventricle especially, but occasionally in the right ventricle and left atrium, are strands of endocardial tissue which cross the chamber from one point to another. In themselves they are probably of no functional significance, but they may at times be responsible for peculiar murmurs.

Pericardium

46. Anomalies of the Pericardium

Anomalies of the pericardium are uncommon, but when present they usually take the form of deficiency in tissue. There may therefore be *absence of the pericardium* or a local deficiency called *defect of the pericardium*. Usually these conditions are of no functional significance, but on rare occasions they may be responsible for mechanical constriction of all or a portion of the heart. In a rare instance of absence of the pericardium, the heart may become strangulated on its base, and in cases of defect of the pericardium, a portion of the heart may herniate through the defect and be constricted by it.

Coronary Vessels

Malformations may affect the coronary venous or arterial system. Significant anomalies of the coronary veins include wide communication with the left atrium or atresia of the right atrial ostium of the coronary sinus.

CORONARY SINUS

47. Atresia of the Right Atrial Ostium of the Coronary Sinus

In this condition the coronary sinus is normally formed but a membrane, probably an adherent valve of the coronary sinus, separates its lumen from the right atrium. Exit of coronary sinus blood is accomplished either through communication of the coronary sinus with the left atrium or through a persistent left superior vena cava. Through the latter coronary sinus blood flows retrograde, ultimately entering the right superior vena cava and the right atrium.

48. Unusually Large Communication of the Coronary Sinus with the Left Atrium

In a rare case the anterior wall of the coronary sinus is deficient near the atrial septum, thereby allowing free communication of the vein with the left atrium. This communication, in effect, functions as though an atrial septal defect were present. Grossly, from the left side of the heart there appears to be an atrial septal defect in the lower part of the septum superior to the posteromedial commissure of the mitral valve. From the right side of the heart no septal defect is present, but the coronary sinus ostium is large and corresponds with the apparent defect when the heart is viewed from the left.

49. Enlargement of the Coronary Sinus

The coronary sinus may be found enlarged under certain circumstances, but this feature is probably always a secondary phenomenon rather than a malformation. This vessel enlarges when a persistent left superior vena cava enters it, when it anomalously receives pulmonary veins, or when the right atrium is greatly enlarged as in tricuspid insufficiency.

50. Absence of the Coronary Sinus

The terminal portion of the left anterior cardinal vein of the embryo becomes, under normal circumstances, the coronary sinus. Therefore, in those cases where a left superior vena cava terminates in the left atrium, no coronary sinus is formed.

51. Coronary Artery—Coronary Sinus Arteriovenous Fistula

Among the fistulous communications in which the coronary arteries may participate is that in which a coronary artery, usually the right, makes gross communication with the coronary sinus or one of its tributaries. As in arteriovenous fistulas in any part of the body, the arteries and veins participating are thick-walled and tortuously dilated.

CORONARY ARTERIES

The significant coronary arterial anomalies (4.6) include: (1) abnormalities in origin from the aorta; (2) abnormal terminations in coronary veins, cardiac chambers, or the pulmonary trunk; and (3) abnormal origin from the pulmonary trunk.

52. Single Coronary Artery

In this condition only one coronary arterial ostium in the aorta exists. Shortly after its origin this may divide into left and right branches, the ramifications of which may follow the usual distribution. In some instances the single coronary artery continues as such in its usual distribution and distally its branches make connection with the distal branches of the coronary artery which does not possess an aortic ostium.

53. Origin of the Left Circumflex Artery from the Right Coronary Artery

As the rubric implies, in this condition the so-called left coronary artery is the anterior descending vessel, and the left circumflex artery takes origin from the right branch shortly after its origin from the aorta. The anomalously arising circumflex branch turns round the posterior aspect of the origin of the aorta and ultimately reaches a normal position in the left atrioventricular sulcus.

54. Origin of Both Coronary Arteries from the Same Aortic Sinus (Valsalva)

This variation is most likely to occur in patients with congenital bicuspid aortic valve. Less commonly it occurs when three aortic cusps are present. Beyond the abnormal origin, the coronary arteries have a normal distribution.

55. Origin of a Coronary Artery from the Pulmonary Arterial Trunk

Several anatomic details are represented when elements of the coronary arterial system arise from the pulmonary trunk.

55.1. ORIGIN OF BOTH CORONARY ARTERIES FROM THE PULMONARY TRUNK. In this rare condition no coronary ostia are present in the aorta and both coronary arteries arise from the pulmonary trunk.

55.2. ORIGIN OF THE LEFT CORONARY ARTERY FROM THE PULMONARY TRUNK. In this rare condition the right coronary artery arises from the aorta and the left arises from the pulmonary trunk. This is the most common variety of major anomalous origin of an element of the coronary arterial system. In the distribution of the left coronary artery, the myocardium may show varying ages of infarction, and over such areas the left ventricular myocardium may be thickened. Death during infancy is common but not universal, some patients reaching adult life.

55.3. ORIGIN OF THE RIGHT CORONARY ARTERY FROM THE PULMONARY TRUNK. In this condition the right coronary artery arises from the pulmonary trunk and the left coronary artery arises from the aorta. This condition is less common than those of reverse origins, and in general the prognosis for survival into adult life is better. Although this has been considered a benign condition, death from coronary insufficiency in early adult life is not uncommon.

55.4. ORIGIN OF AN ACCESSORY CORONARY ARTERY FROM THE PULMONARY TRUNK. In this condition the two standard coronary arteries arise from the aorta. These make communication with one or several accessory coronary arteries arising from the pulmonary trunk. In some instances the accessory artery or arteries are small and probably are not responsible for major functional disturbances. In other instances the communications are wide, as are the main and accessory trunks. In such cases a large left-to-right shunt may occur through the communication between the standard and accessory coronary arteries.

56. Congenital Coronary Arterial Aneurysms

Most or possibly all aneurysms of the coronary arteries that are considered congenital are complications of the enlargement which occurs in arteriovenous-like conditions of the coronary system. These include (1) congenital fistula between a coronary artery and the coronary sinus, (2) communication of a coronary artery with an accessory coronary artery arising from the pulmonary trunk, and (3) communication of a coronary artery with a cardiac chamber.

57. Communication of a Coronary Artery with a Cardiac Chamber

Either of the coronary arteries arising normally from the aorta or one of its branches may make direct communication with any one of the cardiac chambers, usually a right-sided one. As in other arteriovenous fistulous arrangements, the artery proximal to the abnormal communication is wide and tortuous. Such arteries may be the site of one or several saccular aneurysms. Under such circumstances these saccular aneurysms are considered complications rather than primary conditions.

Anomalies of the Ascending Aorta

58. Supravalvular Aortic Stenosis

Obstruction in the ascending aorta, usually termed *supravalvular aortic stenosis*, may take one of the following three forms.

58.1. HOURGLASS STENOSIS. As this term implies, there is an hourglass deformity of the ascending aorta, in which the point of major narrowing lies about 1½ cm or less above the aortic valve.

58.2. DIAPHRAGM TYPE OF STENOSIS. A localized area of fibrous thickening of the lining of the ascending aorta results in a diaphragm-like narrowing. Fibrous adhesions between the fibrous lesion of the aorta and the aortic valve may occur.

58.3. DIFFUSE TYPE OF STENOSIS. The obstruction starts just above the level of the coronary arterial ostia and continues upward to the beginning of the aortic arch. The aortic wall is uniformly thick and there is corresponding narrowing of the lumen. The pulmonary trunk may simultaneously be similarly affected.

59. Origin of the Right Pulmonary Artery from the Ascending Aorta

This is a rare condition in which the right pulmonary artery arises from the right side of the ascending aorta. The site of origin may be at the base of the origin of the innominate artery or below it. Beyond the anomalous site of origin the artery has a normal course and distribution. Focal stenosis may occur in the anomalous artery. The pulmonary venous terminations in the left atrium are normal.

60. Communication of the Ascending Aorta with the Pulmonary Trunk (Aorticopulmonary Septal Defect, Aorticopulmonary Window, Partial Persistent Truncus Arteriosus, 15.21)

Those aspects of the ascending aorta and pulmonary trunk which normally are in contact may be in continuity through a large defect. From the aortic aspect the defect lies just anterior to the ostium of the right pulmonary artery. Both aortic and pulmonary valves are present and each is normally formed. An inordinately high incidence of patent ductus arteriosus occurs in patients with communication between the ascending aorta and pulmonary trunk (4.22).

61. Hypoplasia of the Ascending Aorta

In atresia of the aortic valve, a condition discussed in the section dealing with malformations of the valves, it was indicated that the ascending aorta is hypoplastic. In this segment of the vessel the lumen is narrow, the wall relatively thin, and the external diameter narrow. This condition is secondary to the functional derangement peculiar to aortic valvular atresia.

Lesser degrees of hypoplasia of the ascending aorta occur when there is diversion of part of the full cardiac output from the aorta, as in atrial and in ventricular septal defects with large left-to-right shunts.

Without other malformations a strikingly reduced caliber of the ascending aorta is usually associated with a thick wall and an external diameter greater than that encountered with aortic valvular atresia. Such lesions are probably best classified as representing the diffuse type of *supravalvular aortic stenosis*.

Anomalies of the Aortic Arch System

62. Interruption of the Aortic Arch

There is loss in continuity of the aorta. Most commonly this occurs in the segment between the left common carotid and left subclavian arteries. The proximal segment of the aorta ends by dividing into the innominate and left common carotid arteries, and the descending aorta receives a patent ductus arteriosus and gives rise to the left subclavian artery.

In one variant of this condition both subclavian arteries arise from the descending aorta, the proximal aortic segment ending by bifurcating into the two common carotid arteries. In another variant the left subclavian artery arises from the descending aorta, and the right subclavian artery has no connection with the aorta. Instead, it makes continuity with the right pulmonary artery through a right-sided ductus arteriosus which may be either patent or closed. A rare form of interruption of the aortic arch is that in which the three standard branches of the aortic arch arise from this segment before it ends.

In instances of interruption of the aortic arch there is usually a coexistent ventricular septal defect alone or subaortic stenosis lying above a ventricular septal defect.

63. Tubular Hypoplasia of the Aortic Arch

Occurring either proximal or distal to the left subclavian artery, a segment of the aortic arch may have a cylindrical shape and be uniformly narrow. Some refer to it as *infantile coarctation* or simply as *coarctation*. The preferred term is justified in that the lesion fails to show the characteristic medial deformity of classic coarctation of the aorta.

In tubular hypoplasia the narrow segment may have considerable length, approaching 1 cm in infants. A ventricular septal defect or single ventricle is common but not universal.

64. Coarctation of the Aorta

Localized obstruction of the aorta (4.1) most often occurs in the general region of the junction of the arch and descending aorta. It may lie proximal, opposite, or distal to the ductus arteriosus, which may be patent or closed. Variants include: (1) coarctation just proximal to the left subclavian artery, (2) coexistent stenosis or atresia of the proximal segment of either the right or left subclavian artery, and (3) anomalous origin of the right subclavian artery as the fourth branch of the aorta. In the latter situation the right subclavian artery may arise either proximal or distal to the site of aortic obstruction.

The aortic obstruction is caused by a medial deformity characterized by a peculiar curtain-like infolding of the media

216

toward the lumen. Since all aspects of the aorta except the lower part are involved, the narrow lumen lies eccentrically, near the lower aspect of the aorta. Furthermore, there is at the site of the obstruction a concavity in the superior wall of the aorta, and the external diameter of the vessel is considerably wider than the lumen at this site.

A congenital bicuspid aortic valve is commonly associated with coarctation.

65. Patent Ductus Arteriosus

This is a persistence of the fetal communication between the pulmonary arterial system and the aorta (4.21). Most commonly the ductus arteriosus is a left-sided structure running from the proximal part of the left pulmonary artery to the upper end of the descending aorta.

When malformations of the aortic arch are associated, the systemic site of insertion of the ductus may vary from the normal. It may pass behind the esophagus to insert into the proximal end of the left subclavian artery when the latter vessel arises as the fourth branch of a right aortic arch. It may insert into the base of a left innominate artery in those forms of right aortic arch which possess a left innominate artery.

65.1. RIGHT DUCTUS ARTERIOSUS. This occurs rarely and when present is usually but not universally associated with a right aortic arch. The pulmonary site of insertion of the right ductus arteriosus is the right pulmonary artery. The systemic site of insertion depends upon the nature of the aortic arch. When a right arch is present, a right ductus arteriosus inserts into the arch just beyond the origin of the right subclavian artery. When a left aortic arch is the sole arch, the very rarely occurring right ductus arteriosus inserts either into the origin of the innominate artery or into a right subclavian artery that is the fourth branch of the aorta.

65.2. BILATERAL DUCTUS ARTERIOSUS. A ductus arteriosus occurring on both sides is rare but its presence may be understood from the fact that the embryo's sixth aortic arch, from which the ductus arteriosus is derived, is bilateral. There is a single arch from which one ductus extends to the homolateral pulmonary artery. The opposite ductus extends from the innominate artery to the pulmonary artery on that side. If an innominate artery is absent, the subclavian artery on the side opposite the intact aortic arch arises from the second ductus arteriosus.

66. Absence of a Ductus Arteriosus

This term indicates absence of any vestige of a ductus arteriosus, either patent or occluded (ligamentum arteriosum), on both sides. This absence may occur in any of the conditions wherein there is a ventricular septal defect, a channel through which, in the fetus, right ventricular blood may enter the aorta. Among conditions in which the ductus arteriosus may be absent are the tetralogy of Fallot and persistent truncus arteriosus.

67. Vascular Rings

Vascular rings are malformations of the aortic arch system which interfere with function of the trachea and/or the esophagus. Although many different anatomic patterns are represented, the one feature which each has in common with the other is that part of the major arterial system passes behind the esophagus (4.2). The three common patterns are: (1) double aortic arch, (2) right aortic arch with retro-esophageal segment and left-sided descending aorta, and (3) anomalous origin of the right subclavian artery as the fourth branch of an otherwise normal aorta. The latter condition, though common (occurring in about 1 of 200 in the general population), is much less likely to cause the characteristic effects of a vascular ring than is either of the other two types.

Pulmonary Veins

Anomalies of the pulmonary veins are chiefly those of abnormal termination, of obstruction, and of abnormal communication with the pulmonary arteries.

68. Anomalous Connection of the Pulmonary Veins

Although the term *anomalous drainage* of the pulmonary veins is often used synonymously with *anomalous connection,* it seems preferable to reserve the term *drainage* for a functional definition and *connection* for an anatomic state.

Sites of anomalous termination of the pulmonary veins include the right atrium, the left innominate vein, the superior vena cava, the azygos vein, the coronary sinus, the inferior vena cava, the ductus venosus, and the portal vein of the liver or its tributaries.

68.1. PARTIAL ANOMALOUS PULMONARY VENOUS CONNECTION. This is the condition in which part of the pulmonary venous system terminates normally in the left atrium and part in one of the aforementioned anomalous sites (4.31).

68.2. TOTAL ANOMALOUS PULMONARY VENOUS CONNECTION. This is the condition in which no pulmonary veins join the left atrium but in which instead the entire pulmonary venous system has anomalous termination. Usually there is a single anomalous site of termination, but rarely several sites may be represented (4.30).

69. Pulmonary Venous Stenosis or Atresia

Congenital stenosis may affect any one or all of the normally oriented pulmonary veins, or it may occur in channels that lead to sites of anomalous termination. Rarely is there no channel of exit, either normal or anomalous, from the pulmonary venous system. The pulmonary veins converge to form a blind cul-de-sac. This condition may be termed either *pulmonary venous atresia* or *atresia of the common pulmonary vein.*

70. Pulmonary Arteriovenous Fistula

In this condition there is a direct connection between one or several pulmonary arteries with one or several pulmonary veins. Telangiectasis occurring in other organs is common. A familial tendency is recognized.

A special form of pulmonary arteriovenous fistula is the condition in which a pulmonary artery terminates in the left atrium.

Central Systemic Veins

71. Persistent Left Superior Vena Cava

The most common malformation involving the major systemic veins is the presence of bilateral superior venae cavae, usually called persistent left superior vena cava. The latter vein terminates in the left lateral extremity of the coronary sinus, through which its blood is delivered to the right atrium. The coronary sinus is enlarged. The left superior vena cava receives the hemiazygos vein. The normal venous bridge in the superior mediastinum between the left and right upper venous systems usually occurs, but uncommonly this bridge may be absent. Absence or hypoplasia of the right superior vena cava may occur in association with persistent left superior vena cava.

72. Termination of the Left Superior Vena Cava in the Left Atrium

In cor biloculare, a condition usually associated with agenesis of the spleen, bilateral superior venae cavae are common. However, the left vein terminates in the left side of the common atrium and a coronary sinus is not formed.

Left atrial termination of a left superior vena cava occurs rarely in other circumstances, but it almost never occurs in the absence of an associated intracardiac malformation.

73. Termination of the Inferior Vena Cava in the Left Atrium

This decidedly uncommon condition may appear when there is only one inferior vena cava. It is more likely to occur when there are bilateral inferior venae cavae, in which case the left displays the anomalous termination.

74. Continuity of the Inferior Vena Cava with the Azygos System

The inferior vena cava may fail to take a normal position with respect to the liver and become continuous with the azygos vein, through which inferior vena caval blood is carried to the superior vena cava and the right atrium. The hepatic veins are normal and join one another to form a common hepatic vein. The latter follows the course usually taken by the proximal part of the inferior vena cava, perforates the diaphragm, and enters the right atrium at the usual position of the inferior vena caval orifice.

Rarely the inferior vena cava is left-sided and terminates in the hemiazygos vein. Continuity of the inferior vena cava with the azygos system of veins has a tendency to be associated with partial or total situs inversus, multiple spleens, and partial or total anomalous connection of pulmonary veins with the venous atrium.

16 / Atherosclerotic Coronary Artery Disease

Atherosclerosis involves the coronary arteries directly; the myocardium is involved indirectly if ischemia is produced.

1. Coronary Atherosclerosis

Atherosclerosis (2.3) primarily involves the intima of the coronary arteries; changes in the media and adventitia occur secondarily. The *intimal* lesions may consist of increase of the intimal ground substance with deposition in it of fat droplets, cholesterol-bearing macrophages (foam cells), cholesterol crystals, and other interstitial fatty substances; proliferation of connective tissue with fibrous thickening; development of foci of calcification in the disintegrated lipoid zones; and rarely formation of bone. The *medial* changes which may occur are fraying, fragmentation, and rupture of the internal elastic lamina; destruction or atrophy of muscular fibers and possible fibroblastic reaction with necrosis and calcification. The extent of the medial lesion appears to be proportional to the thickness of the adjacent intimal plaque. In the *adventitia* there may be periarterial lymphocytic infiltration and collagenous thickening.

As a sequel to the degenerative and proliferative alterations in the intima, there is often a rich capillary formation that usually originates from the vasa vasorum and, to a lesser degree, from the endothelium of the coronary artery proper.

The evolution of the intimal plaque may be punctuated by

any one or a combination of the following: deposition of fibrin on the surface with organization; necrosis and pultaceous softening with ulceration; hemorrhage into and occasionally dissection of the ulcerated plaque (Fig. 1); rupture of capillaries with intramural hematoma; intraluminal thrombosis.

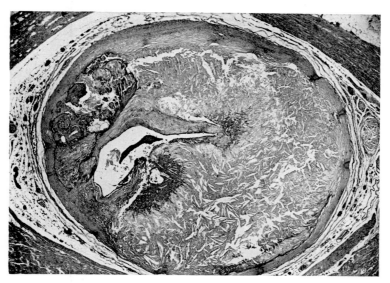

Figure 1.   Cross section of coronary artery. Beginning ulceration of the lipoid plaque with penetration of blood from the lumen of the vessel.

Occlusion of a coronary artery may be gradual or rapid. Gradual occlusion is produced by eccentric or concentric thickening of the intima to which any or all of the foregoing processes, except intraluminal thrombosis, may have contributed at one time or another. Gradual occlusion is not commonly total but may be very nearly so. Rapid occlusion may be caused either by rupture of intramural capillaries in a necrotic lipoid plaque, or by hemorrhage into an ulcerated lipoid plaque, or by intraluminal thrombosis which most commonly but not invariably occurs over an ulcerated plaque into which hemorrhage has taken place (Fig. 2). Less commonly, intra-

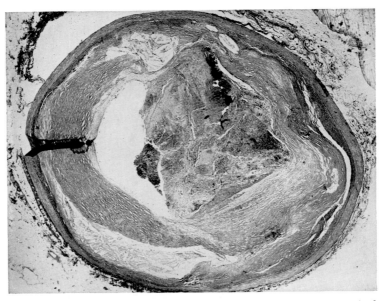

Figure 2. Cross section of coronary artery. Recent thrombus deposited on an ulcerated plaque into which hemorrhage has occurred.

luminal thrombosis may be implanted on a nonulcerated, nonhemorrhagic plaque which has narrowed the lumen of the vessel considerably.

The most severe changes and the common sites of gradual or acute occlusion are found in the anterior descending branch of the left coronary artery, about 2 to 3 cm distal to its orifice; in the right coronary artery within 3 to 5 cm of its origin; in the left circumflex branch just beyond its origin from the main trunk or in its ramus marginis obtusi. At necropsy extensive atherosclerosis is frequently found in several branches of the coronary system, but clinically significant and even fatal atherosclerosis may vary from a small segmental lesion in one coronary artery to diffuse lesions in all of the major branches of the coronary arteries.

Coronary thrombi and the other types of acute occlusion may vary from a few hundred microns to a centimeter or more

in length. If the site of occlusion encompasses no more than
a few hundred microns of the vessel, serial microscopic sections
may be necessary to disclose its presence. A coronary thrombus
may be recent (acute, fresh, subacute) or old (organized,
healed). The former is usually red or grayish-red, but without
microscopic examination it is frequently impossible to differentiate it from hemorrhage into an atheromatous plaque with
thrombosis. In some instances microscopic sections through
one part of the occlusion may show hemorrhage into a plaque,
whereas another part may show intraluminal thrombosis, and
serial microscopic sections may be necessary to establish a
continuity between the two. Old (organized, healed) thrombi
are commonly gray or grayish-white, but, because of blood-
filled channels within the organized core, they may occasionally
appear red (Fig. 3). In some instances many histologic sections

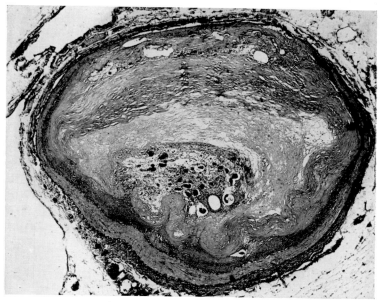

Figure 3.   *Cross section of coronary artery. Old and completely organized
thrombus in the eccentrically displaced lumen. The blood-filled re-
canalized channels in the central core were responsible for the red
appearance of this old thrombotic occlusion.*

may prove necessary for differentiation between organized thrombi, organized hemorrhage into a plaque, and a more gradual type of occlusion. Occasionally, even the study of such sections will fail to establish this differentiation.

Alterations of the myocardium in atherosclerotic coronary artery disease are produced directly or indirectly by a compromised coronary circulation. These are infarction of the myocardium; rupture, fibrosis, or aneurysm secondary to infarction; and hypertrophy.

2. Infarction of the Myocardium

The area of ischemic necrosis or infarction of the heart may vary from focal and microscopic to diffuse and massive. Most infarcts which are grossly visible are between 1 and 5 cm in maximum width. Gross infarcts do not ordinarily involve the myocardial wall uniformly throughout their extent. The same infarct may be transmural in one area and subendocardial or intramural in another. When the infarct involves the pericardium, it may be followed by fibrinous pericarditis, and when it involves the endocardium, it may be followed by mural thrombosis.

Infarcts may be recent (acute, fresh, hemorrhagic, necrotic, subacute) or old (fibrotic, organized, ancient, healed). Differentiation between a recent and an old infarct is clear and unequivocal. Within some limitations, identification of the approximate age of a recent infarct by its color and consistency is generally possible. Gross changes ordinarily do not develop until five or six hours after an acute attack. The earliest change is a loss of luster of the necrotic muscle and a diminution in its firmness. This muscle soon becomes pale, dry, and somewhat swollen. Within a day or two the infarct assumes a clay color if diffuse, or a streaked yellow appearance if patchy. During the subsequent week or two, the involved area may become sharply circumscribed, may be uniformly light tan and dry, or may show dark red, purple, yellow, and white mottling. Generally, the process does not involve all of the muscle fibers within a circumscribed area, nor is the involvement uniform in age. Hence, there is commonly a mixture of healthy and dead or dying muscle; fatty change from infiltrated leukocytes; condensation of reticulum and blood-filled capillary and venous channels where necrotic muscle fibers have been resorbed; and focal hemorrhages. Shrinkage following removal of necrotic muscle begins between the first and second week, and then the border of the infarct becomes depressed. Young granulation tissue appears. In the next few weeks this is replaced by fibrous tissue. The lesion becomes a white scar within two or three months.

The histologic findings reflect the age of the infarct. In recent infarcts it is uncommon to find a uniform histologic picture throughout, or indeed even in the same microscopic field. Lesser ischemic damage commonly causes swelling and vacuolation of myofibers (Fig. 4). In frank infarction necrosis

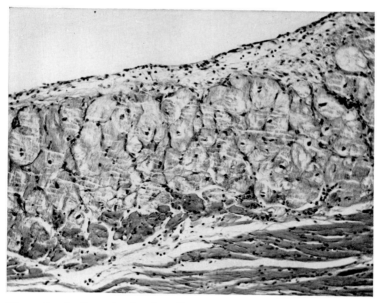

Figure 4. Section of subendocardial left ventricular myocardium. The subendocardial tissue shows swelling and vacuolation of myofibers.

does not become evident for five or six hours after onset of ischemia. The muscle fibers then become hyaline and take a deeper acid stain. The striations become less evident and the nuclei undergo pyknosis or karyolysis. Infiltration of polymorphonuclear leukocytes begins between and surrounding the necrotic fibers at about five hours after arrest of circulation (Fig. 5). Within 24 hours degeneration of the leukocytes begins, and within a few days they become necrotic and gradually disappear. Eosinophilic polymorphonuclear leukocytes are seen by the end of the first week and may persist for another week or two. Removal of the necrotic muscle fibers (Fig. 6), condensation of the supporting stroma, and formation of granulation tissue are initiated by the fourth or fifth day. Phagocytes engulf the necrotic muscle fibers and may contain lipo-

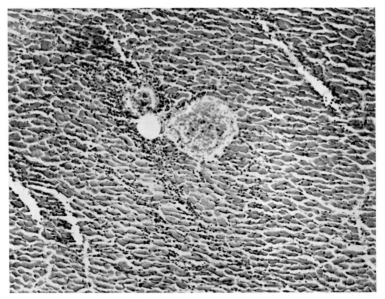

Figure 5. Section of left ventricular myocardium in acute infarction. Necrosis of muscle fibers with disappearance of their nuclei and loss of striations. Infiltration with polymorphonuclear leukocytes between and surrounding necrotic muscle fibers.

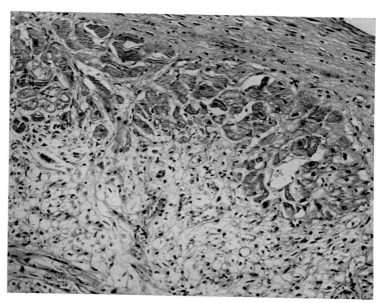

Figure 6.   Section of left ventricular myocardium in the subendocardial zone. The muscle immediately beneath the thickened endocardium shows swelling and vacuolation of myofibers. Beneath this, necrotic muscle fibers have been removed and condensation of supporting stroma has begun.

fuscin pigment or hemosiderin. Proliferation of fibroblasts and ingrowth of new blood capillaries begin about the end of the first week. In about ten days the granulation tissue may be abundant, the fibroblasts numerous, the eosinophils, plasma cells, and lymphocytes prominent. Toward the end of the first week removal of necrotic muscle at the periphery of the infarct begins. In the third week collagen appears, which increases in abundance by the fourth to sixth week, and the vascularity diminishes. Subsequently there is condensation of the collagen (Fig. 7), and uncommonly there is deposition of calcium. It is re-emphasized that commonly all portions of the infarct will not simultaneously have reached the same stage in their evolution.

Infarcts occur most often in the apical portion of the an-

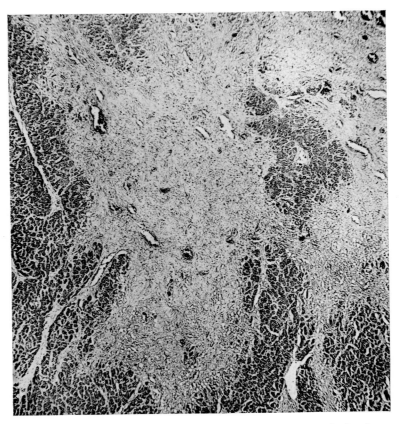

Figure 7. Healed infarct of myocardium. The necrotic muscle has been replaced by fibrous tissue which ramifies irregularly. In places it encloses groups of living muscle bundles. The scar tissue is relatively acellular but still contains numerous thin-walled blood channels. Note the loss of bundle outlines.

terior wall and the contiguous portion of the ventricular septum as a result of obstruction of the anterior descending branch of the left coronary artery; in the basal posterior wall and contiguous septum as a result of obstruction of the right coronary artery; and in the lateral wall of the left ventricle as a result of obstruction of the left circumflex artery. Cardiac infarction usually involves some portion of the left ventricle or the ventricular septum. Rarely, infarction may be confined to the right ventricle alone or to one or the other of the atria. Even in conjunction with left ventricular infarction, only 5 percent of hearts will show right ventricular infarction, and about 15 percent will show infarction of the atria, the right more often than the left.

3. Fibrosis of the Myocardium

Myocardial fibrosis in atherosclerotic coronary artery disease is a stage in or a sequel to myocardial infarction rather than an independent phenomenon. Whether the size or distribution of the myocardial fibrosis is microscopic, minute, focal, in strands, in patches, subendocardial, transmural, or massive, it is a manifestation of previous acute ischemic myocardial necrosis.

4. Rupture of the Myocardium

Rupture occurs only as a sequel to myocardial infarction. It is encountered in about 10 percent of fatal recent myocardial infarcts. Rupture is most common during the first week and may occur as early as the second day or as late as the fourth week. Dissection of the muscular wall may be present. The site of rupture is usually in the anterior or posterior wall of the left ventricle; more rarely it may be limited to the ventricular septum or to a papillary muscle. The line of rupture varies. Sometimes it is ragged and irregular, resembling a traumatic rupture, sometimes cleanly cut and regular like an incised wound, and at other times tortuous through the heart wall with small internal and external openings.

5. Hemopericardium

Hemopericardium occurs in atherosclerotic heart disease most often as the result of rupture of a recent myocardial infarct.

It may, however, be a sequel to recent myocardial infarction without rupture, most often but not exclusively in patients who have received anticoagulants.

6. Aneurysm of the Heart

Aneurysms vary in size from a few centimeters to as large as half of the left ventricle. Often a thrombus adheres to the wall of the ventricle and may partially or completely fill the pouch. In many instances, however, the lining is white, smooth or corrugated, and glistening. Pericardial adhesions often form. Rupture of a cardiac aneurysm is rare.

Microscopically, the wall of the aneurysm consists of dense scar, with occasional groups or bands of muscle fibers, and thickened endocardium.

7. Rupture of the Papillary Muscle

As a sequel to recent myocardial infarction, the posterior papillary muscle ruptures twice as often as the anterior.

8. Mural Thrombosis

Mural thrombi often form in relation to an infarct, but may occur independent of an infarct, usually in the left ventricular apex, as a consequence of cardiac failure.

9. Hypertrophy of the Myocardium

In atherosclerotic heart disease without hypertension, hypertrophy of the myocardium is most often a sequel to the larger healed infarcts, some with cardiac insufficiency, and less often is the consequence of calcific aortic stenosis, atrial fibrillation, or complete atrioventricular block. Approximately one-third of persons with gross myocardial infarction have cardiac hypertrophy. It is frequently limited to the left ventricle. With long-standing left ventricular failure, the entire heart may participate in the hypertrophy.

10. Dilatation of the Myocardium

Acute dilatation without hypertrophy may occur in recent myocardial infarction. The heart presents a globoid form, the muscle is flabby, and the chambers are enlarged. In the ventricles there is a flattening of the papillary muscles and of the trabeculae carneae, and in the atria there is flattening of the pectinate muscles.

17 / Hypertensive Heart Disease

In its pure form the spectrum of structural findings in heart disease due to systemic diastolic hypertension is narrow. Although alterations resulting from this type of hypertension are commonly joined by those that are the result of atherosclerosis, the picture presented by unmixed hypertensive heart disease is so sharply different as to demand separate attention.

The distinctive feature of the purely hypertensive heart lies in the simplicity of its anatomy, i.e., hypertrophy that is chiefly or solely left ventricular, without other myocardial, coronary, or valvular disease.

1. Hypertrophy of the Myocardium

Systemic diastolic hypertension is the most common cause of cardiac hypertrophy. Except for aortic valvular disease, it is responsible for the greatest degree of left ventricular hypertrophy. Before congestive heart failure has supervened, hypertrophy of the concentric type, without dilatation, will be observed. Only the left ventricle is involved. In long-standing cases, however, there may occur hypertrophy of the right ventricle that is slight unless there is chronic left ventricular failure. With congestive heart failure, the entire heart participates in the hypertrophy, although the left ventricle remains the predominantly hypertrophied chamber.

Histologically, the finding is hypertrophy of muscle fibers without increase in number. The change is especially noticeable in the increased average transverse diameter of the muscle cells. There is also some increase in the length of the fibers due to increase in sarcoplasm as well as myofibrils. The nuclei are enlarged, have blunt ends, and may be hyperchromatic. There may be inadequate capillary blood supply to the hypertrophied myocardial fibers because of failure of the capillaries to increase in number proportionately.

2. Dilatation of the Myocardium

In hypertensive heart disease acute dilatation without hypertrophy occurs in acute glomerular nephritis. It is associated with a congested circulation. The dilatation may be largely or solely left ventricular and associated with pulmonary edema, or there may be dilatation of the entire heart with signs of right and left ventricular failure.

Acute dilatation with hypertrophy is characteristic of long-standing hypertension, death being due to acute left ventricular failure. The gross morphologic characteristics of acute dilatation differ from those of chronic dilatation primarily in the greater degree of flattening of the papillary muscles and trabeculae carneae of the ventricles found in the former.

Chronic dilatation with hypertrophy is the cardinal finding in heart failure due to long-standing hypertension.

3. Necrosis and Fibrosis of the Myocardium

Although hypertrophy without other myocardial alterations is characteristic of hypertensive heart disease in its pure form, necrotic and fibrotic lesions of the myocardium are not uncommon. In most instances a causal connection with atherosclerotic changes in the supplying arteries of the affected area is evident. However, death of scattered muscle strands and their replacement by islets and reefs of fibrous tissue, for which no adequate vascular obstruction can be detected, identifies the process as that of pure hypertensive heart disease. It is unknown whether these lesions result from relative ischemia that accompanies the progress of hypertrophy or from some humoral mechanism in hypertensive disease.

Signs of gross myocardial infarction are rarely seen in the hearts of hypertensive patients without significant coronary atherosclerosis. Most often, infarction of the myocardium in these patients owes its existence to atherosclerosis of the coronary arteries, and, except for the hypertrophy, the changes in the coronary arteries and myocardium are identical with those of ischemic atherosclerotic heart disease in nonhypertensive patients (16.2, 3).

4. Coronary Arterial Lesions

There are no characteristic or distinctive alterations of the large or medium-sized coronary arteries in hypertensive heart disease. The involvement of these arteries differs only in frequency from that of atherosclerotic heart disease without hypertension. The small coronary arteries and arterioles in hypertensive heart disease show, at the most, only slight intimal hyalinization and medial hypertrophy. As a rule, they, almost alone among the small arterial channels, fail to show the severe regressive changes which are the fate of such vessels elsewhere in hypertensive disease.

5. Valvular Lesions

Valvular lesions occur in hypertensive heart disease, but they are rarely distinctive or unique. The valvular lesions of rheumatic etiology are coincidental. In the hypertensive patient the aortic valvular lesions of calcific nature do not differ qualitatively from those that occur in the normotensive subject.

18 / Pulmonary Heart Disease

Pulmonary heart disease (cor pulmonale) is distinguished anatomically by hypertrophy or dilatation of the right ventricle or both, and by the presence of disease affecting the function or anatomy of the lungs or both.

Lesions that are responsible for pulmonary heart disease may involve the air-bearing parenchyma, the pulmonary vascular system, or the neuromuscular or skeletal systems of the respiratory apparatus.

1. Acute Pulmonary Heart Disease (Acute Cor Pulmonale)

In some instances of acute pulmonary heart disease (acute cor pulmonale) it may not be possible at post mortem examination to detect right ventricular dilatation of very recent origin. In other instances the right ventricle is soft and moderately dilated. The pulmonary arterial trunk may also be abnormally distended. Exploration of its major branches reveals an occlusion of a large percentage of their lumina. The most common cause of this extensive pulmonary vascular obstruction is massive embolization from thrombosed veins in the lower extremities. Less common causes are the sudden perforation of an aortic aneurysm into the pulmonary artery and multiple fat emboli from traumatic fractures of the long bones.

2. *Chronic Pulmonary Heart Disease (Chronic Cor Pulmonale)*

This type is readily demonstrable at autopsy. The heart weight is increased by approximately 40 percent to 130 percent of normal. Cardiac enlargement is caused principally by conspicuous hypertrophy of the right ventricular wall and relative dilatation of its chamber. The muscular response is dependent upon the duration, constancy, and degree of the hypertension in the lesser circulation. The earliest changes of right ventricular hypertrophy are found about the pulmonary outflow tract. In the more advanced disease the trabeculae carneae are prominent, and there is an increase in the muscle mass of the wall. Exclusive of epicardial fat and trabeculae carneae, the wall has an average thickness of 5 mm or more (normal: 2 to 3 mm) by direct measurement. A more accurate determination is obtained by weighing the excised free wall of the right ventricle. In chronic cor pulmonale it usually exceeds 80 gm in adults. The weight ratio of the left ventricle plus septum to the right ventricle is always less than 2:1 in isolated right ventricular hypertrophy.

In far-advanced cases with long-standing right heart failure the annulus of the tricuspid valve may be stretched, and the right atrial chamber may be increased in size and its wall moderately hypertrophied. The right atrial appendage contains an adherent or organized mural thrombus in approximately 15 percent of autopsied cases with cor pulmonale.

The pulmonary arterial trunk and its larger branches may develop nonulcerating atheromatous plaques, and the smaller divisions may show both intimal thickening (Figs. 8 and 10) and medial hypertrophy (Fig. 9).

Microscopic examination of sections prepared from the right ventricle may reveal nothing remarkable. When hypertrophy is pronounced, an increase in the transverse diameter of the fibers, mild anisonucleosis, and nuclear hyperchromatism are present.

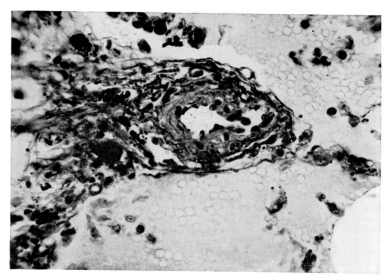

Figure 8. *Arteriolar intimal thickening of a precapillary pulmonary arteriole. Note the circumferential fibrosis of the intima with moderate narrowing of the lumen. (× 300)*

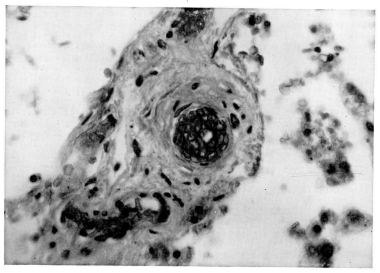

Figure 9. *Pulmonary arteriolar medial hypertrophy. The large nuclei in the wall are those of hypertrophied smooth muscle elements. Intimal changes are minimal. (× 300)*

239

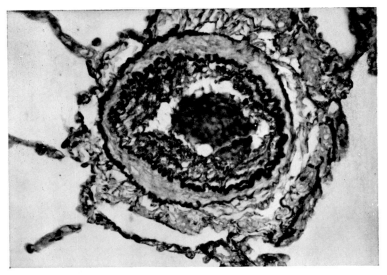

Figure 10. Pulmonary arteriosclerosis. The intima of this very small pulmonary artery is thickened by a reduplication of the internal elastic lamella and the proliferation of elastic fibers in a fibrous tissue matrix. (× 240)

The most common pathologic processes found in the lungs in chronic cor pulmonale are (1) pulmonary emphysema, usually associated with chronic bronchitis and bronchiolitis; (2) chronic bronchitis and bronchiolitis alone; (3) pneumoconiosis (particularly anthracosilicosis); (4) pulmonary tuberculosis when it is associated with distortion of the chest wall (surgical), fibrothorax, or massive fibrosis; (5) pulmonary sarcoidosis; (6) kyphoscoliosis; (7) diffuse interstitial pulmonary fibrosis (Hamman-Rich syndrome); (8) chronic recurrent diffuse pulmonary embolism. Less common lesions found in the lung are the types produced by schistosomiasis, scleroderma, multiple congenital cysts (cystic fibrosis), carcinoma with pulmonary lymphangitic metastases, and sickle-cell anemia.

19 / Rheumatic Heart Disease

It is a widely accepted concept that the anatomic lesions of rheumatic heart disease are the consequences of an antecedent hemolytic streptococcal infection. There is also an impressive body of evidence that points to a recessive genetic trait as being responsible for susceptibility to this disease. The pathogenesis of the lesions, whether by hypersensitivity, direct toxicity of certain streptococcal products, or other means, is not well understood.

The basic tissue alteration in acute rheumatic fever is swelling and fibrinoid degeneration of the collagenous ground substance seen in the fibrous tissue of the myocardium, heart valves, joints, and other tissues. The swollen collagen loses its wavy, fibrillar structure and becomes homogenous, hyaline, and strongly eosinophilic. Other important and perhaps fundamental morphologic changes are the degeneration and necrosis of cardiac muscle fibers and the necrotizing and inflammatory lesions that occur in blood vessels.

1. Rheumatic Myocarditis

The anatomic hallmark of rheumatic heart disease is the Aschoff nodule. This is a focal, granulomatous lesion occurring in close proximity to blood vessels and consisting of a central core of swollen collagen surrounded by large, often multi-nucleated basophilic cells with large vacuolated nuclei having a prominent nucleolus (the so-called Aschoff cells), a sprinkling of smaller mononuclear cells, and occasionally a few polymorphonuclear leukocytes (Fig. 11). Evolutionary changes occur with the passage of time. The nodule is gradually replaced by connective tissue (Fig. 12) and after several months becomes a fibrous scar.

Aschoff nodules are usually most abundant in the myocardium of the left ventricle and interventricular septum, and less common in the right ventricle. They also occur in the atrial myocardium and have been observed with surprising frequency in auricles removed during surgical procedures on the rheumatic heart, where their presence has been interpreted as evidence of rheumatic activity. Lesions morphologically resembling Aschoff nodules have been observed at other sites, such as the valves, pericardium, pleura, periarticular tissues, and in the adventitia of the major blood vessels.

In addition to the pathognomonic Aschoff nodule, active rheumatic myocarditis is characterized by edema of the inter-

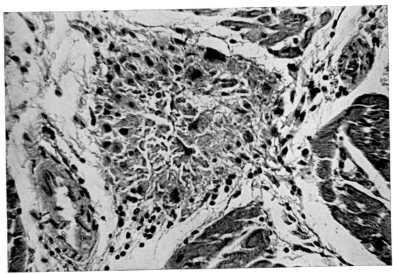

Figure 11. Rheumatic myocarditis. Early Aschoff nodule. In the center is swollen fragmented collagenous tissue; about the periphery are small mononuclear cells and a few Aschoff cells.

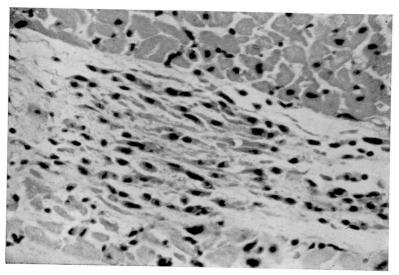

Figure 12.   *Rheumatic myocarditis. Healing Aschoff nodule. The Aschoff cells have become spindle-shaped and resemble connective tissue cells.*

stitial connective tissue and a variable cellular exudate consisting of lymphocytes, polymorphonuclear leukocytes, Anitschkow myocytes, and sometimes plasma cells and eosinophils. The cardiac muscle fibers may be the seat of degenerative changes such as swelling, eosinophilia, and occasionally frank necrosis. These changes are of particular importance, for they are in all likelihood the anatomic changes responsible for the cardiac dilatation and failure often seen in acute rheumatic heart disease. As the acute stage of the process subsides, the edema and cellular infiltrate disappear, leaving behind small, focal interstitial and myocardial scars.

2. Rheumatic Valvulitis and Endocarditis

During the acute phase of rheumatic heart disease, tiny, wart-like nodules (verrucae), 1 to 3 mm in size, may be seen along the line of closure of the valvular leaflets. These are firm and usually translucent and occur singly, in clusters, or in a continuous chain (Fig. 13). Being strongly adherent, they do not easily become emboli. The mitral valve is most frequently affected, followed closely in frequency by the aortic. The tricuspid valve is involved less frequently and less severely, and the pulmonic valve is affected only rarely. Verrucae may be present along the chordae tendineae, which become swollen and fused. The affected leaflets are edematous and often adhere to each other.

Microscopically, the vegetations consist of small platelet and fibrin thrombi deposited on damaged proliferated endocardial cells. The underlying valvular tissue is edematous and contains a cellular infiltrate (Fig. 14). The verrucae undergo or-

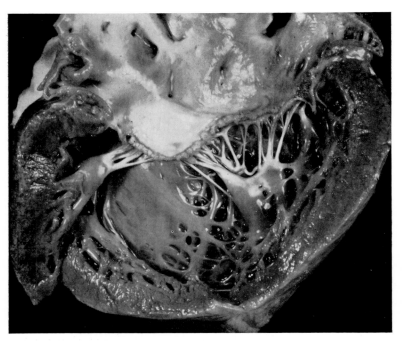

Figure 13. *Acute rheumatic endocarditis. Mitral valve. A continuous chain of verrucae along line of closure.*

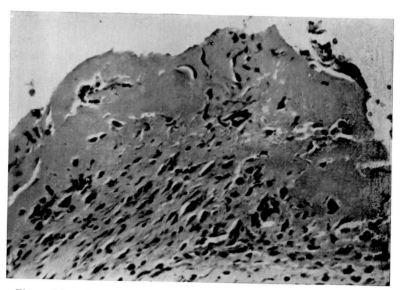

Figure 14.   Rheumatic endocarditis. Mitral valve. A healing vegetation composed of eosin-staining material with ingrowth of connective tissue at base.

ganization with an ingrowth of connective tissue cells, and the surface becomes covered by a smooth layer of endothelium. Within the leaflet and in the valve ring there is also a concomitant diffuse, inflammatory process characterized by edema, an ingrowth of capillaries, and the presence of polymorphonuclear cells and occasionally Aschoff bodies (Fig. 15). Subsidence of this interstitial valvulitis is followed by an increase in connective tissue and an ingrowth of new blood vessels.

The repetition of the acute insults to the valves with recurrent attacks of rheumatic carditis leads to progressive scarring and deformity (Fig. 16). The leaflets become fused, retracted, thickened (often grotesquely so), vascularized, and calcified. The edges of the aortic valve cusps become thickened and rolled, and the fusion of the cusps may be so extensive as to give the valve a bicuspid appearance. The chordae tendineae also become fused, thickened, and shortened, thus add-

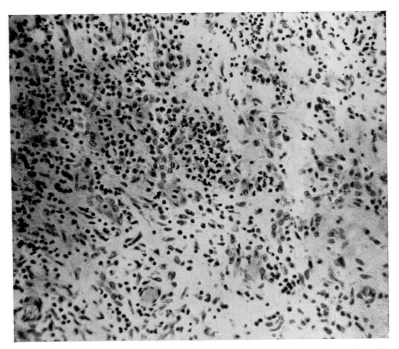

Figure 15. *Rheumatic valvulitis. The substance of the leaflet is heavily infiltrated by polymorphonuclear leukocytes and lymphocytes. Fibroblasts and capillaries are increased in the leaflet.*

ing to the mechanical deformity of the valve. Microscopic examination of the valves at this stage reveals masses of hyaline fibrous tissue, numerous thick-walled blood vessels, irregular collections of calcium, and foci of lymphocytes and monocytes, particularly in the annulus. These structural alterations in the leaflet lead to stenosis of the orifice and insufficiency of the valve and to the hemodynamic changes that ensue therefrom.

Some thickening and vascularization of the mitral valve, slight fusion and thickening of the chordae tendineae, and slight fusion of the commissures of the cusps of the aortic valve are not infrequent incidental postmortem findings in older

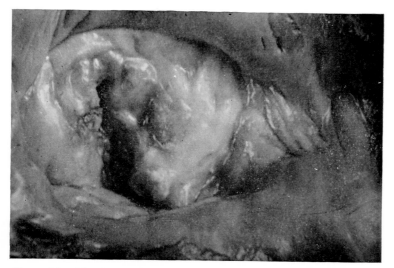

Figure 16. *Mitral stenosis due to rheumatic endocarditis. The mitral valve assumes the appearance of an irregular diaphragm with the orifice reduced to a slit-like space. The knobby excrescences are areas of calcification.*

patients. These changes are often referred to as "stigmata of rheumatic heart disease," although there is usually no history of rheumatic fever, and there were no murmurs or other evidence of rheumatic heart disease detected during life. The changes are the anatomic sequelae of a long-past inflammatory process affecting the valves and chordae, and in many cases are very likely the result of mild attacks of rheumatic heart disease. Whether they are all due to rheumatic infection or whether other disease processes are implicated is not clear at the present time.

3. Rheumatic Endocarditis of the Atrium

The endocardium of the left atrium just above the posterior leaflet of the mitral valve is often the seat of a lesion that in most respects is comparable to that in the valves. There is proliferation of the endocardial cells and sometimes the development of verrucae. There is swelling and cellular infiltration of the underlying atrium which elevate the surface and produce a rounded, plaque-like area (MacCallum's patch, Fig. 17). They are usually several centimeters across, although they may cover a large part of the endocardial surface of the atrium.

4. Rheumatic Pericarditis

Involvement of the pericardial surfaces occurs commonly in rheumatic heart disease. The parietal and visceral pericardial

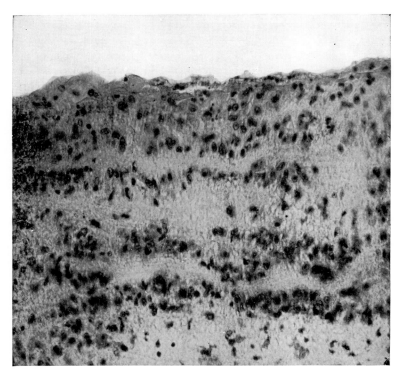

Figure 17. *Rheumatic endocarditis of the left atrium. There is infiltration of the endocardium by mononuclear cells. These are collected in rows perpendicular to the swollen collagenous fibrillae.*

surfaces may be covered extensively with fibrin, or only small focal areas may be affected. The earliest changes consist of proliferation of the mesothelial lining cells, some of which may become multinucleated, and swelling of the subepicardial connective tissue fibers with areas of fibrinoid change. Exudation into the pericardial sac may occur with a variable amount of fluid containing leukocytes, a few red cells, platelets, and fibrin. There may be a diffuse reaction in the subepicardial connective tissue with fibrinoid degeneration, inflammatory cells, and lesions closely resembling Aschoff bodies. The exudate may be rich in fibrin which plasters the pericardial surfaces firmly together. As the process subsides, granulation tissue replaces the exudate, resulting in stringy, fibrous adhesions or in extensive scarring that obliterates the pericardial cavity.

5. Rheumatic Vasculitis

Important changes in both the large and small arteries and veins occur during the course of rheumatic fever. Not infrequently there are lesions of the aorta that appear grossly as discrete reddish or yellow raised areas of the intima or as intimal ridges extending across the vessel just above the aortic valve. Similar lesions may also be seen in the pulmonary artery. On histologic examination, the elastic fibers are disrupted, the fibrillar material of the intima is edematous, and about the affected area there is a collection of large basophilic mononuclear cells and variable numbers of polymorphonuclear leukocytes (Figs. 18, 19). When healing supervenes, the lesion is represented by an avascular scar. Acute lesions may also be present in the media, particularly about the penetrating vessels. The elastic fibers may be destroyed and the muscle fibers often show hydropic degeneration. The adventitia of the larger blood vessels may contain a variety of rheumatic changes, including edema, fibrinoid degeneration, arteritis of the nutrient vessels, and Aschoff nodules.

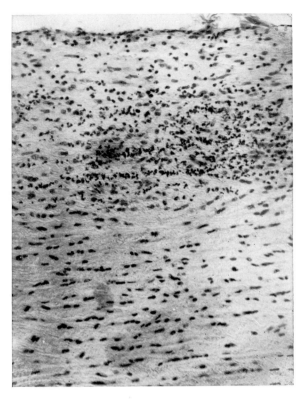

Figure 18. *Rheumatic aortitis. The lesion is limited to the inner third of the media and is characterized by a dense leukocytic infiltration.*

Focal lesions of the small arteries, arterioles, and even capillaries are present in many cases of rheumatic infection. These may be seen in the coronary arteries and also in the vessels of the pancreas, kidney, lung, and other tissues. The acute lesion consists of swelling of the endothelium, a fibrinous exudate beneath the endothelium, fragmentation and disruption of the internal elastic membrane, and thickening, fibrinoid swelling, and hyalinization of the media (Fig. 20). The lesion may be patchy or involve the entire circumference of the vessel. The degree of cellular reaction varies considerably;

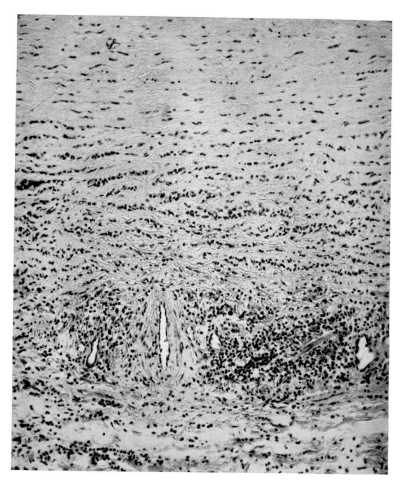

Figure 19. *Rheumatic aortitis. The inflammatory reaction involves the outer third of the media with a pronounced cellular infiltration by polymorphonuclear leukocytes. Large mononuclear cells are held in rows by the elastic lamellae.*

thus it may be quite sparse in some instances and exuberant in others, resembling the exudative necrotizing arteritis seen in polyarteritis nodosa. The lumen of the affected vessel is usually narrowed and may be completely occluded by fibrin

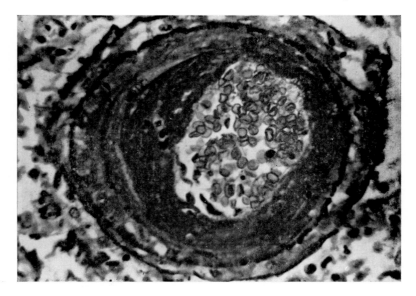

Figure 20. *Rheumatic arteritis. The acute lesion shows a thick layer of fibrin beneath the endothelium; the elastica is beaded and fragmented, and the lumen is patent.*

thrombi or by leukocyte-platelet aggregates. A type of verrucous endarteritis has also been observed in acute rheumatic fever, with irregular nodules of granular or hyaline material protruding into the lumen (Fig. 21).

Following the acute stage, the healed lesion resembles an obliterating endarteritis (Fig. 22). There may be extensive musculo-elastic hyperplasia of the intima with narrowing of the lumen. The wall of the vessel may be thickened or partially or completely replaced by a hyaline scar. In healed, inactive rheumatic heart disease, there is usually extensive fibrosis of the adventitia, and wide bands of adventitial fibrosis are often present about the smaller coronary arteries.

Lesions similar to those of rheumatic arteritis may occasionally be seen in the veins. A distinctive type of phlebitis affecting the coronary sinus has been described in rheumatic fever that is not associated with thrombosis and that histologically resembles rheumatic endocarditis.

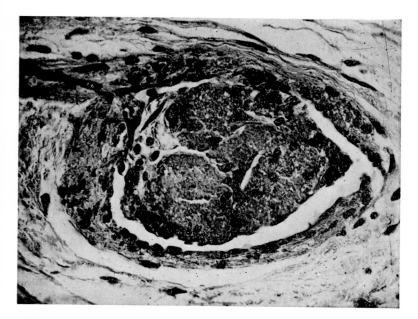

Figure 21. *Verrucous endarteritis. A mass of granular material covered by endothelium is attached to the intima and almost fills the lumen.*

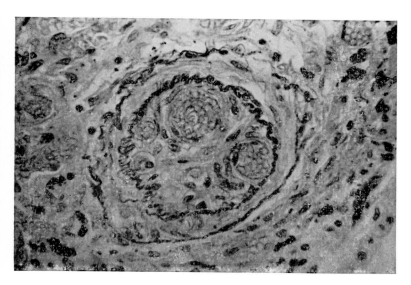

Figure 22. *Rheumatic arteritis, healed. The fibrin has been replaced by connective tissue and new channels have been formed.*

253

20 / Syphilis of the Heart and Aorta

Syphilis of the cardiovascular system chiefly affects the aorta itself, but the process may extend to the aortic valves, to the tissues around the coronary orifices, and rarely to the myocardium. The pulmonary arteries are seldom involved.

1. Syphilitic Aortitis

This is most frequent in the ascending portion and arch of the aorta, and is less common in the thoracic part and rare in the abdominal segment. The vessel wall is thickened and inelastic. The lumen may be dilated. The intima contains well-defined, pearly white, hyaline, smooth-surfaced elevations of variable size. Longitudinal wrinkling of the intima is frequent. The advancing edge of the lesion may be sharply demarcated. Atheromatous deposits in the intima may complicate and obscure its appearance to the naked eye. The intimal plaques may encroach upon and obstruct the orifice of any arterial branch, including the orifice of either or both coronary arteries.

Histologically (Fig. 23), there is an increase of connective tissue in the adventitia, thickening and endothelial proliferation in the vasa vasorum, and perivascular infiltration of lymphocytes and plasma cells. The media is penetrated at intervals by thin-walled vascular channels and collections of lymphocytes and plasma cells, usually situated in areas of

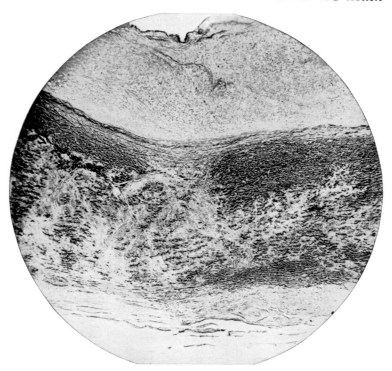

Figure 23. *Syphilitic aortitis. Van Gieson and Weigert's elastic tissue stain. The fibrous overgrowth of the intima is marked. The media is considerably reduced in thickness and the continuity of dark-staining elastica is interrupted in many places by irregular scars.*

scarring where the elastic lamellae are ruptured and the smooth muscle cells are replaced by collagen. Occasionally the larger cell aggregates show miliary gummas with central areas of necrosis (Fig. 24). Rarely a few multinuclear, foreign-body, giant cells may also appear. The intima is irregularly thickened by proliferation of connective tissue.

Treponema pallidum cannot usually be demonstrated in the lesions, although presence of the organism has been described. Spontaneous rupture, without aneurysm, has been reported but is extremely rare.

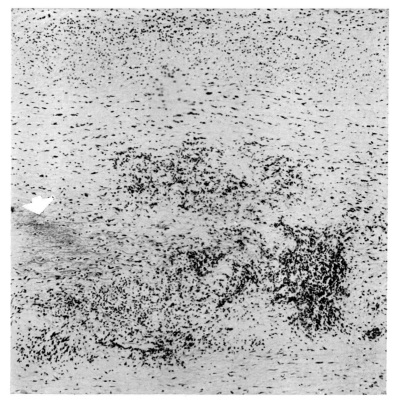

Figure 24. *Syphilitic aortitis. Chronic inflammation of the media and of the thickened adventitia, which shows in the lower part of the photograph. Many small foci of lymphocytes and plasma cells are scattered throughout. In the area indicated by the arrow, a portion of the media has undergone gummatous necrosis.*

2. Syphilitic Aneurysm of the Aorta

Most aneurysms of the aorta are caused by syphilis. They may be saccular or fusiform, single or multiple. The most common sites in order of frequency are the ascending, transverse, and descending thoracic aorta. Syphilitic aneurysms of the abdominal portion are rare.

Saccular aneurysm is the more common type; its diameter may vary from a few centimeters to 20 cm or more. It is usually connected with the lumen of the vessel by a single, well-formed stoma. Its lining may be smooth, wrinkled, ulcerated, or covered by a thrombus. The latter may be laminated by successive deposits of blood elements, the superficial layers being the newest. At the junction of the thrombus and the wall of the sac, evidence of organization may be seen. There may be several such aneurysms of varying size and age in a single aorta. The adjacent periaortic structures are subject to erosion, compression, obstruction, or displacement. More than half of all such aneurysms rupture. Rupture leads to hemorrhage, the distribution of which depends on the site of the tear.

Fusiform or diffuse dilatation of the aorta due to syphilis is also common in the thoracic portion and may be associated with saccular aneurysm in some other part. Its extent is variable. Thrombosis in this type is rare.

Histologically, the wall of a sac is composed of dense, hyalinized connective tissue which sometimes calcifies and may even ossify. The layers of the original vessel wall may be lacking and the specific character of the syphilitic lesion obscured except at its mouth or in sections from the adjacent aortic wall. The sac is lined by endothelium or organizing thrombus. In fusiform aneurysm remnants of the original vessel wall usually persist and syphilitic changes are still detectable.

3. Involvement of the Aortic Valve (Syphilitic Valvulitis)

This is found in one-third of all cases of syphilitic aortitis. The leaflets are cicatrized and incompetent as a result of inflammatory change in the underlying aortic wall and dilatation of the ring. The lateral parts of the aortic cusps may coalesce with the intima of the aorta, leading to further separation of the commissures. Hyaline plaques in these areas denote underlying commissural scars. In more advanced cases the margins of the cusps show thickening and rolling toward the ventricular aspect. This sclerosis is mechanical. Further cicatrization may reduce the cusps to cord-like structures and increase their incompetency. Dilatation of the aortic ring and supravalvular portion of the aorta without changes in the cusps occasionally leads to incompetency of the valve. Primary syphilitic valvulitis probably does not exist.

Rarely, the anterior leaflet of the mitral valve is affected by extension from syphilitic aortitis. Myocardial gummas occasionally involve valves by direct contiguity, especially the aortic valve.

Microscopic examination of the affected leaflets and of the aortic ring and root of the aorta shows, in addition to fibrous proliferation, endothelial proliferation in the vasa vasorum and perivascular infiltration by lymphocytes and plasma cells in the adventitia of the aorta near the ring.

4. Coronary Artery Involvement in Syphilitic Aortitis

This frequently causes stenosis or almost complete obliteration of the orifices. Complete occlusion rarely occurs. Syphilitic coronary arteritis without syphilitic aortitis is rare.

Microscopic sections of the stenosed portion of such coronary arteries usually reveal intimal fibrous proliferation. The site of the original lumen may be demonstrated only by elastic tissue stains. In some cases there is extension of the aortic lesion into the artery. The thickened intima and even the media may contain granulation tissue. There is also overgrowth of the adventitial connective tissue, obliteration of the vasa vasorum, and perivascular infiltration of lymphocytes.

Active stages of syphilitic inflammation of the coronary arteries may be found in any stage of syphilitic aortitis.

5. The Myocardium in Syphilis

The main effects of syphilis on the myocardium are produced by lesions in the aorta, particularly coronary ostial stenosis.

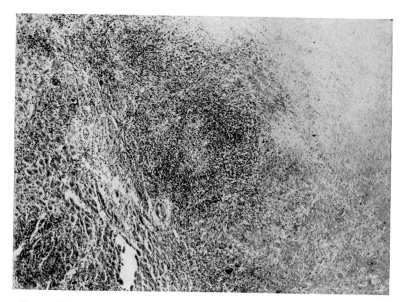

Figure 25. *Gummatous myocarditis. Low-power view shows the muscle bundles terminating at the edge of a necrotic acellular zone.*

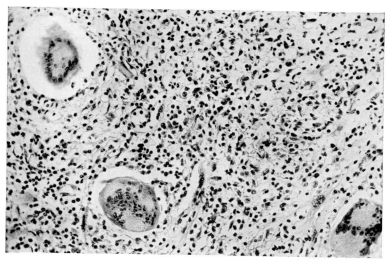

Figure 26. *Gumma of myocardium. Granulation tissue present at margin of gumma; also present are multinucleated giant cells, lymphocytes, plasma cells, and large mononuclear cells.*

Gummas, solitary or multiple, have been described but are rare. They may be found anywhere, but are most frequent in the walls of the left ventricle near the base or in the ventricular septum. In the latter site they sometimes involve the bundle of His and cause complete heart block. Rarely, they may result in a myocardial aneurysm. Diffuse interstitial myocarditis has been noted in patients dying in the secondary stage of syphilis. These instances are so rare as to be considered curiosities.

Microscopically, myocardial gummas (Fig. 25, 26) replace the muscle bundles or produce pressure atrophy of adjacent muscle fibers.

6. Congenital Syphilis of the Heart and Great Vessels

This may occur in syphilitic infants who are stillborn, die shortly after birth, or live for an indefinite period. Spirochetes are frequently present in large numbers with or without anatomic lesions. They are unusually abundant in the macerated fetus. Myocarditis, coronary arteritis, and aneurysm have been recorded. In myocarditis there may be edematous fibrotic areas overrun with spirochetes. Associated with these lesions there may be fibrosis of the endocardium.

21 / Other Diseases of the Aorta and Pulmonary Artery

The aorta and the pulmonary artery are subject to the same diseases, but the larger vessel is involved more frequently and to a greater degree. Much of the difference in incidence and severity is due to the significantly higher blood pressure within the aorta and to the respective locations of these two vessels in the vascular system.

Arteriosclerosis is the general name given to a group of degenerative diseases which cause a hardening of the arterial wall. Two of these pathologic conditions are found in the aorta, and one involves the pulmonary artery.

1. Atherosclerosis of the Aorta

Atherosclerosis of the aorta is a variable combination of the focal accumulation of lipids, complex carbohydrates, blood and blood products, fibrous tissue, and calcium deposits. The degree of atherosclerosis varies with age and sex. The earliest gross changes consist of small, soft, yellow, slightly raised, ovoid or irregularly shaped intimal deposits. Initial foci measure several millimeters in diameter; larger lesions form by fusion. In children and young adults the disease has an affinity for that segment of the aorta just distal to the valve, and for the posterior wall of the descending thoracic aortic limb, particularly about the orifices of the intercostal arteries. These early changes constitute a form of lipoidosis and are reversible. The gross manifestations of the disease become more pronounced and variable with advancing age. Some plaques still appear yellow, many are yellow-gray in color, and some have the pearly grey hue of fibrosis. Hemorrhage into a lesion gives it a rusty tint. Dystrophic calcification causes the degenerative process to become brittle. Although a well-developed focus (the "impingement plaque") may be found at the junction of the ascending limb and the aortic arch, the disease is concentrated in the abdominal aorta; it is most severe just proximal to the bifurcation. Elsewhere in the vessel, pronounced lesions occur about the orifices of its branches and at points of fixation to surrounding structures.

Microscopically, the early lesion consists of an accumulation of fine intra- and extracellular lipid droplets in the aortic intima. There is also an increase of mucopolysaccharides in the subendothelial connective tissue. As the plaque enlarges, its content is transformed into amorphous eosinophilic debris. Cholesterol clefts, intact red blood cells, and hemoglobin pigment are common findings. Fine granules of calcium are deposited in and about the central nidus. Older lesions show vascularization and peripheral fibroblastic proliferation. There is an exudative cellular response of varying intensity throughout the life span of the disease. It is composed principally of lymphocytes with a smaller number of monocytes and plasma cells; a few neutrophils are seen during the necrotic stage. The overlying media may be compressed and scarred, or it may actually be destroyed by the penetration of lipid material from the subjacent plaque. The tensile strength of the aortic wall is lessened by the expanding lesion.

The complications of atherosclerosis, which have a definite pathogenic relationship, include the following.

1.1. ULCERATION. This follows the rupture of a degenerating plaque through the thin subendothelial hyaline layer into the vascular lumen. This untoward development is common and usually causes no detectable difficulty unless the excavated grumous material assumes the role of an embolus and lodges in a vessel of critical importance such as the superior mesenteric or a renal artery. The rough base of the ulcer, however, does provide a favorable site for thrombosis.

1.2.   THROMBOSIS.   When an adherent, mural blood clot forms high in the aorta, it rarely increases sufficiently in size to obstruct the lumen. Serious complications do occur if a thrombus forms at the aortic bifurcation and obstructs the lumina of the common iliac arteries (Leriche's syndrome). Mural thrombi at any level are potential sources of peripheral emboli. Disengaged fragments cause serious damage if they are carried to nearby vessels supplying the gastrointestinal tract, kidneys, or lower extremities.

1.3.   ANEURYSM.   Aneurysm is also directly related to the ulceration of the initial plaque. Medial weakening by the destruction of elastic tissue and muscle cells, operating in concert with a frequently elevated intraluminal blood pressure, force the aortic wall to dilate locally. This abnormal enlargement is usually saccular in shape, but it may also be fusiform or cylindrical. It is found most frequently in the abdominal aorta between the origin of the renal arteries and the bifurcation. Atherosclerotic aneurysms are multiple in approximately 5 percent of the cases. Secondary complications, including erosion of the vertebrae, leakage of blood, creation of a "false aneurysm," and frank rupture, may follow the enlargement of the lesion. Perforation of the aneurysmal wall with massive hemorrhage into the retroperitoneal space or peritoneal cavity is a frequent cause of death. At autopsy the tear is found in the widest, and consequently the thinnest, portion of the pathologic dilatation; it rarely occurs at the ends or margin.

2. Calcification of the Aorta

This type of arteriosclerosis occurs much less frequently than atherosclerosis of the aorta. The calcium deposits are metastatic rather than dystrophic; the involved tissue is initially undamaged. The following two distinct variations of the lesion have been described.

2.1. SUBINTIMAL CALCIFICATION. This rare type is characterized by the lodgment of finely divided calcium granules in close relation to the internal elastic lamina. There is usually an associated hypercalcemia caused by hyperparathyroidism, osteitis fibrosa cystica, or osteomalacia. This form of vascular lesion has also been described in other secondary bone diseases, as, for example, in chronic nephritis with bone resorption ("renal rickets"). The intima may appear intact on gross examination, or it may present transverse or circumferential ridges over the calcific deposits. Small thrombi may form and adhere to these sites. Microscopically, the elastic fiber appears to be the focus about which basophilic amorphous or plate-like deposits of calcific material are placed. Ruptured strands may be impregnated with the salt. Secondary fibrosis and even metaplastic bone formation may occur in long-standing lesions. The media appears normal.

2.2. MEDIAL CALCIFICATION. This type is most frequently found in older individuals. The aorta shows some degree of senile ectasia with mild intimal thickening and moderate atrophy of the medial muscle cells. The elastic fibrils are separated and abnormally stretched. The definitive features of the lesion are best seen histologically (Fig. 27). Finely divided calcium granules are dispersed irregularly throughout the middle third of the media. They occur independently of other degenerative diseases and bear no relationship to any known inflammation.

3. Atherosclerosis of the Pulmonary Artery

Atherosclerosis is the most common lesion of the main pulmonary artery. Mild examples are prevalent in later life. When it occurs before the age of 40, it is usually associated with a

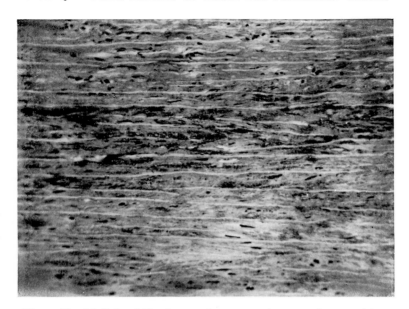

Figure 27. *Medial calcification of the aorta. Fine granules of calcium precipitate are deposited in the middle third of the media. Where these are most abundant, the tissue appears dark-staining. The unstained elastic fibers can be seen to course through the calcified portion and are themselves not involved.*

cause of elevated blood pressure within the lesser circulation. Although both the gross and microscopic findings in the pulmonary artery and its major branches are similar to those seen in the aorta, they are much milder in degree. True plaque formation is exceptional, and ulceration is rare. The pathologic changes have little functional significance. No constant relationship has been found between the extent of pulmonary arterial atherosclerosis and the thickness of the right ventricle.

4. Medial Necrosis

This is a degenerative disease that involves the aorta with moderate frequency and the pulmonary artery rarely. The aortic lesion is much the more important because of its grave complications. The pulmonary arterial lesion has been described as an incidental finding at necropsy in patients with Marfan's syndrome. Gross examination of the aorta in *medionecrosis aortae idiopathica cystica,* as the disease is also called, may reveal pale blue intimal discolorations with puckering of the endothelial surface. On cross section it is sometimes possible to identify a thin translucent media containing small cysts that are surrounded by fibrous tissue.

Microscopic study of damaged areas reveals an accumulation of a homogenous, pale-staining, basophilic, cellular material in slit-like interlamellar spaces (Fig. 28). Most authors believe that the amorphous material arises from degenerating elastic tissue and collagen; there is also an associated destruction of

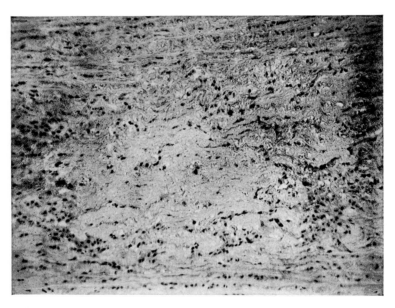

Figure 28. *Medial degeneration of the aorta. There is an irregular gap in the media filled with mucoid substance and depleted of nuclei. The cells at the margins of this lesion are irregularly arranged without any inflammatory cellular infiltration.*

muscle cells. This abnormal substance reacts positively to most metachromatic tissue dyes and shows an affinity for fat strains.

The cause of medial necrosis is unknown. The lesion has been classified as a form of senile involution, because the disease occurs with increasing frequency in older age groups. It is more common in patients with elevated blood pressures. Special studies have shown a reduced number of arteriolar branches from the vasa vasorum within the degenerated areas. Their lumina are narrowed by intimal hyperplasia and medial hypertrophy.

The following complications may occur.

4.1. DISSECTING ANEURYSM.   This is caused by a forceful penetration of blood between the tissue layers of the damaged arterial wall. In the opinion of some authors, the initial injury is caused by hemorrhage from the vasa vasorum into a medial cyst. Subsequent expansion of the intramural hematoma leads to its rupture through the aortic intima. This break provides the opening wedge for a more dynamic extension of the lesion with the systemic blood pressure as a driving force. On gross examination of the aorta, the tear is located most frequently in the proximal 3 cm of its ascending portion. The defect is usually transverse or circumferential and measures from 1 to 4 cm in length. Subsequent dissection may progress for short distances in either direction, or it may continue throughout the entire length of the artery. The column of blood characteristically separates the outer third from the inner two-thirds of the media. The path of dissection may end as an opening into the pericardial sac, pleural space, peritoneal cavity, mediastinum, or retroperitoneum. The resulting massive hemorrhage is usually fatal. Infrequently, the aneurysm reopens into the main aortic lumen to form a "double-barreled aorta." This artificially created channel may remain functional and become endothelialized, or it may close by thrombus formation and fibrosis. In those instances where the dissection continues throughout the entire length of the aorta, the smaller branches of the artery, such as the intercostals, may be severed; larger divisions, such as the renal vessels, may be restricted by a continuation of the pathologic process within their walls. The latter development can cause fatal uremia if the patient survives his vascular accident.

Microscopically, the tissue changes about the primary site of rupture are those of cystic medial necrosis heavily overshadowed by interstitial hemorrhage. Evidence of medial degeneration can also be found in parts of the aorta that are not involved by the aneurysm. If the arterial lesion is not immediately fatal, histologic examination at a later date usually shows the residua of old hemorrhage, endothelial proliferation, thrombosis with organization, and extensive fibrosis of the aortic wall. Pathologic findings in the heart and in the kidneys suggest a high incidence of associated systemic hypertension.

4.2. RUPTURE OF THE AORTA. Rupture most frequently takes the form of a restricted dissecting aneurysm, although it can result from trauma and may rarely complicate congenital malformations such as coarctation and hypoplasia of the aorta. In the most common type of lesion, medial necrosis is also the underlying defect. After gaining entrance into the area of degeneration, the column of blood forcefully penetrates the remaining layers of the aortic wall directly. Grossly, the aorta away from the lesion may appear normal to naked-eye examination, or it may show characteristic atrophy of the media with cyst formation. In its size, shape, and location, the intimal tear resembles that found in the much more extensive type of dissecting aneurysm. There is, however, minimal lateral extension of the lesion through the media. The adventitial layer and the aortic reflection of the pericardium are disrupted. The pericardial tissues are infiltrated with blood, and the cavity is distended by massive hemorrhage. The microscopic picture is identical to that seen in dissecting aneurysm. Death occurs from cardiac tamponade. Anatomic evidence of pre-existing hypertension is frequently found at autopsy.

5. Granulomatous Giant Cell Arteritis

This is a widespread, nonsuppurative inflammation in which there is a peculiar destruction of elastic fibers with a resulting giant cell formation. The lesions are characteristically found in the temporal arteries, but autopsy studies have shown involvement of the aorta and pulmonary artery. The cause of the disease is unknown. On gross examination the pathologic alterations are usually difficult to detect. The microscopic changes are characteristic. Elastic fibers are swollen, fragmented, or completely destroyed. The damaged fragments are engulfed by large multinucleated giant cells; this finding is pathognomonic. There is a diffuse inflammatory response by monocytes, lymphocytes, and lesser numbers of eosinophils and neutrophils. The pathologic process spreads to destroy adjacent muscle cells. The intima may be initially involved and the lesion may extend into the adventitial layer of the vessel. Healing takes place by granulation tissue formation and fibrosis. Granulomatous giant cell arteritis occurring in the aortic arch near the origin of the innominate, carotid, or subclavian artery is one of the causes of the "aortic arch syndrome."

6. Thrombosis of the Pulmonary Artery

Indigenous thrombus formation within the pulmonary arterial trunk or its major divisions from any cause is an uncommon postmortem finding. Pulmonary artery thrombosis as a consequence of intrinsic disease involving the vessel wall is a pathologic rarity. This exceptional absence of primary blood clot production is due in large part to the failure of pulmonary atherosclerosis to form plaques and to ulcerate. When mural thrombi do form, they are most frequently secondary to the involvement of the artery by a malignancy or spreading pulmonary tuberculosis. In the latter instance, the thrombi may contain viable tubercle bacilli and give rise to septic emboli. Retrograde coagulation of blood behind a large nonfatal embolus of peripheral origin is not considered to be true primary thrombosis of the pulmonary artery. Organization and recanalization of the adherent clot have been described in unusual cases.

7. Embolism of the Pulmonary Artery

Only massive emboli lodge in the main arterial segment or its larger branches. They generally arise in the great veins of the lower extremities, and their release is one of the more serious complications of congestive heart failure, postoperative states, and chronic debilitating conditions. Emboli of this magnitude are rarely compatible with life. At autopsy more than 60 percent of the vascular canal is obstructed by the elongated clot, which is usually curled upon itself and firmly wedged into the arterial lumen. The involved lung may be remarkably free of sequelae; there is insufficient time for infarction to develop.

22 / Other Diseases of the Coronary Arteries

1. Arteritis (Endarteritis, Mesarteritis, Periarteritis)

This disease of the coronary arteries may be found in such conditions as rheumatic fever, scarlet fever, and septicemia, or it may be part of a generalized vascular reaction. Inflammation may involve the intima primarily, with secondary extension to the media. More rarely, all coats may be involved, resulting in abscess or mycotic aneurysm, sometimes with rupture and hemorrhage. Periarteritis may be seen when an abscess of the myocardium or a suppurative pericardial lesion is in proximity to the coronary vessels; the lesion may eventually involve all coats of the arterial wall.

The microscopic picture varies according to the causative agent, e.g., toxins, bacteria, or emboli. The injury to the vessel wall may be slight or severe.

The lesion attributed to the toxins of infectious agents shows endothelial proliferation and fat in the injured cells; less often it shows "fibrinoid" change, or necrosis. In lesions caused by bacteria, the response is usually suppurative. Necrosis with lack of cellular response is also seen in some lesions, and mycotic aneurysm may ensue. An embolus containing bacteria may occupy the lumen. In some instances a secondary thrombus may surround the original embolus, and in other instances thrombosis may be incidental to the arteritis. Microorganisms may be identified in the lesion.

2. Polyarteritis Nodosa (Essential Polyangiitis, Periarteritis Nodosa, Panarteritis Nodosa)

This condition may involve the coronary arteries, particularly the secondary branches (9.10). The outstanding features of the disease are inflammation of all coats with conspicuous medial and adventitial involvement and perivascular infiltration, leading only occasionally to the formation of visible nodules. Thrombosis of the coronary arteries, with infarction of the myocardium and aneurysm, or rupture of a necrotic artery with hemorrhage into the adventitia or epicardium, may occur. These lesions are readily seen grossly.

Histologically, in the *acute* stage there is dense infiltration of the media and adventitia by polymorphonuclear neutrophils, eosinophils, lymphocytes, and plasma cells (Fig. 29). The elastic lamellae are frequently fragmented or destroyed.

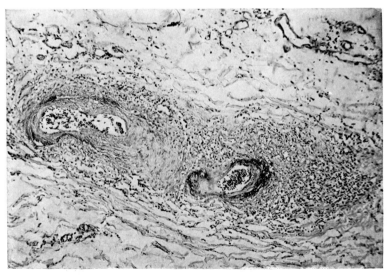

Figure 29. *Acute polyarteritis nodosa. The adventitial cellular infiltration is pronounced. The media of one vessel is necrotic and dark-staining. The lumina are still patent.*

"Fibrinoid" degeneration and necrosis in the medial and adventitial layers are characteristic features. The intima is frequently involved, and secondary occlusion of the lumen by thrombosis may occur. The periarterial connective tissue may become edematous and infiltrated by leukocytes and erythrocytes. Later, there is proliferation of fibroblasts from the adventitia into the inflammatory zone, with an increase in lymphocytes, plasma cells, and sometimes eosinophils in large numbers. Granulation tissue and, subsequently, connective tissue replaces the destroyed components of the wall, including the interrupted elastic tissue. Ultimate canalization of thrombi occurs.

Aneurysm, a rather common sequel of segmental destruction of the arterial wall, may, in association with periarterial cellular infiltration of connective tissue, produce a visible nodule.

In some cases both fresh and healed lesions occur together. Occasionally, however, only a healed stage of polyarteritis nodosa is found. Scars in the myocardium representing healed infarcts may be the only naked-eye finding. The vessels may be tortuous and studded with bluish-white nodules, not unlike those seen in acute stages of the disease. The lumina may be greatly reduced or obliterated. Periarterial mantles of scar tissue are characteristic of the end stage.

Histologically, the *healed* stage of polyarteritis (Fig. 30) is characterized by connective tissue replacement of the arterial wall with stenosis of the lumen. The intima may be variously deformed, depending upon previous thrombosis, organization, and canalization, or there may be simple fibrous thickening. There is interruption of elastic fibers by scars in the media. The vessel appears embedded in a dense mass of contracted and sometimes hyalinized connective tissue. Occasionally, sections may display small aneurysmal pouches.

3. Thromboangiitis Obliterans

Although this disease of unknown cause usually affects the vessels of the extremities (9.9), a few authentic reports of coro-

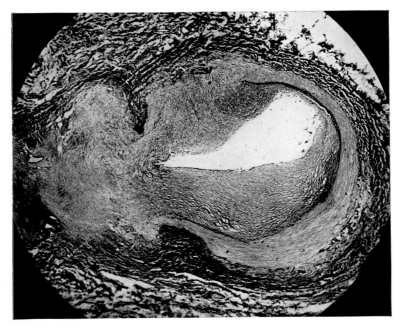

Figure 30. *Healed polyarteritis nodosa with aneurysm.*

nary involvement are on record. Advanced coronary atherosclerosis, with thromboangiitis obliterans elsewhere, may
present difficulties in differential diagnosis. To justify the
diagnosis, features of the lesion in the coronary vessels should
correspond with those in the vessels of the extremities. The
myocardium may show recent or old infarcts.

4. Aneurysm

Aneurysm of a coronary artery is rare. It is usually single,
varies from 1 to 2 cm in diameter, and is ruptured in approximately half of the cases which come to autopsy. The proximal
part of the left coronary artery is most often involved.

Microscopically, the elastic and muscular fibers of the media show fragmentation. The intima and media may display foci of necrosis or the entire wall may be necrotic.

Following are the several types of aneurysm.

4.1. MYCOTIC–EMBOLIC. This type may be secondary to bacterial endocarditis. It may show partial or complete occlusion of the lumen by a plug in minor stages of organization or by acute inflammation of the vascular wall.

4.2. ATHEROSCLEROTIC. The majority of cases show an advanced degree of atherosclerosis, occasionally with dissection of the wall by hemorrhage.

4.3. COMPLICATING CONGENITAL COMMUNICATION OF A CORONARY ARTERY WITH A CARDIAC CHAMBER OR WITH THE PULMONARY ARTERY. This type is saccular, may be multiple, and may develop atherosclerosis secondarily (15.55, 56, 57).

4.4. DISSECTING. This type is usually the result of extension from a dissecting aortic aneurysm. Rarely, it begins in and may be localized to a coronary artery.

5. Embolism

Embolism of the coronary arteries is rare. The most common sources are bacterial vegetations on the aortic valves. These emboli often initiate inflammatory lesions at their point of lodgment. Rarely, atheromatous material from aortic valvular deposits may break off and cause coronary embolism.

6. Rupture (Spontaneous)

Spontaneous rupture of the coronary arteries is rare. Mycotic-embolic aneurysms, and especially the aneurysms that accompany polyarteritis nodosa, may precede rupture of the arterial wall. Rarely, rupture of the wall due to dissecting aneurysm may be seen. The histologic findings are those of the underlying disease, e.g., atherosclerosis, arteritis, polyarteritis nodosa, or dissecting aneurysm.

275

23 / Other Diseases of the Endocardium and Valves

This section deals with anatomic changes that occur in the valves and in the lining of the cardiac chambers as a result of bacterial action, in association with systemic diseases (lupus erythematosus, rheumatoid arthritis), or as a result of causes yet unknown (**19**.1–5).

1. Bacterial Endocarditis

Septic vegetations occur on the cusps and chordae of the valves, and occasionally also on the adjacent atrial and ventricular endocardium. Bacterial endocarditis may be classified on clinical, bacteriologic, and morphologic grounds into two main groups—acute and subacute—but clinically the division is in part arbitrary (**3**.24). Because of its greater incidence, subacute bacterial endocarditis will be considered first.

1.1. SUBACUTE BACTERIAL ENDOCARDITIS (ENDOCARDITIS LENTA). The great majority of cases are caused by the *Streptococcus viridans,* although occasionally the gonococcus, *Hemophilus influenzae,* enterococcus, or one of the yeasts or fungi may be the responsible organism. Subacute bacterial endocarditis is usually engrafted upon valves previously affected by rheumatic heart disease or deformed by congenital defects. The valves are the site of a proliferative process containing small granular or large polypoid vegetations. The vegetations vary in color from gray to red to dark brown, depending upon the amount and age of the blood trapped within them, and they are usually irregular in shape and friable, so that small masses may readily be broken off. Direct examinations of smears made from bits of the vegetations will in most instances reveal the presence of bacteria and be helpful in establishing a precise diagnosis. The vegetations are located mainly on the contact surfaces of the valves but they may also be present on the mural endocardium, especially on the left atrium and the upper portion of the left ventricular aspect of the interventricular septum. The left side of the heart is preponderantly involved. The vegetations often extend onto the chordae tendineae and papillary muscles. Occasionally the valve leaflet may be ulcerated and the chordae ruptured, although this occurs more commonly in the acute form of bacterial endocarditis than it does in the subacute.

Microscopic examination of the vegetation (Fig. 31) shows it to consist principally of a central core of necrotic tissue capped by an irregular mass of fibrin in which are imbedded colonies of bacteria, varying numbers of red blood cells, and a few polymorphonuclear leukocytes near the surface. The underlying leaflet is usually thickened and infiltrated with large and small mononuclear cells with granulation tissue and proliferating fibroblasts extending into the vegetation. Foci of interruption in continuity of valvular tissue may occur. There may be varying degrees of organization of the fibrinous mass, occasionally with some calcification.

Since the advent of antibiotic therapy, varying degrees of healing are frequently encountered. The vegetations undergo fibrosis, hyalinization, and occasionally calcification, forming irregular nodular masses and deforming the valve. In some instances aneurysms of the valve leaflets occur. Serious consequences of the active stages, also seen in the healed stage, include perforation or excavation, rupture of the chordae, and fusion of the posterior mitral leaflet to the left ventricular endocardium.

1.2. ACUTE BACTERIAL ENDOCARDITIS (INFECTIVE, VEGETATIVE, ULCERATIVE).   The bacteria usually responsible are the hemo-

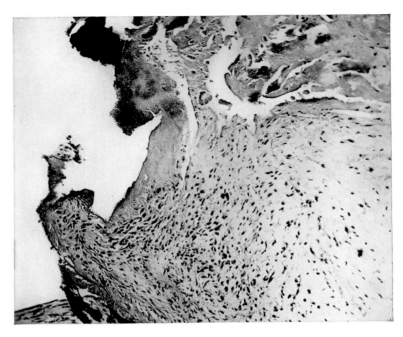

Figure 31. Subacute bacterial endocarditis. The ulcerated surfaces are covered by fibrin, platelets, and masses of bacteria. The substance of the leaflet is heavily infiltrated by large hyperchromatic mononuclear cells.

lytic streptococcus, pneumococcus, and *Staphylococcus aureus,* although cases due to the gonococcus, meningococcus, salmonella, and other organisms are occasionally encountered. Acute bacterial endocarditis is often a secondary complication of a primary bacterial infection elsewhere in the body, as, for example, lobar pneumonia or septicemia.

The vegetations are generally large and exuberant. They may or may not be superimposed on a previously diseased or congenitally deformed valve. Destruction of a portion of the valve leaflet or of the chordae occurs more frequently in acute than in subacute endocarditis. Microscopically (Fig. 32), these lesions resemble those seen in subacute bacterial endocarditis except that there is generally a more florid acute inflammatory

278

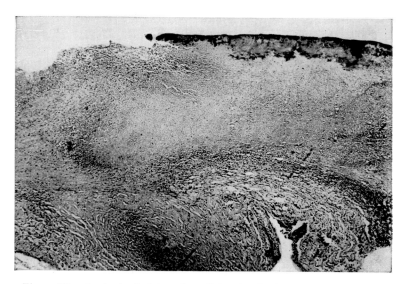

Figure 32. *Acute bacterial endocarditis of mitral valve due to hemolytic streptococcus. The swollen leaflet is necrotic in places and is heavily infiltrated by fragmented polymorphonuclear leukocytes. The endothelial surfaces are ulcerated and partly covered by surface growth of dark-staining bacterial colonies.*

reaction in the valve itself and less evidence of healing. With the use of chemotherapeutic agents, various stages of healing may be observed, and in such cases the pathologic, like the clinical, distinction between acute and subacute endocarditis may be difficult.

2. Nonbacterial Endocarditis (Indeterminate Endocarditis)

The lesions in this category of endocarditis resemble those of bacterial endocarditis in many respects. They differ from the latter in that they may be engrafted on a previously normal valve and contain no bacteria upon either direct examination or culture (3.25).

2.1. NONBACTERIAL THROMBOTIC ENDOCARDITIS (MARANTIC ENDOCARDITIS, NONRHEUMATIC VERRUCOUS ENDOCARDITIS, ENDOCAR-

DITIS SIMPLEX, TERMINAL ENDOCARDITIS). This type of endocarditis is seen most frequently in individuals succumbing after chronic wasting diseases, including malignancies with metastases and nutritionally depleted states. The pathogenesis of the lesion is not clear. Grossly, the lesion consists of firm, gray, yellow, or pink, flat or raised nodules along the line of closure of the mitral valve and occasionally of the aortic valve; they resemble in some aspects the lesions of rheumatic endocarditis. They are, however, often larger than rheumatic verrucae and occasionally may be seen as quite large polypoid or pedunculated vegetations. The underlying valves may show some degenerative change. The mural endocardium and the chordae tendineae are usually not involved. Microscopically, the vegetations consist largely of agglutinated platelets and an admixture of red blood cells and fibrin, often with some evidence of organization at the periphery. Polymorphonuclear leukocytes are only rarely found in the lesion (Fig. 33). There

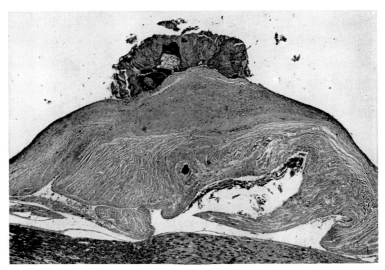

Figure 33. *Nonbacterial thrombotic endocarditis. An agglutinated mass of platelets with entrapped red cells is implanted upon the valvular surface. There is minimal cellular reaction.*

is a striking paucity of inflammatory reaction at the base, and bacteria are not present. Embolic phenomena are not infrequently associated with this type of endocarditis.

2.2. ATYPICAL VERRUCOUS ENDOCARDITIS. This type is a pathologic entity occurring in association with disseminated lupus erythematosus (3.25). The lesions may vary in size from small verrucae to large vegetations, frequently located on the ventricular aspect of the valves and extending in some cases onto the neighboring mural endocardium. The mitral and tricuspid valves are most often involved, the pulmonic and aortic valves less so. Perforation of the valve and rupture of the chordae have not been described with the lesion. Microscopically, the verrucae consist of granular fibrinous masses, in the meshes of which are red and white blood cells. When present, hematoxylin bodies provide a distinctive feature of the lesion. At the base of the verrucae there is infiltration with macrophages and lymphocytes, and occasionally there are plasma cells and evidence of organization.

3. Tuberculosis

Tuberculosis of a valve and of the endocardium is rare, and when present, it is usually associated with miliary tuberculosis.

4. Annular Sclerosis

The annulus fibrosus of the mitral valve and occasionally also that of the aortic valve are commonly the sites of a fibrocalcific deposit in older individuals (Fig. 34). The deposits of calcium may involve as little as a few millimeters to as much as all of the ring. These lesions do not produce stenosis or insufficiency and are not related to antecedent endocarditis. The valves are usually not involved, or only slightly so at their bases, and valvular function remains undisturbed. In rare instances the calcific deposits may affect the conduction system and result in conduction defects. Microscopically, the principal features

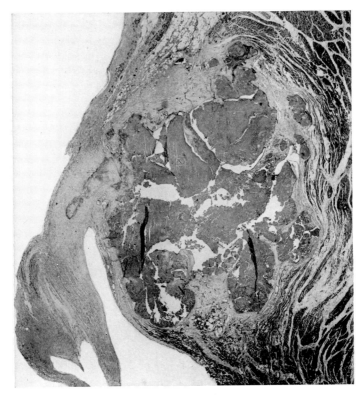

Figure 34. *Calcification of the annulus of the mitral valve. A large mass of calcium, which has become fragmented in preparation, is situated at the base of the valve and extends into the ventricular myocardium. The valve leaflet is shortened and thickened.*

are fibrosis, hyalinization, extensive and irregular calcification, and foci of lipid deposits with cholesterol clefts. Ossification of the lesion may also be present at times. Extensive lesions may extend into the underlying left ventricular myocardium.

5. Valvular Atheroma

Lipid deposits are almost universally present on the ventricular aspect of the anterior leaflet of the mitral valve. The lesions are found even in children and young adults, although they are larger and more extensive in older individuals. Grossly, they consist of soft, irregular yellow patches just beneath the endocardium, and produce only slight deformity of the valve. Microscopically, they consist of focal collections of lipid with varying degrees of fibrosis and calcification.

6. Valvular Sclerosis (Calcific Nodular Valvular Sclerosis, Calcareous Valvular Disease, Mönckeberg's Aortic Sclerosis, Primary Ascending Sclerosis of the Aortic Valve)

In older, nonrheumatic individuals, the aortic cusps may be the seat of sclerotic and calcific changes which produce rigidity and deformity of the valves, accompanied by stenosis of the orifice with or without insufficiency (Fig. 35). Since sclerosis and calcification of the aortic valve are often sequelae of aortic valvulitis, it may occasionally be impossible to differentiate this primary valvular sclerosis from underlying rheumatic disease. In some cases the presence of other stigmas of rheumatic heart disease, such as changes in the mitral valve, may be the only clue to the fundamental background of the process. In the primary form, the fibrosis and calcification usually begin in the sinus of Valsalva and extend up onto the leaflets of the aortic valve. Small irregular calcific nodules, usually first present in the base of the valve leaflets, may in more advanced cases involve a large portion of the valve, including the free margins, and produce variable degrees of thickening, stenosis, and deformity of the cusps. In far-advanced cases there may be fusion of the commissures, producing an appearance that is difficult to distinguish from a congenital bicuspid aortic valve.

Microscopically, the lesion consists of areas of fibrosis and hyalinization and extensive areas of calcification. Occasionally there is metaplastic bone formation and a mild, nonspecific cellular reaction at the periphery.

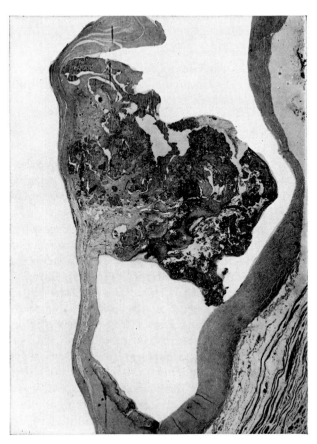

Figure 35. Calcification of the aortic valve. A large mass of calcified material is embedded in fibrous tissue which protrudes into the sinus of Valsalva. The proximal portions of the leaflet and the entire ventricular aspect show little change.

7. Mural Endocardial Fibrosis (Fibroelastosis, Endomyocardial Fibrosis)

Gray or pearly white thickening of the endocardium of either ventricle is seen in infants and young children and occasionally in adults with this disease (3.23). The pathogenesis of the lesion is obscure. In children it is often associated with valvular anomalies and may be congenital in origin (4.9). In cases where there are no other congenital anomalies, the lesion has been attributed to alterations in the blood supply of the endocardium, to nutritional defects, and to infection. However, evidence of inflammatory reaction is usually conspicuously absent. The area of endocardial fibrosis may be quite large. The lesion may be associated with mural thrombi, and it may result in cardiac failure.

Microscopically, the endocardium is enormously thickened, largely as the result of hyperplasia of elastic and collagenous elements.

Endocardial fibrosis may occur in adults in association with malignant carcinoid tumors (2.4). The lesion characteristically involves the right side of the heart, with considerable fibrous thickening of the endocardium of the right atrium or ventricle and in some instances also of the tricuspid and pulmonic valves (Fig. 36). The changes are thought to result from the increased amounts of circulating serotonin known to be present in patients with malignant carcinoid tumors, although this pathogenic relationship has not as yet been clearly established.

8. Rheumatoid Valvulitis

Patients who have suffered from rheumatoid arthritis not infrequently display at postmortem lesions of the valves that are indistinguishable from those of rheumatic heart disease (19.2). In addition, a few cases have been known involving lesions of the valve cusps that microscopically resemble the subcutaneous nodules associated with rheumatoid arthritis (Fig. 37).

9. Mural Thrombosis (Endocardial Thrombosis)

Mural thrombosis may result from inflammation, injury, necrosis and fibrosis (16.8), and slowing and abnormal eddying of

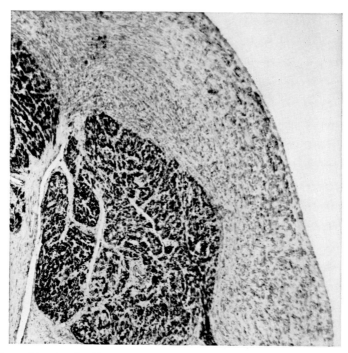

Figure 36. *Carcinoid heart disease. Endocardial thickening demonstrated by Alcian Blue stain. The pale-staining material is brilliantly blue due to the presence of large quantities of interfibrillar ground substance.*

the blood stream. Thrombi may form on the endocardium of any of the cardiac chambers; they are especially frequent in the atrial appendages (auricles).

The marantic thrombus (stasis thrombus) is frequently found in the atrial appendages, most often associated with atrial fibrillation and congestive heart failure (3.27). "Ball" or "globoid" thrombi occasionally lie free in the atrial chambers or may be attached to the endocardium by a thin pedicle (3.46). These may act as ball-valve obstructions by protruding into the atrioventricular orifices. They are most often found in association with stenosis of the mitral or tricuspid valve. Atrial mural thrombosis is encountered in rheumatic heart disease with

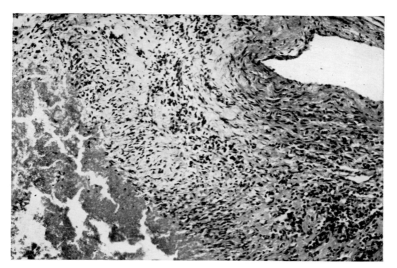

Figure 37.   Rheumatoid valvulitis. A zone of necrosis is surrounded by palisaded mononuclear cells in a fashion resembling the subcutaneous nodule. Section is of the base of the mitral valve in a patient with disseminated granulomatous lesions.

mitral stenosis and rheumatic endocarditis, and may serve as the nidus for bacterial implantation.

The majority of the mural thrombi in the ventricles form as complications of myocardial infarction, particularly with cardiac failure (3.40; **16.2, 8**). They are found predominantly in the left ventricle, and may be small or may be large enough to fill a third or more of the chamber. In ventricular aneurysms incidental to myocardial infarction, mural thrombosis is common (**16.6**). The large thrombi are attached at their bases, are friable and laminated, and may be organized. Large thrombi may show central liquefaction. On section they vary in color but are predominantly red or gray. They may be the source of systemic or pulmonary emboli.

It is often difficult to distinguish between *antemortem* and *postmortem* thrombi. In general, postmortem thrombi are easily removed; antemortem thrombi are adherent to the underlying surface and when detached leave a roughened area. Histologic study of the site of attachment is necessary in doubtful cases, and will reveal evidence of organization of the thrombus in the case of antemortem thrombi.

10. Endocardial Blood Cysts

These are seen quite frequently in the hearts of new-born infants. They are small, discrete, nodular, dark red, cyst-like lesions usually on the atrial aspect of the mitral and tricuspid valves. They vary in diameter from a pinpoint to 1 mm, and may be multiple. Histologically, they appear as simple or multilocular, endothelium-lined spaces filled with blood, and give the appearance of blood lacunae.

11. Anatomic Signs of Valvular Dysfunction

The main disturbances of function resulting from deformed valves are stenosis, insufficiency, or both. Although rheumatic fever is the most frequent cause, inflammatory and degenerative lesions such as syphilis, sclerosis of valves, bacterial endocarditis (active or healed), and congenital anomalies may also produce deformities with resulting valvular dysfunction.

No satisfactory method of measuring valvular orifices has been established. Tables which give the average normal circumference of the various orifices in the adult heart are unreliable: e.g., aortic, 7 to 8 cm; mitral, 9 to 11 cm; tricuspid, 11 to 13 cm. The diagnosis of stenosis or insufficiency should rest on the anatomic factors described. At times collateral evidence obtained clinically, e.g., cardiac catheterization or angiography, may be necessary for a comprehensive opinion as to the valvular dysfunction that existed during life.

11.1. INSUFFICIENCY (REGURGITATION, INCOMPETENCY) OF A VALVE. This is present when complete closure during life was impossible and the valvular orifice is enlarged. The diagnosis that is often difficult by anatomic means may be made when the altered valves cannot be made to coapt. Insufficiency may be produced by fibrosis and retraction of the semilunar cusps or widening of their commissures, or by flattening of the lateral portions of the cusps due to their adherence to the adjacent intima of the aorta or pulmonary artery, or by fusion and retraction of the chordae with dilatation of the rings of the atrioventricular valves.

Collateral evidence is noted mainly in advanced degrees of valvular dysfunction and consists of the following:

a. Hypertrophy and dilatation of the chamber behind an incompetent semilunar valve and proximal and distal to an incompetent atrioventricular valve.
b. Mural endocardial pockets, often with the openings of the pockets directed toward the incompetent orifice, or patchy fibrosis in similar locations. These pockets are mural endocardial thickenings often found on the wall of the outflow tract of the left ventricle below an incompetent aortic valve and on the left atrium above an incompetent mitral valve. They are small, localized, grayish-white, often shaped like a pocket. Histologically, the lesions consist of thickened fibrous mural endocardium.
c. Perforation of valve leaflets resulting from disease or trauma.

11.2. STENOSIS OF THE ORIFICE OF A VALVE. This is present when fibrosis of a valve has produced fusion and stiffening of the cusps, with narrowing of the valve orifice. Hypertrophy and dilatation of the chamber behind the valvular deformity usually occur and are roughly proportional to the degree of stenosis. Mild grades of stenosis without such secondary changes are seen. Valvular stenosis may be accompanied by insufficiency, but if one dysfunction is severe the other tends to be mild. Additional evidence of insufficiency may be circumscribed endocardial thickenings or pocket formations behind the affected orifice.

24 / Other Diseases of the Myocardium

1. Infectious Myocarditis

Acute myocarditis may occur in association with infectious diseases of bacterial, fungal, rickettsial, viral, or helminthic origin. The lesions may consist of focal abscesses in which specific organisms such as staphylococci (Fig. 38) or fungi (Fig. 39) may be demonstrated; or they may consist of focal or diffuse interstitial infiltration of histiocytes, lymphocytes, or polymorphonuclear leukocytes between the muscle fibers and in the perivascular connective tissue. Varying degrees of myocardial injury from fatty change to frank myofiber necrosis may be observed.

1.1. SPECIFIC GRANULOMATOUS MYOCARDITIS. This may occur in the course of disseminated infection by organisms characteristically evoking a granulomatous response. These include tuberculosis (particularly with massive hematogenous dissemination), fungal infection, and rarely syphilis. Systemic sarcoidosis may similarly involve the myocardium. The lesions consist of interstitial aggregates of mononuclear cells with giant cells and zones of necrosis impinging on and replacing the myofibers. In all but sarcoid, the causative organism is demonstrable within the lesion.

1.2. PARASITIC LESIONS OF THE MYOCARDIUM. Although rare, echinococcus cysts may be visible grossly. They may be mul-

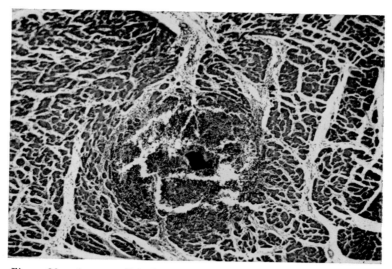

Figure 38. *A myocardial abscess in the center of which is a colony of staphylococci.*

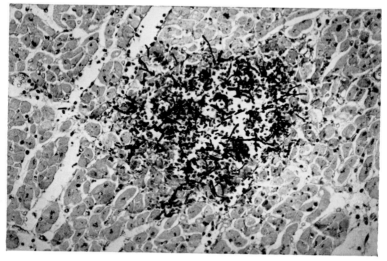

Figure 39. *A myocardial abscess in a patient with disseminated candidiasis. The abscess contains hyphal forms of the fungus.*

tiple in the septum or lodged between columnae carneae. Cysticercosis (*Taenia solium*) is rare; when present, larvae may be found in the myocardium. Infrequently, myocardial granulomas may be encountered in schistosomiasis; hematogenous dissemination of the ova may produce schistosomal "tubercles" of miliary size.

Trichinosis may, in severe cases, induce myocardial lesions. It does not produce changes in the heart muscle that are visible to the naked eye. Although the larvae of the *Trichinella spiralis* almost never develop in the myocardium, they may produce a lesion in which the heart is dilated and soft. The muscle may appear pale brown and show areas of fatty change. Microscopic examination (Fig. 40) may reveal loss of cross striations and sarcoplasm, and various regressive nuclear changes in the muscle fibers. In addition, there may be diffuse infiltration by polymorphonuclear leukocytes, plasma cells, and, in some cases, by eosinophils. The parasites, although

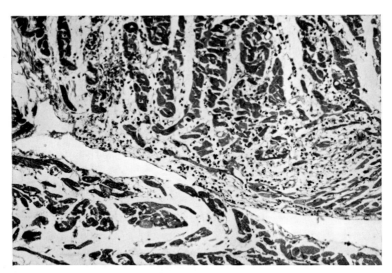

Figure 40. *Myocarditis associated with trichinosis. Degeneration and fragmentation of myofibers is associated with an infiltration of polymorphonuclear leukocytes, plasma cells, and mononuclear cells.*

usually undetectable, may be demonstrated following digestion of a fresh specimen.

In the myocarditis caused by *Trypanosoma cruzi* (Chagas' disease), the protozoa lodge in the muscle, producing necrosis and reactive inflammation in the interstitium (Fig. 41).

Plasmodium, usually *falciparum,* rarely *vivax,* may, in severe cases, produce capillary thrombi with ischemic changes in the muscle. The parasites are visible with the agglutinated erythrocytes in the myocardial capillaries (Fig. 42).

Toxoplasmosis may occur in the myocardium (Fig. 43), producing focal necrosis associated with an eosinophilic and leukocytic infiltration. *Heterophyes* ova may, in rare instances, be found in the valves and myocardium. *Sarcocystis,* a parasite infecting certain animals, may occur in man, producing microscopic cysts in the myocardium. Sarcosporidia, common

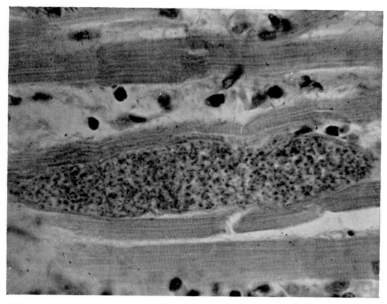

Figure 41.   Chagas' disease (Cruz trypanosomiasis) showing an encysted lesion in the heart muscle. The individual parasites are leishmaniform in nature, resembling Leishman-Donovan bodies.

293

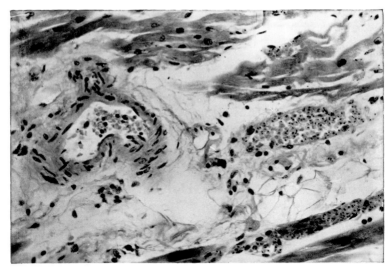

Figure 42. *Myocardium in malaria* (falciparum) *exhibiting slight edema, slight increase in interstitial cells (histiocytes, plasma cells, and Anitschkow myocytes) with parasitized erythrocytes crowding capillaries and venules. (Courtesy of Armed Forces Institute of Pathology; Negative No. 78177, Accession 104175)*

in lower animals, may occur in man, with demonstrable lodgment of the parasites in the myocardium. *Strongyloides* larvae may be found, in severe cases, in the myocardium.

2. Isolated Myocarditis (Fiedler's Myocarditis, Idiopathic Myocarditis)

This is a form of cardiopathy of unknown cause, occurring chiefly in adults, principally males, in the absence of other diseases associated with myocarditis. There is cardiac enlargement and diffuse myocardial inflammation. Grossly, the muscle is flabby and pale gray with zones of hyperemia. Microscopic examination reveals disseminated areas of necrosis of myofibers with histiocytic reaction and areas of replacement fibrosis. Wide bands of lymphocytes, histiocytes, plasma cells, and

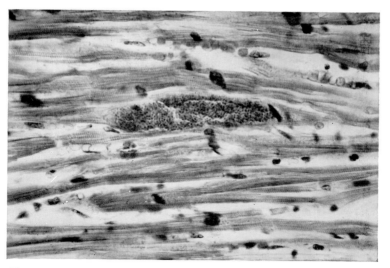

Figure 43. *Pseudocyst (terminal colony) of* Toxoplasma gondii *in a myofiber of a patient with toxoplasma encephalitis. (Courtesy of Dr. Gleb Budzilovich)*

occasionally numbers of eosinophils may separate and replace muscle fibers (Fig. 44).

In some instances of isolated myocarditis the reaction is characterized by the presence of large numbers of giant cells. Some appear to be of muscular origin; others are of the Langhans type. They may make up part of a diffuse reaction or may be arranged in discrete granulomas in association with lymphocytes and mononuclear cells arrayed about variably sized areas of necrosis. No organisms are demonstrable. The terms *nonspecific granulomatous myocarditis* and *giant cell myocarditis* are also employed to designate this form of the disease.

3. Myocarditis Associated with Hypersensitivity Reactions

Acute interstitial myocarditis with or without accompanying vascular lesions may occur in association with sensitivity reac-

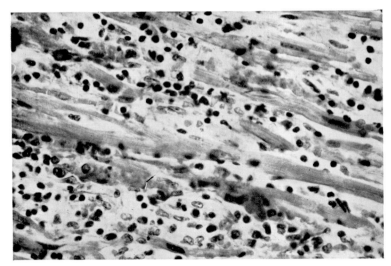

Figure 44. *Isolated myocarditis (Fiedler's myocarditis). Lymphocytes, histiocytes, and plasma cells separate the myofibers and surround the areas of necrosis.*

tions to drugs or heterologous serum. Eosinophils may predominate or the reaction may consist principally of histiocytes and neutrophils.

In patients dying with acute or subacute diffuse glomerulonephritis, there is observed a form of myocarditis characterized by interstitial edema and infiltration of lymphocytes, mononuclear cells, and occasional plasma cells.

4. Metabolic Heart Disease

4.1. NONSPECIFIC METABOLIC CARDIOMYOPATHY. This is seen in a group of conditions characterized by a deficiency in or an inability to utilize oxygen and substrate. These include anemia, beriberi, and hypovolemic shock. Grossly, the heart may be enlarged, dilated, and flabby, with fatty change visible through the endocardium as transverse yellow markings, so-called tabby cat appearance or tigering. The microscopic lesions in all conditions are similar, consisting of fatty change (Fig. 45), hydropic degeneration (Fig. 46), and swelling of the myofibers. In the advanced form, this damage may progress to actual necrosis.

Other causes of myofiber necrosis, when examined at the level of the energy-producing system of the muscle, may reveal themselves as metabolic diseases. Thus diphtheria toxin may block the oxidation of succinate. In diphtheritic myocarditis the primary alteration is damage to the myofiber that expresses itself as hyaline, granular, or fatty change, progressing to necrosis and destruction of muscle with a secondary inflammatory response, composed principally of mononuclear cells (Fig. 47). Healing occurs by fibrous replacement of areas of necrosis.

The alterations seen in myocardial ischemia (16.1, 2) may in the last analysis properly be included in the category of metabolic heart disease, since they represent examples of myocardial derangement secondary to a deficiency in oxygen and sub-

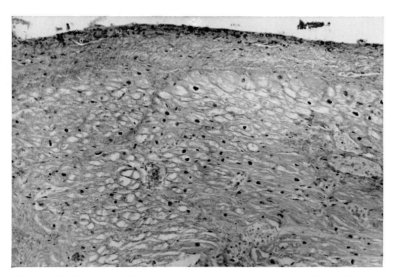

Figure 45. *Hydropic degeneration, fatty change, and swelling of myofibers in severe anemia.*

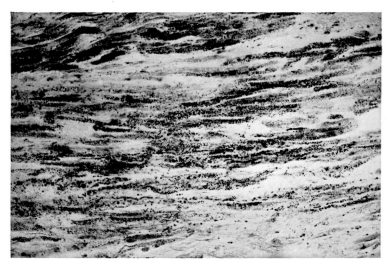

Figure 46. *Fat stains of the myocardium in the case illustrated in Fig. 45. The fat is deposited in droplets arranged in longitudinal array and accounts for only part of the vacuolar swelling seen in the previous figure. Much of the vacuolation is due to Schiff-positive material, which disappears with diastase digestion, indicating that it is glycogen.*

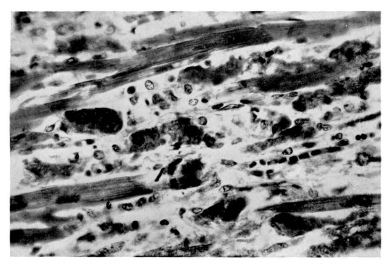

Figure 47. *Myocardium in diphtheria. Necrotic myofibers demonstrate eosinophilic clumping and are surrounded by an infiltration that is principally histiocytic in type.*

strate. Indeed, in areas of lesser damage in atherosclerotic coronary artery disease, there may be seen swelling and hydropic and fatty changes identical with those found in anemia, beriberi, or shock.

4.2. SPECIFIC METABOLIC CARDIOMYOPATHY

a. *Amyloidosis of the heart* may occur as a feature of primary systemic amyloid deposition or as an isolated lesion. In the *systemic* form the small arteries and arterioles may be involved to a degree leading to myocardial ischemia. In addition, there may be interstitial amyloid infiltration. The *isolated* variety is seen in patients dying in the eighth decade or later. The deposit takes the form of minute subendocardial nodules in the atria, where the lesion may be recognized grossly, and also involves the myocardium. In the latter site individual myofibers are surrounded, compressed, rendered atrophic, and eventually replaced by amyloid. Neighboring muscle fibers may be hypertrophied but the weight of the heart is not increased. Extensive involvement of this type may occasionally lead to congestive failure (Fig. 48).

b. *Glycogen disease of the heart* is a rare familial disease that should be differentiated from classic von Gierke's disease in which only a mild excess of glycogen is present in the heart (4.10). This cardiomyopathy is a component of a generalized glycogenosis and is characterized by enormous cardiac enlargement that principally involves the ventricles. The enlarged myofibers consist of cell membranes about clear spaces laden with glycogen and containing few myofibrils.

c. *Nodular glycogen infiltration* (so-called rhabdomyoma) is most often observed in association with tuberous sclerosis. The nodular lesions may occur in the atria or ventricles and are usually multiple. They compress surrounding normal myofibers and are made up of a lacy network of cell membranes encompassing large vacuolar spaces that contain glycogen.

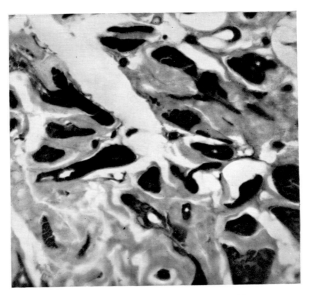

Figure 48. *Amyloidosis of the myocardium. Muscle fibers are surrounded and displaced by deposits of amyloid. There is hypertrophy of myofibers in areas of lesser or absent involvement.*

d. *Calcification of the myocardium* may be dystrophic or metastatic in type. In the former calcium is deposited in scarring, as, for example, in the walls of ventricular aneurysms. Metastatic calcification occurs in association with renal, pulmonary, and gastric calcification in hyperparathyroidism, chronic renal disease, extensive neoplastic destruction of bone, and hypervitaminosis D.

e. *Hypokalemic cardiomyopathy.* An abnormally low level of serum potassium may result in degenerative changes in myofibers followed by necrosis. Swelling and vacuolation are followed by karyolysis and by death of individual fibers accompanied by a lymphocytic response.

f. *Hemochromatosis.* Involvement of the myocardium is common and consists of the accumulation of hemosiderin within the myofibers. This begins as perinuclear deposition and spreads to involve much of the fiber. Rupture of the fiber may occur and is followed by focal scarring.

g. *Adipose infiltration* of the myocardium is seen particularly in obese individuals with excessive epicardial fat. The right ventricle is predominantly involved. Adipose tissue extends into the myocardium, infiltrating between fibers, which in extreme cases may undergo atrophy and extensive replacement (Fig. 49).

h. *Basophilic (mucinous) degeneration* of the myocardium is characterized by swelling of the myofibers due to the accumulation of basophilic material within them. The material is Schiff-positive and resists digestion with both diastase and hyaluronidase (Fig. 50).

5. Myocardial Disease in Familial Myopathies

5.1. FRIEDREICH'S ATAXIA. Myocardial degeneration without pericardial or valvular disease has frequently been found in

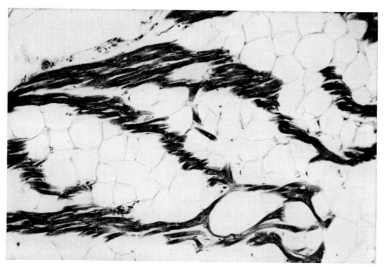

Figure 49. *Adipose infiltration of the myocardium in a strikingly obese patient. The right ventricular myofibers are separated and compressed by adipose tissue and are undergoing atrophy and replacement.*

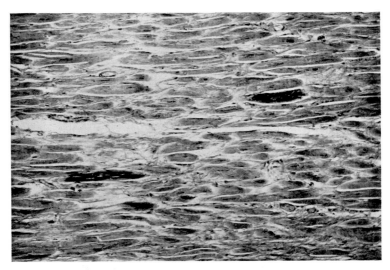

Figure 50. *Schiff-positive fibers in the myocardium in an instance of basophilic degeneration. This material stains blue in the standard hematoxylin and eosin stains. The material is resistant to digestion with both diastase and hyaluronidase.*

Friedreich's ataxia. It consists of cardiac enlargement with focal destruction of myofibers, replacement fibrosis, and hypertrophy of intact fibers. Focal interstitial myocarditis characterized by lymphocytic infiltration and occasionally polymorphonuclear leukocytes may be observed. The conduction system may be involved in this process. (Fig. 51).

5.2. PROGRESSIVE MUSCULAR DYSTROPHY. This disease may display myocardial degeneration characterized by a heart that may be diffusely yellow-brown with grossly visible patchy scarring. Microscopically, areas of fibrous replacement are seen. Residual atrophic myofibers are encompassed by the fibrous tissue. Other muscle fibers are hypertrophied.

5.3. FAMILIAL CARDIOMEGALY (HEREDITARY CARDIOVASCULAR DYSPLASIA). This entity, characterized by cardiac hypertrophy and myocardial fibrosis, displays a familial tendency frequently

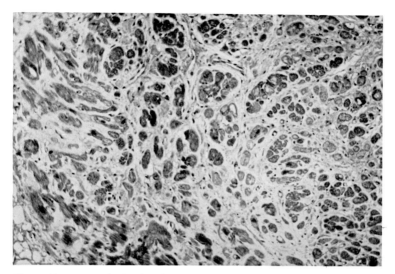

Figure 51. *Interstitial fibrosis and focal replacement of myofibers by fibrous tissue in a patient with Friedreich's ataxia. There is little or no inflammatory reaction in this area.*

traceable over several generations. Hypertrophy is not due to any of the generally accepted causes of this lesion. Microscopically, there is a transition from hypertrophied myofibers to disintegration with fibrous replacement. No associated inflammatory reaction is observed. Organizing ventricular mural thrombi may be seen.

6. Idiopathic Ventricular Hypertrophy

In persons dying after a period of congestive failure or, occasionally, dying suddenly, there is observed advanced ventricular hypertrophy and dilatation which is predominantly left-sided. No evidence of hypertension, significant coronary sclerosis, valvular disease, or myocardial inflammatory reaction can be found. Some of these persons may represent instances of familial cardiomegaly, but in many of them no familial

303

association can be identified. Microscopically, the primary alteration is myofiber hypertrophy. There may, in addition, be varying degrees of degenerative change in the muscle, including necrosis and patchy fibrosis. These latter alterations are predominantly subendocardial in location and are most frequently associated with mural thrombosis.

7. Atrophy of the Heart

This is characterized by diminution in the size of the muscle fibers. It is found in starvation, in association with wasting diseases, and in senility. It may be accompanied by an increase in paranuclear lipochrome pigment within the myofibers, imparting a dark mahogany color to the myocardium, the so-called *brown atrophy*.

25 / Other Diseases of the Pericardium

1. Acute Infectious Pericarditis

This type of pericarditis may be produced by bacterial or viral agents. Bacterial infection may be secondary to septicemia or regional (pulmonary, pleural, mediastinal) inflammation. In the former the hemolytic streptococcus is usually involved, and in the latter the pneumococcus.

Pericarditis may result from penetrating wounds of the chest, or injury to the esophagus by swallowed foreign bodies such as chicken bones or toothpicks. It may be secondary to descending infection originating in the neck. Sometimes it is associated with interstitial emphysema. Mixed bacterial infection is often found and the character of the pericarditis varies accordingly, but purulent types of exudate are commonly present.

Acute infectious pericarditis may be classified according to the nature of the exudate.

1.1. SEROFIBRINOUS. The pericardial fluid is increased and slightly turbid due to flakes of fibrin. Histologically, eosinophilic filaments of fibrin cover the mesothelial cells. The latter are often unusually well preserved, although swollen.

1.2. FIBRINOUS. The fibrin deposits are abundant and the pericardial surfaces may have a granular, dull yellowish-gray or a shaggy, ragged appearance. Histologically, the fibrin is

305

often compressed, its fibrillar characteristics lost, and solid irregular masses of deeply eosinophilic material are noted. Hyperemia is observed in the adjacent connective tissues.

1.3. SUPPURATIVE OR PURULENT. Disintegration of the leukocytes in the exudate is noted and leukocytic exudate predominates over fibrin.

1.4. ORGANIZING. A zone of young capillaries and fibroblasts, together with mononuclear leukocytes, forms a layer of granulation tissue at the junction between the exudate and the underlying pericardium. The newly formed blood vessels are often placed at right angles to the surface. The epicardial fat is usually relatively unaltered. As healing proceeds, new connective tissue is laid down. The exudate is resorbed and fibrous adhesions of varying extent may cause permanent union between the two pericardial layers. Occasionally, these may have the appearance of slender bands or synechiae.

2. Acute Nonbacterial Pericarditis

2.1. RHEUMATIC. This type almost always occurs in conjunction with the myocardial and endocardial lesions of rheumatic fever (**19**.4).

2.2. UREMIC. This type usually occurs terminally in chronic renal diseases in the form of a mild fibrinous inflammation. In more extreme lesions the exudate may be hemorrhagic and partly organized. The inflammatory reaction is nonspecific histologically, and the identification of the uremic origin of the lesion depends upon the demonstration of a renal lesion of sufficient extent to cause renal insufficiency or failure.

2.3. FOLLOWING MYOCARDIAL INFARCTION. The pericarditis is usually limited to the epicardial surface over the zone of infarction and is often fibrinous in character (**16**.2, 5). It may occasionally be diffuse. In extensive myocardial infarction a hemorrhagic exudate may cover the entire pericardium. Local or diffuse fibrous adhesions form on healing.

3. Acute Nonspecific Pericarditis (Benign, Idiopathic, Viral)

A benign form is recognized clinically (3.54). It occurs chiefly in young adults and is not associated with other demonstrable heart disease, but is commonly associated with pneumonitis and pleuritis. In infants, children, and young adults the Coxsackie B virus has been isolated from pericardial fluid and from stools. Death from this infection is rare in adults and children, but in newborn infants, in whom myocarditis usually also occurs, it is not uncommon. Although nonspecific pericarditis leaves no apparent injury to the pericardium, recurrences are common.

4. Granulomatous Pericarditis

4.1.   TUBERCULOUS. The pericardium may be involved by extension of pulmonary or pleural foci, from caseous mediastinal lymph nodes, or in the course of miliary tuberculosis. Tuberculous pericarditis may vary from a few scattered miliary tubercles to extensive pericardial thickening, caseation and obliteration of the pericardial sac by tuberculous granulation tissue. Large effusions may be encountered. Healing is often accompanied by calcification and may result in constrictive pericarditis.

Histologically, the lesion is similar to tuberculous lesions seen elsewhere. The tubercles consist of epithelioid cells and Langhans' giant cells, and may show central caseation. They may be miliary in size or they may be large and conglomerate. Often the tubercles are poorly defined and may be entirely lacking in later stages when tuberculous granulation covers the entire epicardial surface. Nevertheless, the tuberculous character can be recognized by the presence of large numbers

307

of epithelioid cells and occasional multinuclear giant cells as well as by foci of caseation in the granulation tissue. Identification of the nature of the lesion depends upon the demonstration of the organisms, since other forms of granulomatous lesions of the pericardium may simulate tuberculosis.

4.2. ACTINOMYCOSIS OF THE PERICARDIUM. This is the only fungal infection that involves the pericardium with any frequency. It usually develops as a result of direct extension from a pulmonary lesion. The pericardial lesions consist of multiple abscesses separated from each other by granulation tissue. As a rule, only localized areas of the pericardium are involved. Irregular sinus tracts leading into the adjacent mediastinum and into the myocardium occur frequently.

The histologic characteristics of the inflammatory reaction are not specific, and the presence of the ray fungus discloses the nature of the lesion. The latter may be distinguished from bacterial colonies by the presence of eosin-staining radiation or clubs at the periphery, and in gram stains by the presence of branching gram-positive filamentous structures within the mass.

5. *Chronic Pericarditis*

5.1. CONSTRICTIVE. This form is recognized by obliteration of the pericardial sac by thick fibrous tissue and calcific material resulting from previous inflammation. The nature of the original lesion is not always discoverable, nor is it always possible to correlate clinical manifestations of pericardial constriction with anatomic findings.

5.2. ADHESIVE. This is a form that does not cause constriction of the heart and may also be termed *nonconstrictive pericarditis*.

5.3. ASSOCIATED WITH SYSTEMIC DISEASE. Chronic pericarditis may be associated with such systemic diseases as lupus erythematosus, scleroderma, rheumatoid arthritis, and polyserositis or Pick's disease. Usually the recognition of the nature of such lesions depends upon the finding of characteristic lesions in other organs. In lupus erythematosus the fibrous tissue may have a gelatinous appearance and may stain metachromatically.

6. Parasitic Disease of the Pericardium

The most common lesion seen is echinococcus cyst of the pericardium.

7. Hemopericardium

This condition may be post-traumatic or may follow rupture of dissecting or saccular aortic aneurysms or of myocardial infarcts. It may also complicate organizing pericarditis of the various acute types. If the parietal layer is intact, free bleeding into the sac rapidly causes fatal tamponade of the heart. Epicardial hemorrhage is common in those conditions with hemorrhagic tendencies.

8. Hydropericardium

This condition may occur in any disease in which extracellular fluid is increased, as in congestive heart failure or renal failure. It is sometimes associated with mediastinal masses such as metastatic bronchogenic carcinoma or lymphoblastoma. In these conditions fluid accumulations may be due to local compression of veins or to direct invasion of the pericardium.

9. Adipose Changes in the Pericardium

The epicardial adipose tissue may be excessive in obese persons and may cover the entire epicardium. In some instances it may even extend into the right ventricular myocardium. The epicardial fat may undergo serous atrophy in wasting diseases. Such atrophic fat has a watery appearance, and, histologically, the interstices between the shrunken adipose cells are filled with an eosinophilic granular protein precipitate, indicating that watery fluid has replaced the fat. The fat cells become fusiform and several droplets instead of one may be identified in the cytoplasm.

10. Neoplasm of the Pericardium

Primary neoplasms of the pericardium are extremely rare, although tumors within the mediastinum, especially bronchogenic carcinoma, may invade the parietal pericardium directly. Tumors which metastasize to the pericardium as a group are most commonly derived from bronchogenic carcinoma, occasionally from carcinoma, and from the lymphomas. A secondary tumor in the myocardium, especially malignant melanoma, may extend into the pericardium. The latter is often but not always recognizable by the presence of melanin in the tumor cells.

26 / Diseases of the Conduction System

Physiologic evidence has established that certain structures in the heart constitute a specialized conduction system: the sino-atrial (S–A) node, the atrioventricular (A–V) node and bundle; the right and left bundle branches and the peripheral Purkinje fibers.

These structures have common characteristics which differentiate them from the myocardium: (1) a lesser number of myofibrils, and (2) a greater amount of elastic tissue.

Each subdivision of the system has further characteristics of its own. The bundle of His and the bundle branches possess a mesothelium-lined sheath surrounding a space, or bursa. The S–A node is characterized by the small diameter of most of its fibers, arranged in a plexiform manner, and by a relatively large number of collagenous fibers. The A–V node is a reticulated structure, and the diameter of its fibers is small. The A–V bundle displays small fibers arranged in a lobulated fashion. The left bundle branch is characterized by the large diameter of its fibers (Purkinje fibers) in its distal four-fifths, and by the sharp reticular component of its basement membrane. The right bundle branch is divided into three recognizable portions. The first has fibers with diameters smaller than, the second equal to, and the third larger than the fibers of the ventricular myocardium.

With advancing age, all of these structures show an increase in collagenous and elastic fibers, in fat, and in density of the reticular component of the basement membranes.

Normally, there are present in some hearts paraspecific fibers (of Mahaim) joining the distal part of the A–V node, the A–V bundle, and the left bundle branch to the ventricular myocardium. Neural ganglia are present around and in the periphery of the S–A node and around the A–V node. Nerves are present in the S–A and A–V nodes, in the A–V bundle, and in limited number in the beginning of the bundle branches.

In infants under 6 months of age, there may be occasional muscular connections between the atrial and ventricular myocardium.

Pathologic changes in the conduction system have been described in congenital, rheumatic, syphilitic, and atherosclerotic heart disease, and with myocarditis and tumors of the heart. Degenerative changes may be noted in various other diseases. The presence of morbidity does not necessarily mean that a functional conductive disturbance is also present.

1. Congenital Disease

Any part of the specialized conduction system may be abnormally placed or interrupted in continuity. In addition, accessory structures may be present, either accompanying or replacing the normal structures.

1.1. ABNORMALLY PLACED STRUCTURES. In mixed levocardia with atrial inversion, the bundle branches are similarly inverted. In common atrioventricular canal and persistent ostium primum, the A–V node is displaced posteriorly. The bundle of His may be longer than normal, and the left bundle branch may show abnormality (Fig. 52). In isolated ventricular septal defect, the conduction system is variably involved, depending upon the location of the defect. When the defect is in the pars membranacea and the anterior muscular ventricular septum, the A–V bundle usually lies on the posterior wall of the defect (Fig. 53). If there is considerable overriding of the aorta, the bundle may lie to the left of the summit of the

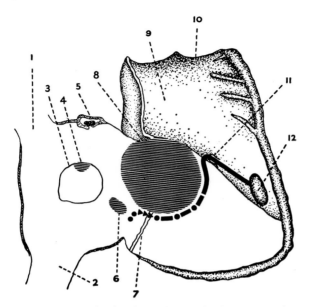

Figure 52. *Diagrammatic sketch of the conduction system in common atrioventricular orifice. Right atrial and ventricular view. Dots indicate A–V node; triangles, penetrating portion of the A–V bundle; dots and dashes, branching portion of the atrioventricular bundle; solid line, right bundle branch. (1) Superior vena cava; (2) inferior vena cava; (3) limbus; (4) patent foramen ovale; (5) cut edge of atrial appendage; (6) entry of coronary sinus; (7) base of tricuspid valve; (8) combined patency of atrial and ventricular septa; (9) conus; (10) base of pulmonary valve; (11) muscle of Lancisi; (12) cut edge of moderator band. (Courtesy of A.M.A. Arch. Path. 65: 174, 1958)*

posterior wall of the defect. In the tetralogy of Fallot, the A–V bundle is usually on the left side of the summit of the posterior wall of the defect (Fig. 54).

1.2. INTERRUPTION OF STRUCTURES. In isolated ventricular septal defect, in mixed levocardia with ventricular septal defect, in persistent ostium primum, and in some cases of otherwise normally formed hearts, there may be interruption of the junction of the A–V node and bundle or of the bundle itself to produce persistent complete or incomplete atrioventricular

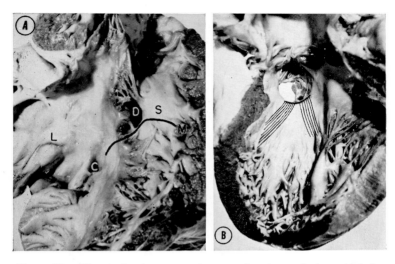

Figure 53. *The conduction system in one type of ventricular septal defect. A. Right atrial and right ventricular view. The course of the A–V node, bundle, and right bundle branch is diagrammatically depicted by the dark line. (C) Coronary sinus; (D) ventricular septal defect; (S) septal band of the crista; (M) moderator band; (L) limbus fossae ovalis. B. Left ventricular view. Dark line depicts the branching bundle. Fine lines depict the left bundle branch. (Courtesy of A.M.A. Arch. Path. 70:529, 1960)*

block. Similarly, occasional interruption of the right bundle branch may be present, or rarely the right bundle branch may be absent. Secondary fibrosis with interruption of the A–V node and bundle may occur.

1.3. ACCESSORY COMMUNICATIONS. An A–V nodal structure may occasionally be present in the anterior portion of the atrial septum near the aorta, and proceed to form a bundle which may be present in the anterior aspect of a ventricular septal defect. This nodal structure may take the place of the normal A–V node or it may accompany the normal A–V node. Accessory muscular atrioventricular communications may be present in the right and, less commonly, in the left atrioventricular ring. These may be present in congenital heart disease or in otherwise normally formed hearts.

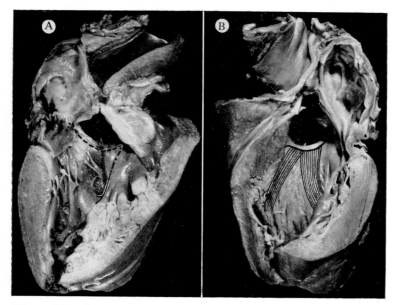

Figure 54. *The course of the conduction system in the tetralogy of Fallot. Atrial and ventricular septa of a specimen of the tetralogy of Fallot. The parietal walls of the heart have been removed to allow a better view of the ventricular septal defect.*

A. *Right ventricular view. Dots represent the A–V node; dashes, the bundle of His present on the left side of the septum; dots and dashes, the right bundle branch within the myocardium; solid line, the right bundle branch subendocardially.*

B. *Left ventricular view. Dense line represents the bundle of His and the beginning right bundle branch. Fine lines represent the anterior and posterior radiations of the left bundle branch. (Courtesy of A.M.A. Arch. Path. 67:572, 1959)*

2. Rheumatic Disease

The conduction system may be involved in both the acute and healed phases. In the acute phase the reaction is said to be as in the myocardium itself, consisting of myocarditis, fibrositis, and arteritis. This involves the A–V node and bundle to produce mild degrees of atrioventricular block. In the healed phase extension of a fibrous process from the aortic valve or the aortic leaflet of the mitral valve may produce partial or complete interruption of the A–V node or bundle, or more commonly the right or left bundle branches.

3. Syphilitic Disease

The A–V node, A–V bundle, and bundle branches may be involved in gummatous or nonspecific myocarditis. In addition, there may be extensions of lesions from the aortic valve or from the sinuses of Valsalva to produce fibrosis with or without interruption.

4. Atherosclerotic Disease

Narrowing of the ostial region of the right main coronary artery, before the origin of the ramus ostii cavae superioris, may produce pathologic change in the S–A and A–V nodes, the A–V bundle, and the bundle branches. If narrowing of the right main coronary artery is distal to the origin of the ramus, the S–A node may be spared. Narrowing of the posterior descending coronary artery may produce changes in the posterior radiation of the left bundle branch. Narrowing of the anterior descending coronary artery before the origin of the second perforating branch may produce changes in the right bundle branch and anterior radiation of the left bundle branch. Narrowing of the anterior descending coronary artery distal to the above point may produce changes in the anterior radiation of the left bundle branch alone. It is possible to have narrowing of only the ramus septi fibrosi supplying the A–V node and bundle. The reduced arterial lumina may be associated with severe degeneration, necrosis (Fig. 55), and fibrosis (Fig. 56) of any of the above structures. This may or may not be associated with functional changes such as atrioventricular or bundle-branch block.

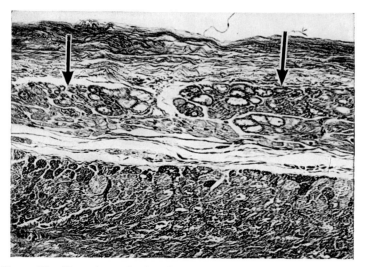

Figure 55. Necrosis of the left bundle branch (upper part) in atherosclerotic heart disease. Hematoxylin-eosin stain. Arrows point to the left
bundle branch. (× 150)

5. Myocarditis

The conduction system may be involved in myocarditis of
viral (Fig. 57) or pharmacologic origin (sulfonamides), and in
myocarditis secondary to diphtheria, scarlet fever, pneumonia,
influenza, typhus, tuberculosis, mumps, measles, German measles, malaria, and amebic hepatitis. Usually involvement is
progressively more severe distally. The most severe myocarditis, however, can occur in any part of the conduction
system. It is not known whether the conduction system can be
involved without also involving the rest of the myocardium.

6. Neoplasms

A lymphangio-endothelioma, a primary tumor of the A–V
node, may produce atrioventricular block. Any tumor, such as
myxoma, fibroma, or angioma, may compress part of the conduction system with resultant functional disturbance.

317

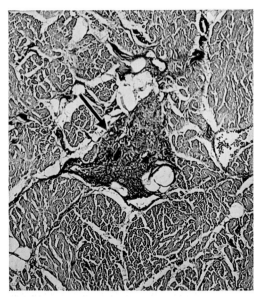

Figure 56. *Fibrosis and elastosis of the right bundle branch (second portion) in atherosclerotic heart disease. Weigert–van Gieson stain. Arrow points to the right bundle branch. (× 80)*

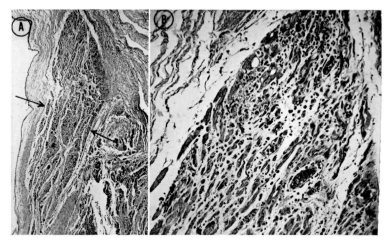

Figure 57. *Acute inflammation involving the A–V bundle and the beginning of the left bundle branch in acute myocarditis. Arrows point to the bundle. A. Hematoxylin-eosin stain (× 30). B. Part of the area depicted in A. (× 100) (Courtesy of A.M.A. Arch. Path. 60:502, 1955)*

318

7. Other Involvement of the Conduction System

Fibrosis, with or without *calcification,* of the mitral annulus with involvement of the central fibrous body and the pars membranacea may occur unrelated to coronary disease. Calcification of the base of the aorta may spread to the pars membranacea and produce fibrosis. In either instance there may be involvement of the A–V node, the A–V bundle, and the left bundle branch. *Adipose infiltration* may involve the approaches to the A–V node. Such change may also be present in the A–V node itself, in the A–V bundle, and in the bundle branches. *Fatty degeneration* may occur in toxic and inflammatory states and be of functional import. *Hemorrhage and leukemic infiltration* are usually functionally unimportant. Complete atrioventricular block in *hemochromatosis* has been ascribed to pigmentary changes in the conduction system. It is not known whether the conductive changes in azotemia are related to morbidity in the conduction system or to chemical abnormalities exclusively.

Part IV | The Roentgenologic Diagnosis

27 / Criteria for Roentgenologic Techniques

Roentgenologic examination of the heart enables the examiner to observe the contour, size, and position of the heart and of its individual chambers. The usual methods of roentgenologic examination are: (1) roentgenoscopy (fluoroscopy), (2) teleroentgenography, and (3) orthodiagraphy. Special methods include: (4) roentgenkymography, (5) angiocardiography, and (6) angiography.

Generally speaking, radiation hazards are slight but nevertheless must be considered in each instance against the anticipated gains achieved through the most precise diagnosis. Suitable shielding devices must protect the observers as well as the patient.

1. Roentgenoscopy (Fluoroscopy)

Roentgenoscopy is the direct examination of the patient behind the fluorescent screen. The closeness of the heart to the target of the roentgen tube results in an exaggeration of its size. Thus this technique is unsatisfactory for measurements. To determine the size of the cardiac shadow more exactly, teleroentgenography or orthodiagraphy must be used.

The cardiac contour should be studied fluoroscopically not only in the postero-anterior position but also in various degrees of rotation so that depth may be estimated. The patient should be turned sufficiently so that the border to be examined appears clear of the shadow of the vertebrae. The amount of rotation needed to effect this is usually about 50 degrees to the right or left but may be more or less, depending upon whether the chest is of the hypersthenic or hyposthenic type, upon the presence of emphysema, scoliosis, or kyphosis, and upon the degree of enlargement of the cardiac chambers. Abduction of the arms or elevation of the scapula may be used to clear the field of vision. The standard positions are:

Postero-anterior (P–A): patient facing the screen (Fig. 1, p. 335).

Right anterior oblique (RAO): patient facing the screen but turned so that the right shoulder is toward the screen (Fig. 2, p. 335).

Left anterior oblique (LAO): patient facing the screen but turned so that the left shoulder is toward the screen (Fig. 3, p. 335).

The normal cardiac configuration may be altered by displacement of the heart or by enlargement of one or more of its chambers. It is possible to observe the outline of the individual chambers of the heart. In the oblique positions the barium-filled esophagus and the bifurcation of the trachea serve as aids in determining enlargement, particularly of the left atrium. These positions reveal the character and timing of the pulsations of the individual chambers and of the great vessels, and the localization of the interventricular septum and groove. The oblique views may reveal enlargement of one or more chambers when the usual postero-anterior view shows a normal configuration.

Considerable experience is needed to judge the range of normal variation. The best procedure is to combine roentgenoscopic examination of the individual cardiac chambers with teleroentgenograms, including oblique views, although orthodiagrams may serve as well. The value of permanent records for purposes of comparison is obvious.

2. Teleroentgenography

Teleroentgenography is the technique of taking thoracic roentgenograms with the tube at a standard distance, usually 2 meters, from the film. At such a distance the divergent rays which delineate the borders of the cardiac shadow exaggerate its size from 4 to 12 percent. For the P–A view, the patient's sternum is in contact with the film cassette. The target of the roentgen tube is centered at the level of the sixth thoracic vertebra. Synchronization of the exposure with systole or diastole may at times make a significant difference, but the most important condition in the determination of heart size is that the exposure must be made with the diaphragm in a standard position. Exposures should be made *at the end of a normal inspiration;* otherwise standards cannot be applied.

Roentgenograms taken in the right and left oblique positions are desirable and are recommended as supplements to the P–A view and the roentgenoscopic findings. Certainly detail in the lungs is better portrayed on films than on fluoroscopy. Lateral views have the value of being taken in a position that is reproducible for serial records, but they do not give as much information about the size and shape of the different cardiac chambers and of the aorta as do the oblique views.

For measurement of the P–A view, a vertical line is drawn approximately through the spinous processes of the lower dorsal vertebrae. The perpendiculars from this line to the most distant point of the right and left cardiac borders are added together to make the transverse diameter. The ratio between the transverse diameter of the heart and the transverse diameter of the thorax (the cardiothoracic ratio) is an unreliable index of cardiac enlargement and should not be used as such.

Tables of normal cardiac measurements and their variation within physiologic limits as affected by height, weight, and age are available (Tables I and II, pp. 326–328). The disadvantage of prediction formulas applied to teleroentgenography and to orthodiagraphy is that they do not always give a correct separation between hearts of normal and of abnormal size. Measurements smaller than the predicted normal are sometimes obtained from hearts with evident enlargement of individual chambers. Conversely, a value 10 percent greater

Table 1. Prediction Table for Average Normal Transverse Diameters of the Heart Silhouette Based on the Teleroentgenogram*

T.D. of Heart, mm	HEIGHT																		
	5'0"	1"	2"	3"	4"	5"	6"	7"	8"	9"	10"	11"	6'0"	1"	2"	3"	4"	5"	6"
100	83	85	86	87	89	90	92	95	100										
101	85	86	88	89	91	92	93	97	102										
102	87	88	90	91	92	94	95	99											
103	88	90	92	93	94	96	97	99											
104	90	92	93	95	96	98	99	101											
105	92	93	95	96	98	99	101	103	104	106									
106	94	95	97	98	100	101	103	105	106	108									
107	95	97	99	100	102	103	105	107	108	110	111								
108	97	99	100	102	104	105	107	109	110	112	113								
109	99	101	102	104	106	107	109	111	112	114	115	117							
110	101	102	104	106	108	109	111	113	114	116	118	119	121						
111	103	104	106	108	109	111	113	115	116	118	120	121	123	125					
112	105	106	108	110	111	113	115	117	118	120	122	124	125	127	129				
113	106	108	110	112	113	115	117	119	121	123	124	126	128	129	131	133			
114	108	110	112	114	115	117	119	121	123	125	126	128	130	132	133	135	137		
115	110	112	114	116	117	119	121	123	125	127	129	130	132	134	136	138	140	141	
116	112	114	116	118	120	121	123	125	127	129	131	133	134	136	138	140	142	144	146
117	114	116	118	120	122	124	125	127	129	131	133	135	137	139	141	143	144	146	148
118	116	118	120	122	124	126	128	129	131	133	135	137	139	141	143	145	147	149	151
119	118	120	122	124	126	128	130	132	134	136	138	140	142	143	145	147	149	151	153
120	120	122	124	126	128	130	132	134	136	138	140	142	144	146	148	150	152	154	156
121	122	124	126	128	130	132	134	136	138	140	142	144	146	148	150	152	154	156	159
122	124	126	128	130	132	134	136	138	140	143	145	147	149	151	153	155	157	159	161
123	126	128	130	132	134	136	139	141	143	145	147	149	151	153	155	157	160	162	164
124	128	130	132	134	137	139	141	143	145	147	149	152	154	156	158	160	162	164	166
125	130	132	134	137	139	141	143	145	147	150	152	154	156	158	160	163	165	167	169
126	132	134	137	139	141	143	145	148	150	152	154	156	159	161	163	165	167	170	172
127	134	137	139	141	143	146	148	150	152	154	157	159	161	163	166	168	170	172	175
128	136	139	141	143	146	148	150	152	155	157	159	161	164	166	168	171	173	175	177
129	139	141	143	146	148	150	152	155	157	159	162	164	166	169	171	173	176	178	180

	130	131	132	133	134	135	136	137	138	139	140	141	142	143	144	145	146	147	148	149	150	151	152	153	154	155	156	157	158	159	160	161	162	163	164
130	141	143	145	147	150	152	154	156	159	161	163	166	168	170	173	175	178	180	182	185	187	190	192	195	198	200									
131	143	145	148	150	152	155	157	159	162	164	166	168	171	173	176	178	181	183	185	188	190	193	196	198	201	203	206								
132	145	148	150	152	155	157	160	162	164	167	169	171	174	176	179	181	184	186	189	191	193	196	199	201	204	206	209								
133	147	150	152	155	157	159	161	164	167	169	172	174	177	179	182	184	187	189	192	195	198	200	202	205	208	211	213	216							
134	150	152	155	157	160	162	164	166	169	172	173	176	178	181	184	187	189	192	194	198	201	204	206	209	213	216	219	221	224						
135	152	154	156	159	161	163	166	168	170	173	175	178	180	182	185	187	190	192	195	198	200	203	206	209	212	215	219	222	225	228					
136	154	157	159	161	164	166	168	171	173	176	179	181	183	186	189	190	193	195	198	201	203	206	209	212	215	218	222	225	228	231					
137	156	159	161	164	167	168	171	174	176	179	181	183	186	189	192	193	195	198	201	204	207	210	213	216	219	222	225	228	231	234					
138	159	161	164	167	169	170	173	176	179	182	185	188	191	194	196	196	198	201	204	207	210	213	216	219	222	225	228	231	234	237					
139	161	164	166	169	173	173	176	178	181	185	188	191	194	196	199	199	201	204	207	210	213	216	219	222	225	229	231	234	237	240					
140	163	166	168	170	173	175	178	180	182	185	187	190	192	195	198	201	204	207	210	213	216	219	222	225	228	231	234	237	240	243					
141	166	168	171	173	176	178	180	183	185	188	190	193	196	199	201	204	207	210	212	215	218	221	224	227	230	233	236	240	243	247					
142	168	171	174	176	178	180	183	185	188	191	192	196	199	202	204	207	210	213	216	219	221	224	227	230	233	236	239	243	246	250					
143	170	173	176	179	182	182	185	188	192	195	195	199	202	205	207	210	213	216	219	222	224	227	230	234	237	240	243	246	249	253					
144	173	176	178	181	185	185	188	191	195	198	198	201	204	207	210	213	216	219	222	225	227	230	234	237	240	243	246	249	253	257					
145	175	178	180	181	184	187	189	192	196	199	198	201	204	207	210	213	216	219	222	225	228	231	234	237	240	243	247	250	253	257	260				
146	178	180	183	183	186	189	192	195	198	201	201	204	207	210	213	216	219	222	225	228	231	234	237	241	244	247	250	254	257	260	264				
147	180	183	185	186	189	192	195	198	201	204	204	207	210	213	216	219	222	225	228	231	234	237	240	244	247	250	253	257	260	263	267				
148	182	185	188	189	192	195	198	201	204	207	207	210	213	216	219	222	225	228	231	234	237	240	243	247	250	253	256	260	263	267	270				
149	185	188	191	192	195	198	201	204	206	210	210	213	216	219	222	225	228	231	234	237	240	243	246	250	253	256	260	263	267	270	274				
150	187	190	193	196	198	200	203	206	209	212	212	215	219	222	225	228	231	234	237	240	243	247	250	253	257	260	263	266	270	274	277				
151	190	193	196	199	201	203	206	209	212	215	215	218	222	225	228	231	234	237	241	244	247	250	254	257	260	264	266	270	273	277	281				
152	192	196	199	202	204	206	209	212	215	218	218	221	224	228	231	234	237	241	244	247	250	253	257	260	263	267	270	273	277	280	284				
153	195	198	201	204	207	209	212	215	218	221	221	224	227	231	234	237	240	244	247	250	253	256	260	263	267	270	273	277	280	284	288				
154	198	201	204	207	210	212	215	219	221	224	224	227	230	234	237	240	244	247	250	253	256	260	263	267	270	274	277	280	284	287	291				
155	200	203	206	209	213	215	218	221	224	227	227	230	233	237	240	243	247	250	253	256	259	263	266	270	273	277									
156		206	209	212	216	218	222	225	228	231	230	233	236	240	243	247	250	253	257	260	263	266	270	273	277	281									
157					219	221	224	228	231	234	233	236	239	243	246	250	253	257	260	263	267	270	273	277	280	284									
158						224	227	231	234	237	236	239	243	246	249	253	256	260	263	267	270	273	277	280	284	288									
159						229	230	234	237	240	239	242	246	249	253	256	260	263	267	270	274	277	280	284	287	291									
160													245	249	252	256	259	263	266	270	274	277	280	284	287										
161															255	259	263	266	270	273	277	281													
162																262	266	270	273	277	280	284													
163																	269	273	276	280	284	288													
164																		276	280	284	287	291													

* Refer to paper entitled "A Study of the Transverse Diameter of the Heart Silhouette with Prediction Table Based on the Teleroentgenogram" presented to the Association of Life Insurance Medical Directors of America by Dr. Harry E. Ungerleider of the Equitable Life Assurance Society and Dr. Charles P. Clark of the Mutual Life Insurance Company. From Am. Heart J. 17:92, 1939, by permission of The C. V. Mosby Company.

Table II. *Prediction Table for Average Normal Orthodia-graphic Measurements of the Transverse Diameter of the Heart.**†

Predicted T–D = + 0.1094 × A − 0.1941 × H + 0.8179 × W + 95.8625

	I				II		
Stature		Area, Sq Cm	Transverse Diameter, Mm	Weight		Area, Sq Cm	Transverse Diameter, Mm
Cm	Inches			Kg	Pounds		
150	59	66.7	66.74	50	110	17.00	40.90
151		67.57	66.55	51	112.2	17.34	41.71
152	60	68.44	66.36	52	114.4	17.68	42.53
153		69.31	66.16	53	116.6	18.02	43.35
154		70.18	65.97	54	118.8	18.36	44.17
155	61	71.05	65.77	55	121	18.70	44.98
156		71.92	65.58	56	123.2	19.04	45.80
157		72.79	65.39	57	125.4	19.38	46.62
158	62	73.66	65.19	58	127.6	19.72	47.44
159		74.53	65.00	59	129.8	20.06	48.26
160	63	75.40	64.80	60	132	20.40	49.07
161		76.27	64.61	61	134.2	20.74	49.89
162		77.14	64.42	62	136.4	21.08	50.71
163	64	78.01	64.22	63	138.6	21.42	51.53
164		78.88	64.03	64	140.8	21.76	52.35
165	65	79.75	63.83	65	143	22.10	53.16
166		80.62	63.64	66	145.2	22.44	53.98
167		81.49	63.45	67	147.4	22.78	54.80
168	66	82.36	63.25	68	149.6	23.12	55.62
169		83.23	63.06	69	151.8	23.46	56.44
170	67	84.10	62.86	70	154	23.80	57.25
171		84.97	62.67	71	156.2	24.14	58.07
172		85.84	62.47	72	158.4	24.48	58.89
173	68	86.71	62.28	73	160.6	24.82	59.71
174		87.58	62.09	74	162.8	25.16	60.52
175	69	88.45	61.89	75	165	25.50	61.34
176		89.32	61.70	76	167.2	25.84	62.16
177		90.19	61.50	77	169.4	26.18	62.98
178	70	91.06	61.31	78	171.6	26.52	63.80
179		91.93	61.12	79	173.8	26.86	64.61
180	71	92.80	60.92	80	176	27.20	65.43
181		93.67	60.73	81	178.2	27.54	66.25
182		94.54	60.53	82	180.4	27.88	67.07
183	72	95.41	60.34	83	182.6	28.22	67.89
184		96.28	60.15	84	184.8	28.56	68.70
185	73	97.15	59.95	85	187	28.90	69.52
186		98.02	59.76	86	189.2	29.24	70.34
187		98.89	59.56	87	191.4	29.58	71.16
188	74	99.76	59.37	88	193.6	29.92	71.98
189		100.63	59.18	89	195.8	30.26	72.79
190		101.50	58.98	90	198	30.60	73.61
191	75	102.37	58.79	91	200.2	30.94	74.43
192		103.24	58.59	92	202.4	31.28	75.25
193	76	104.11	58.40	93	204.6	31.62	76.06
194		104.98	58.21	94	206.8	31.96	76.88
195		105.85	58.01	95	209	32.30	77.70
196	77	106.72	57.82	96	211.2	32.64	78.52
197		107.59	57.62	97	213.4	32.98	79.34
198	78	108.46	57.43	98	215.6	33.32	80.15
199		109.39	57.23	99	217.8	33.66	80.97
200	79	110.20	57.04	100	220	34.00	81.79

NOTE: To find normal transverse diameter for a given individual, add T–D figure for stature to T–D figure for weight and to this total add 1 than the prediction figure may occasionally be obtained from a normal heart. This lessens the usefulness of the tables in the borderline group, in which a decisive answer would be most desirable. In spite of this fact, prediction formulas are the best available method for differentiating normal from abnormal. Borderline examples will be encountered in which neither measurement by any method nor by fluoroscopic study of the contours will determine whether enlargement is present or not.

Measurements are used chiefly for comparison of serial roentgenograms in individual cases. In advanced cardiac enlargement, the exact estimation of size is useful in following progression or regression of disease. It may, however, be more important to ascertain which chambers participate in the enlargement and to what degree. Such information cannot be obtained easily by measurement and is probably best obtained by fluoroscopy.

3. Orthodiagraphy

Orthodiagraphy utilizes central parallel rays of the fluoroscope to outline the cardiac contour, thereby enabling the examiner to make a drawing closely approximating in size and shape the outline of the heart in the plane under observation. The outlines of the diaphragm and of the median line are similarly drawn. All are made during quiet or shallow respiration. The lower contour of the heart and the upper contour at the base should not be attempted, as the opacity of the liver and of the vertebrae interferes. To determine the presence of enlargement, the transverse diameter or the surface area is compared with prediction formulas based upon age, height, and weight (Table II). The orthodiagraphic method is subject to only

---

mm for every decade of age; e.g., height, 6 feet; weight, 187 pounds; age, 50 = 134.86 mm T–D or 60.34 + 69.52 + 5.

* From P. C. Hodges and J. A. E. Eyster: *Arch. Int. Med.* 37:711–713, 1926.

† The figures of this table are valid for orthodiagrams and for male subjects. The hearts of female subjects of same stature, weight, and age are slightly smaller in size. Bainton has suggested subtracting 0.8 cm for T–D of female.

slight error in skilled hands. The interpretation of the tracing is subject to the same difficulties as those encountered in tele-roentgenography.

4. Roentgenkymography

Roentgenkymography is a technique by which pulsations of the borders of the heart are registered graphically. This is accomplished by means of roentgen rays directed at a moving film in contact with a stationary grid having vertical or horizontal slits (conventional method), or by the use of a photoelectric cell, amplification, and appropriate shielding and recording devices (roentgenelectrokymography).

5. Angiocardiography

Angiocardiography is the method of visualizing radiographically the cardiac chambers and great vessels by the rapid intravenous injection of a radiopaque substance (*general or intravenous angiocardiography*).

When the radiopaque contrast substance is injected through a needle or catheter into one of the heart chambers or into one of the great vessels, regional opacification takes place (*selective angiocardiography*).

Serial roentgenograms are taken at rapid or appropriate intervals. In cineangiocardiography the whole opacifying process is recorded on rapidly moving film.

6. Angiography

Angiography is the term used for the same method when applied to the visualization of arteries (arteriography) or veins (venography). Depending upon the vessel or vascular system studied and the details of injection, angiography may, for example, be specified as aortography, renal arteriography, cerebral arteriography, peripheral arteriography, splenography.

28 / Nomenclature for the Roentgenologic Diagnosis

1. NORMAL HEART
    1.1. Horizontal heart
    1.2. Vertical heart
    1.3. Oblique or globular heart

2. LEFT VENTRICLE
    2.1. Enlargement in length, outflow tract
    2.2. Enlargement in width and length, inflow tract
    2.3. Concentric hypertrophy
    2.4. Localized ventricular bulge (ventricular aneurysm)
    2.5. Localized impairment of contraction

3. RIGHT VENTRICLE
    3.1. Enlargement in length, outflow tract
    3.2. Rotation of the heart on its vertical axis
    3.3. Enlargement in width and depth, inflow tract

4. LEFT ATRIUM
    4.1. Posterior or horizontal enlargement
    4.2. Vertical or upward enlargement
    4.3. Enlargement toward the right
    4.4. Enlargement toward the left

5. RIGHT ATRIUM
    5.1. Enlargement of the auricle (auricular appendix)
    5.2. Enlargement posteriorly

6. SYMMETRICAL CARDIAC ENLARGEMENT

7. DISPLACEMENT OF THE HEART

8. CALCIFICATION, INTRACARDIAC
    8.1. Valvular
    8.2. Annuli fibrosi
    8.3. Coronary arteries
    8.4. Myocardium
    8.5. Endocardium

9. PERICARDIUM
    9.1. Effusion
    9.2. Adhesions
    9.3. Constriction
    9.4. Calcification
    9.5. Cysts

10. AORTA
    10.1. Elongation and dilatation
    10.2. Calcification
    10.3. Hypoplasia
    10.4. Right aortic arch
    10.5. Coarctation

11. ANEURYSM OF THE AORTA
    11.1. Saccular
    11.2. Fusiform
    11.3. Dissecting hematoma

12. WIDENING OF THE BRACHIOCEPHALIC ARTERIES

13. DILATATION OF THE SUPERIOR VENA CAVA

14. PULMONARY ARTERY
    14.1. Dilatation of the trunk and primary branches

14.2. Dilatation of the secondary or hilar vessels
14.3. Narrowing of the pulmonary artery and its
branches

15. PULMONARY FIELDS
15.1. Hilar dilatation
15.2. Pulmonary stasis: chronic, acute, localized, diffuse
15.3. Pleural involvement

29 / Criteria for the Roentgenologic Diagnosis

1. Normal Heart

The outline of the shadow of the heart can be divided into portions or curves, each due to an individual heart chamber or to a great vessel.

In the postero-anterior (P–A) view (Figs. 1, 7, 8) on the right side, the curve of the right atrium is immediately above the diaphragm, and above this is the curve formed by the ascending aorta. An indentation frequently separates the two. On deep inspiration, a small triangular shadow sometimes may be seen between the diaphragm and the lower contour of the right atrium. It is due to the inferior vena cava and is not to be mistaken for pleuropericardial adhesions. Above the ascending aortic arch, the less dense, vertical shadow of the superior vena cava often is seen extending parallel with and close to the spine.

Three curves are noted on the left side. Highest is the convex knob of the aortic arch as it turns backward and to the left. Immediately below this is the outline of the pulmonary artery, normally straight, concave or slightly convex, often called the pulmonary artery segment. Occasionally the left auricle may occupy a position between the pulmonary artery above and the left ventricle below. When normal, it rarely can be recognized except by electrokymography. Lowest on this border, between the pulmonary artery above and the diaphragm below, is the lateral contour of the left ventricle.

The direction of the systolic pulsation of the left border

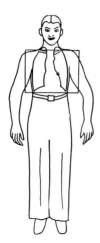

Figure 1. *Postero-anterior (P–A) position. Fluoroscopic screen against the anterior chest wall.*

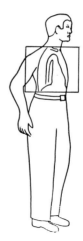

Figure 2. *Right anterior oblique (RAO) position. Arms may be abducted, or elevated and held on top of the head.*

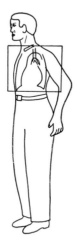

Figure 3. *Left anterior oblique (LAO) position.*

335

of the cardiac shadow is inward over the left ventricle, and outward and upward over the pulmonary artery segment. *A point or area of adjacent opposite pulsations can thus be identified.* The lower border of the heart, even when viewed in deep inspiration, cannot ordinarily be seen below the dome of the left side of the diaphragm. In the cardiodiaphragmatic angle a triangular shadow less dense than the left ventricle or the diaphragm is frequently seen and is due to epicardial fat (Fig. 4).

In the right anterior oblique (RAO) position (Figs. 2, 5), immediately above the diaphragm, the anterior border of the cardiac shadow is formed by the anterior portion of the left or right ventricle, depending upon the degree of rotation. Above this is the shadow of the pulmonary artery, and highest is that of the ascending aorta. The latter is continuous above with a foreshortened view of the transverse portion of the aortic arch. The descending limb of the aorta often may be noted between the posterior surface of the heart and the spinal column, particularly during inspiration and in patients with kyphosis or emphysema. The posterior contour of the heart is formed below by the inferior vena cava and a portion of the right atrium, and above this by the left atrium.

The column of air in the trachea and in the right bronchus can be seen between the shadow of the descending portion of the arch of the aorta and the outline of the upper portion of the heart. The esophagus lies between the anterior surface of the descending aorta and the posterior surface of the heart. When filled with a thick barium paste, its course is seen to be essentially vertical, forming a shallow curve posteriorly. The continuity of its anterior contour is broken above by the normal indentations of the transverse part of the aorta, below this by the right bronchus, and finally by the constriction of the diaphragm. Filling of the esophagus with barium paste should be a part of a routine roentgenoscopic examination.

In the left anterior oblique (LAO) position (Figs. 3, 6), the anterior outline is formed from below and upward by the right ventricle, the right atrium and its auricle, and the as-

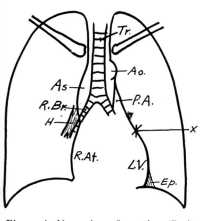

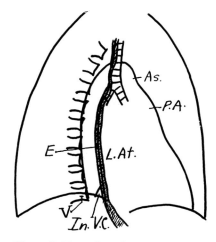

Figure 4. *Normal configuration (P–A).*
X, point of opposite pulsations; Tr.,
trachea; R.Br., right bronchus; As.,
ascending aorta; H., hilar (secondary)
branch of the pulmonary artery; Ao.,
aortic knob; P.A., pulmonary artery;
Ep., epicardial fat; L.V., left ventricle;
R.At., right atrium.

Figure 5. *Normal configuration (RAO).*
E., esophagus; V., vertebral column;
In.V.C., inferior vena cava; L.At., left
atrium; As., ascending aorta; P.A.,
pulmonary artery.

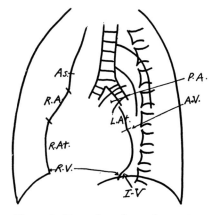

Figure 6. *Normal configuration (LAO).*
As., ascending aorta; R.A., right auri-
cle; R.At., right atrium; R.V., right
ventricle; P.A., pulmonary artery;
L.At., left atrium; A–V., atrioven-
tricular groove; I–V., interventricular
groove.

337

cending aorta. The contour of the right ventricle and the right atrium is vertical; the right auricle may slope obliquely toward the aorta. The ascending limb of the aortic arch is seen to curve upward and posteriorly, and is continuous with the transverse portion of the arch. The latter curves downward into the descending limb of the arch and the thoracic aorta, both of which partly overlap the shadow of the spinal column. The posterior outline of the heart is formed by the left ventricle below and the left atrium above. A shallow indentation, the atrioventricular groove, may separate the two. The pulsations of the left ventricle are of greater amplitude. At or near the junction of the left ventricle with the diaphragm, an indentation may be observed which is clearest in systole during deep inspiration. This is due to the interventricular groove and has a movement of its own, the direction of which is independent of the chambers to either side of it.

The bifurcation of the trachea is seen within and below the density of the aortic arch. The right bronchus appears foreshortened, whereas the course of the left bronchus is more vertical than horizontal and forms an interior angle of less than 45 degrees with the line of the trachea, a magnitude which varies with the degree of rotation. The left branch of the pulmonary artery occasionally may be seen as a shadow, less dense and smaller than the aorta, arching over the left bronchus. It originates arteriorly in a density within the heart shadow which represents the bifurcation of the trunk of the pulmonary artery. The brachiocephalic vessels mounted on top of the aortic arch form the shadow anterior to the trachea.

The appearance of the cardiac shadow in all views is greatly influenced by the level of the diaphragm.

1.1. HORIZONTAL HEART. In hypersthenic individuals the heart lies horizontally on an elevated diaphragm, the anatomic apex of the heart is displaced to the left, and the lower portion of the left border is often obscured by the diaphragm (Fig. 7A). Relatively more of the contour of the left ventricle and less of the pulmonary artery segment can be seen.

338

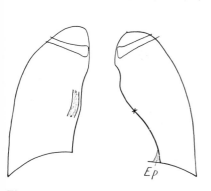

Figure 7A. *Horizontal heart. X, point of adjacent opposite pulsations; Ep., epicardial fat.*

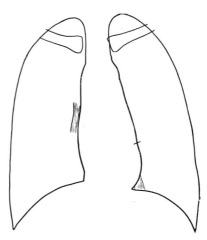

Figure 7B. *Vertical heart.*

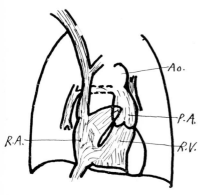

Figure 8A. *Angiocardiogram in the P–A position. Right-sided structures are opacified. R.A., right atrium; Ao., aorta; P.A., pulmonary artery; R.V., right ventricle.*

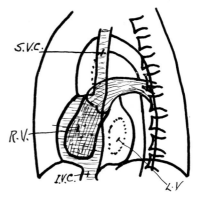

Figure 8B. *Angiocardiogram in the LAO position. S.V.C., superior vena cava; I.V.C., inferior vena cava; L.V., left ventricle (not opacified); R.V., right ventricle.*

339

1.2. VERTICAL HEART.   In asthenic individuals the position of the heart is vertical; it appears long and narrow (Fig. 7B). In extreme forms it appears suspended and is drop-shaped or pear-shaped (hypoplastic). The pulmonary artery forms the larger part of the left contour below the aortic knob. In the RAO position the pulmonary artery is prominent either in length or in degree of convexity, so that in asthenic individuals this appearance does not necessarily indicate enlargement of the right ventricular outflow tract.

1.3. OBLIQUE OR GLOBULAR HEART.   Between the extremes of horizontal and vertical hearts is the oblique position seen in sthenic individuals. The relative length of the pulmonary artery contour and that of the left ventricle may be more or less equal.

In infants the shape of the heart is usually globular. It is centrally located and its borders reach about an equal distance to the left and to the right.

2. Left Ventricle

Anatomically and functionally the left ventricle can be subdivided into two portions, the outflow and inflow tracts.

2.1. THE OUTFLOW TRACT.   This extends from the apex to the aortic valve and is the first portion of the left ventricle to become enlarged. This enlargement is manifested roentgenologically by elongation of the left ventricular segment below the point of opposite pulsation. Elongation may be recognized within the left diaphragmatic density, or within accumulations of gas in the stomach or colon, or by an increase in the convexity of the upper portion of the left ventricle immediately below the point of opposite pulsation (Fig. 10). Differentiation from a horizontally placed normal heart is accomplished by observing the effect of deep inspiration; in a normal heart the unusual convexity should disappear.

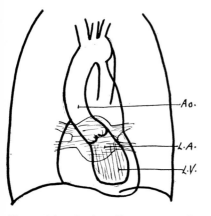

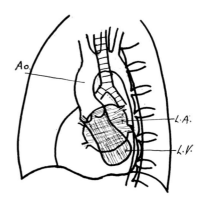

Figure 9A. *Angiocardiogram of the left heart chambers, P–A position. L.A., left atrium; Ao., aorta; L.V., left ventricle.*

Figure 9B. *Same in the LAO position.*

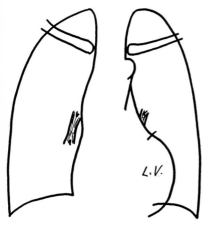

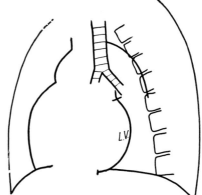

Figure 10. *Enlargement of the left ventricle (L.V.) by elongation and rounding of the upper left ventricular contour and by extension of the left ventricular density below the diaphragm.*

Figure 11. *Enlargement of the inflow tract of the left ventricle. Early elongation of this portion is shown by increased rounding in the LAO position. The interventricular groove is not seen because it is displaced downward and anteriorly.*

341

2.2. THE INFLOW TRACT. This extends from the mitral valve to the apex of the left ventricle. Its enlargement occurs later than that of the outflow tract. The enlargement of the inflow tract is recognized roentgenologically by an increase in length and width of the left ventricular segment when viewed in the LAO position (Fig. 11). It changes from a shallow curve to a longer and more convex segment and bulges posteriorly. The interventricular groove is displaced downward into the density of the infradiaphragmatic structures and cannot be identified.

With marked enlargement when viewed in the P–A position, the left ventricular border is displaced toward the left lateral chest wall. The rounding occupies the lower two-thirds or more of the left contour and may extend below the dome of the diaphragm. In the LAO position the left ventricular contour extends more posteriorly (Fig. 14), so that with the usual rotation it will overlap the shadow of the spine. The diagnosis of left ventricular enlargement should ordinarily be possible before this stage is reached.

2.3. CONCENTRIC HYPERTROPHY. When viewed in the P–A position, this will appear as a rounding of the left ventricular contour without elongation of that segment.

2.4. LOCALIZED VENTRICULAR BULGE (VENTRICULAR ANEURYSM). This is an abnormal bulging of the contour of the left ventricle due to thinning of a portion of the wall. The most frequent site is at the apex and, if slight, it is best seen on fluoroscopy and in deep inspiration. Other common sites are high on the lateral wall (Fig. 15) and on the posterior wall. Obviously, examination in the oblique as well as in the anterior positions is necessary.

At the site of the aneurysm (bulge) there may be pericardial adhesions or an increase in density due to an intraventricular mural thrombus. Calcification is rarely present. Thinning of the entire wall of the left ventricle occasionally occurs and is difficult to differentiate from massive left ventricular enlarge-

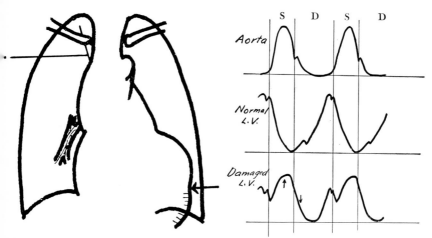

S   D   S   D

Aorta

Normal L.V.

Damaged L.V.

Figure 12. *Left ventricular enlargement plus area of paradoxical pulsation. High left ventricular rounding. The arrow points to a slight indentation best noted on fluoroscopy when the normal segment above this indentation moves inward during systole while the portion below moves outward (area of paradoxical pulsation). In., innominate artery.*

Figure 13. *Electrokymogram. In systole the aorta moves outward (up in the diagram). The normal portion of the left ventricle moves inward (down). In diastole (dicrotic notch indicating closure of the aortic valve), the aortic motion is inward, that of the normal left ventricle outward. In the damaged portion of the left ventricle, there is expansion in systole (outward motion, first arrow) and inward recoil in diastole (second arrow). S, systole; D, diastole.*

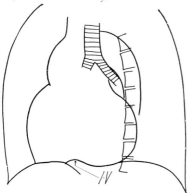

Figure 14. *Enlargement of the inflow tract of the left ventricle. It overlaps the spine posteriorly and displaces the interventricular groove (I–V) anteriorly. The curvature (elongation) of the ascending aorta is increased, and the anterior and posterior limbs of the aortic arch are separated, indicating elongation of the transverse portion.*

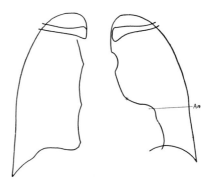

Figure 15. *Ventricular aneurysm (An). This site of localized bulge is uncommon and is much less frequent than in the lower portion of the left ventricular contour.*

ment except by electrokymography. Bulges occur rarely in the right ventricle or in the atria, and diagnosis of such lesions is possible only when the involved areas are on a demonstrable border of the cardiac silhouette.

2.5. LOCALIZED IMPAIRMENT OF CONTRACTION. This is manifested either by a localized diminution of the amplitude of pulsation or by an actual reversal in the direction of pulsations (paradoxical pulsations) (Figs. 12, 13). Either may indicate an area of acute myocardial disease or actual thinning of the wall due to scarring.

3. Right Ventricle

The right ventricle can also be divided into an outflow tract and an inflow tract.

3.1. ENLARGEMENT OF THE OUTFLOW TRACT. The earliest right ventricular enlargement occurs in the outflow tract (except in congenital cardiac defects in which intrinsic deformities modify this portion considerably). This tract extends from the apex of the right ventricle to the pulmonic valve. When viewed in the P–A position, the first noticeable change is a straightening or an increased prominence of the pulmonary artery on the left border. In the RAO position there may be a bulge of the pulmonary artery into the retrosternal space, a bulge made even more prominent by elongation of the conus (infundibular portion) of the right ventricle.

In certain forms of congenital heart disease, the outflow tract may enlarge in the absence of dilatation of the pulmonary artery. Under such circumstances recognition of the enlargement is difficult and may require special techniques such as angiocardiography. Sometimes, when viewed in the RAO position, an anterior bulge of the infundibular portion of the right ventricle may be seen at a lower level than the pulmonary artery.

3.2. ROTATION OF THE HEART ON ITS VERTICAL AXIS. This occurs when the work of the right ventricle is increased out of proportion to that of the left ventricle. Anterior structures move toward the left to form the left lateral contour, and posterior structures such as the left atrium appear on the right contour and may be seen within the right portion of the heart shadow as an added or double density. The pulmonary artery segment increases in size, the prominence of the aortic knob diminishes, and the left ventricular contour becomes shorter and straighter (Figs. 19A, 20A). In certain congenital cardiac defects, notable exceptions occur (4, 15).

3.3. ENLARGEMENT OF THE INFLOW TRACT. The inflow tract is that portion of the chamber extending from the tricuspid valve to the apex. Its enlargement produces increased depth of the chamber and is best seen in the LAO position. In this position the diaphragmatic portion of the heart, chiefly the right ventricle, increases in length, displacing the interventricular groove posteriorly and upward. During deep inspiration the diaphragmatic border remains elongated instead of diminishing as in the normal horizontal heart. The bulge of the anterior contour toward the anterior chest wall is increased. Marked enlargement of the outflow and inflow portions may occur without enlargement to the right in the P–A view (Figs. 16B, 17, 18).

4. Left Atrium

In the P–A view the body of the left atrium normally does not appear. The tip of the left auricle approaches and, to a slight extent, helps form the left contour between the pulmonary artery and the left ventricle, but it rarely projects to form a definite contour of its own.

4.1. POSTERIOR OR HORIZONTAL ENLARGEMENT. When minimal, this is best recognized by its encroachment upon the

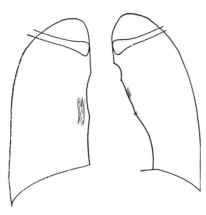

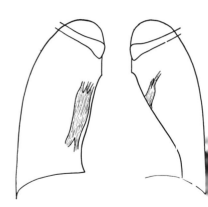

Figure 16A. *Vertical heart (associated with bronchiectasis, emphysema, and pulmonary ventilatory insufficiency) before enlargement of the right ventricle.*

Figure 16B. *Enlargement of the right ventricle. Same heart in right-sided failure. Note the disappearance of the aortic knob (rotation) and straightening of the left upper contour. Note also the increased width of the right hilar branch of the pulmonary artery.*

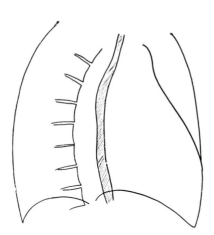

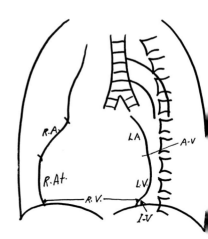

Figure 16C. *Same in the RAO position. Note partial obliteration of the retrosternal space by the enlarged right ventricular outflow tract plus dilated pulmonary artery.*

Figure 16D. *Enlargement of the right ventricular inflow tract and also of the right auricle (formerly termed the right auricular appendage). Note the upward displacement of the interventricular groove. Increase in the length of the diaphragmatic portion indicates inflow tract enlargement.*

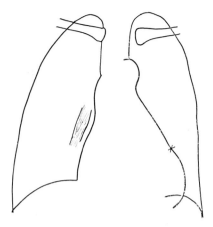

Figure 17. *Right ventricular enlargement secondary to left ventricular enlargement and failure in a patient with hypertensive heart disease.*

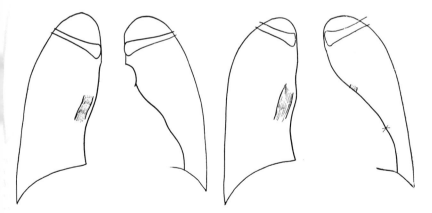

Figure 18. *Progressive stages in the enlargement of the right ventricle leading to rotation of the heart with disappearance of the aortic knob.*

347

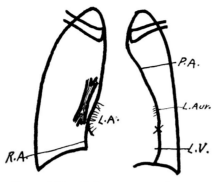

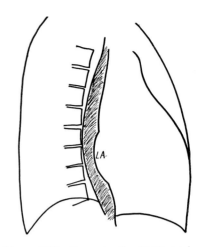

Figure 19A. *Enlargement of the outflow tract of the right ventricle. Note the decrease in convexity at X, indicating that the left ventricle does not participate in the enlargement. The increased density of the left atrium (L.A.) appears on the right contour. Four curves are present in the left contour. Above is the indistinct aortic knob, then P.A. (pulmonary artery), L.Aur. (auricle of the left atrium), L.V. (left ventricle). R.A. is the right atrium.*

Figure 19B. *Same in the RAO position. The pulmonary artery and the right ventricular outflow tract bulge into the retrosternal space. The barium-filled esophagus is indented by the enlarged left atrium.*

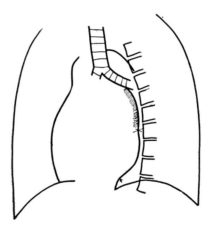

Figure 19C. *Same in the LAO position. Only slight right ventricular outflow tract enlargement. The left main bronchus is elevated by left atrial enlargement.*

retrocardiac space. It is visualized in the RAO position as an arched density projecting toward the spine, situated in the middle portion of the posterior cardiac contour just below the tracheal bifurcation. The extent of this posterior enlargement can be inferred by the compression or displacement of the barium-filled esophagus (Figs. 19B, 20B). One must be sure, however, to distinguish such displacement from that due to the esophagus being pulled to the left and backward by adhesions to an elongated aortic arch or to other mediastinal structures (Fig. 28A, B, C, D). When the esophagus is pulled away from its usually intimate relationship with the posterior surface of the heart, it can no longer be used as a guide to left atrial enlargement.

4.2. VERTICAL OR UPWARD ENLARGEMENT. Superiorly, the left atrium lies in relation to the main bronchi below the bifurcation of the trachea. Vertical or upward enlargement of the left atrium can be observed in its successive stages in the LAO position by a disappearance of the free space between the two main bronchi and an elevation of the left main bronchus. Finally, there is compression as well as displacement of the left bronchus upward and to the left (Figs. 20C, 22C).

4.3. ENLARGEMENT TOWARD THE RIGHT. Enlargement of the left atrium may extend far enough to the right to appear in the middle portion of the right contour of the heart in the P–A position (Figs. 19A, 20A). There may then be two more or less distinct curves on the right border, the lower being the right atrium and the upper the left atrium. Not infrequently, the density of the body of the left atrium may be visualized within the upper central portion of the heart (this is the so-called double density). The rotation of the heart associated with right ventricular enlargement accentuates this displacement of the left atrium toward the right.

4.4. ENLARGEMENT TOWARD THE LEFT. Enlargement of the left auricle does not appear on the left cardiac border at an

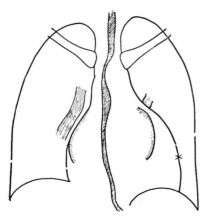

Figure 20A. *Enlargement of the left atrium in an advanced case of mitral stenosis. In this P–A view, the left atrium is noted as an area of increased density, forming the upper part of the right cardiac contour (double density). The barium-filled esophagus is indented by the aorta; below this the left atrium displaces the esophagus slightly to the right. Note the small length of the left ventricular contour.*

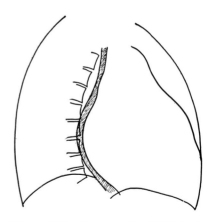

Figure 20B. *Same in the RAO position. Posterior left atrial enlargement. Anterior bulging into the retrosternal space due to right ventricular outflow tract enlargement plus pulmonary artery dilatation.*

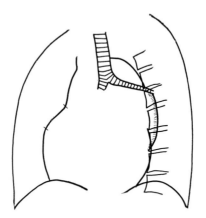

Figure 20C. *Same in the LAO position. The left main bronchus is elevated and compressed. The left ventricular contour is not enlarged. Thus cardiac enlargement in the P–A view (Fig. 20A) is due not to left ventricular enlargement but to displacement of this ventricle to the left by the enlarged right ventricle.*

early stage because it is obscured by the usually coincident enlargement of the pulmonary artery. At a later stage a segment
of a greatly enlarged left atrium may extend farther to the
left than the pulmonary artery and form a recognizable contour of its own. It may be identified by its characteristic atrial
pulsations. At this stage the left atrium may well be called a
giant left atrium.

5. Right Atrium

Enlargement of the right atrium occurs early in the trabec-
ulate portion, which lies anterior and lateral, and quite late
in the rest of the atrium.

5.1. ENLARGEMENT OF THE AURICLE (AURICULAR APPENDIX).
Early enlargement is recognized by elongation of the right
auricle, a contour best seen in the LAO position (Figs. 16D,
21). Characteristic venous type pulsations may occasionally
serve to identify this segment. With massive right atrial enlargement, this segment becomes less oblique and may even
become horizontal (Fig. 22C).

5.2. ENLARGEMENT POSTERIORLY. The posterior smooth portion of the atrium shows enlargement late. It may be noted in
the RAO position when a posteriorly convex shadow of increased density projects into the lower retrocardiac space, immediately above the diaphragm, replacing the former triangular density of the inferior vena cava. Because of the position
of the right atrium to the right of the esophagus, the barium-
filled esophageal density may be noted within the shadow of
the enlarged right atrium (Fig. 22B), in contrast to the posterior displacement of the esophagus that occurs when left
atrial enlargement occurs. Enlargement to the right in the
P–A view is not a reliable criterion for enlargement of the
right atrium in adults. Even a moderate-sized atrium may be
displaced to the right by a greatly enlarged right ventricle.

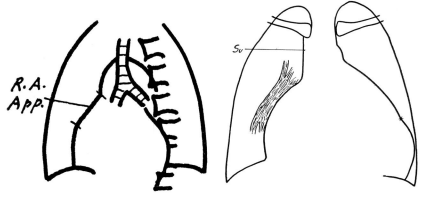

Figure 21. *Enlargement of the right auricle (R.A.App.). LAO position. Elongation of the oblique segment lying between the ascending aorta and the lower anterior contour, the latter composed of right atrium above, right ventricle below.*

Figure 22A. *Right atrial enlargement. A prominent right contour may be due to actual enlargement of the right atrium, to displacement of the right atrium by right ventricular enlargement, or to a combination of the two, as in this instance. Su, dilated superior vena cava.*

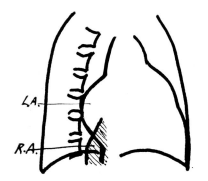

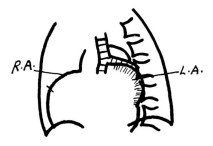

Figure 22B. *Enlargement of the right atrium posteriorly, RAO position. This portion is shaded and seemingly is transected by the barium-filled esophagus, which actually is displaced posteriorly by the only heart chamber in contact with it, the greatly enlarged left atrium.*

Figure 22C. *Advanced right auricular (old terminology: right auricular appendage) enlargement. This segment is practically horizontal. Note also the elevation and compression of the left main bronchus by the markedly enlarged left atrium (L.A.).*

352

6. Symmetric Cardiac Enlargement

In the majority of cases of organic heart disease, more than one chamber is enlarged. This is termed *multiple chamber enlargement*. Enlargement of all the chambers is termed *generalized cardiac enlargement*. When the enlargement of all the chambers is more or less symmetric, a uniformly acting systemic agent is usually found to be the cause, e.g., anemia, metabolic disorder.

Detailed anatomic inferences should not be made from "characteristic" configurations. Terms such as *mitralization, duck-shaped heart,* or *sabot-shaped heart* are undesirable, for they do not give the information obtained from a systematic description of the various chambers.

7. Displacement of the Heart

Slight displacement toward one side may simulate enlargement in this direction, especially if it is associated with a scoliosis of the spine in the opposite direction. Gross displacement of the heart may occur with pneumothorax, pleural effusion, atelectasis, and pulmonary fibrosis. Downward displacement, at times to one side, may occur with large aortic aneurysms or with an enlarged substernal thyroid gland. The contours of the heart often cannot be distinguished from the shadow of dense surrounding structures. Roentgenoscopic examination is necessary, particularly in the oblique positions, with an attempt made to visualize the contours of the individual chambers. Angiocardiography is particularly valuable in differentiating displacement from enlargement.

Deformity of the thoracic spine, if it is convex toward the right, displaces the heart into the left chest, rotating it so that in the P–A view the anterior surface tends to appear on the left border and the posterior surface on the right border. If the scoliosis is convex toward the left, the opposite displacement and rotation occur. Elevation of a portion of the diaphragm by gas, eventration, or abdominal fluid, or herniation of abdominal contents through the diaphragm may also displace and distort the heart contours.

Depression of the sternum (pectus excavatum), if severe, may compress the heart from the front, flattening it by diminishing the anteroposterior thoracic diameter, and displacing and rotating the heart into the left chest. This simulates what occurs with scoliosis of the spine convex to the right (Fig. 23A, B, C).

Emphysema may cause enlargement of the outflow tract of the right ventricle, which, combined with a vertical position of the heart, may greatly increase the prominence of the pulmonary artery (Fig. 16A). Elevation of the heart and mediastinum from its diaphragmatic attachment, due to bilateral upper lobe pulmonary fibrosis, is occasionally seen.

8. Calcification, Intracardiac

8.1. CALCIFICATION OF THE HEART VALVES. ⎫
8.2. CALCIFICATION OF THE ANNULI FIBROSI. ⎬ Both conditions may be noted on roentgenography or roentgenoscopy. With good accommodation, the latter is the more reliable method. Synchronous with cardiac pulsations, dense intracardiac linear or circular shadows may be seen moving up and down or from side to side (in aortic valvular involvement) or in rotary fashion (in mitral involvement). These movements are best noted in the RAO position.

8.3. CALCIFICATION OF THE CORONARY ARTERIES. This is rarely visualized. A double row of linear densities with motion synchronous with cardiac pulsations may be visualized in regions where the main coronary arteries may be expected. The most common site of such calcification is below and anterior to the ascending aorta in the RAO position.

8.4. CALCIFICATION OF THE MYOCARDIUM. This may occur at

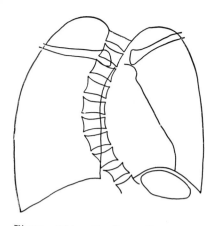

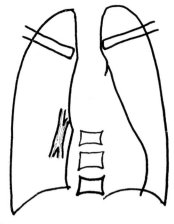

Figure 23A. Cardiac displacement (scoliosis of the spine). The heart is displaced into the left chest and is also rotated. Frequently, due to associated emphysema, right ventricular outflow tract enlargement and pulmonary artery prominence may be demonstrated.

Figure 23B. Cardiac displacement (funnel chest deformity). Variable degrees of cardiac displacement to the left. The lower dorsal vertebrae are often visualized even without proper roentgen techniques, presumably because of lesser opacification in the A–P diameter.

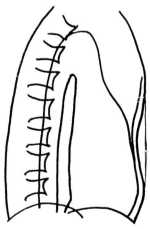

Figure 23C. Same in the RAO position. Note the narrowing of the A–P diameter, particularly at the site of the funnel-shaped depression.

355

sites of extensive myocardial necrosis, as, for example, with ventricular aneurysm.

8.5. CALCIFICATION OF THE ENDOCARDIUM. A rare condition, this represents the secondary deposition of calcium on a previously injured endocardium. It is almost always on the posterior wall of the left atrium and is best recognized in the RAO position.

9. Pericardium

9.1. EFFUSION. Pericardial effusion causes a generalized enlargement of the cardiac area and a disappearance of the usual curves of the outline in the P–A position (Fig. 24). Diminution of pulsations is variable, depending upon the amount of effusion. Filling the stomach with air may reveal absent or diminished pulsations of the inferior contour of the heart. An increase in the acuteness of the right cardiodia-

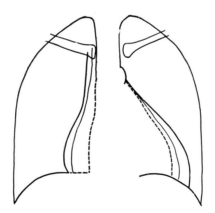

Figure 24. *Pericardial effusion. The broken lines show the normal cardiac silhouette. The two lateral contours indicate degrees of pericardial and superior vena caval distention. Note the loss of individual chamber contours and the increased acuteness of the right cardiohepatic angle.*

phragmatic angle is common. In the RAO position filling of the right postero-inferior recess in the vicinity of the inferior vena cava may be observed early in the course of the effusion. The superior vena cava is often dilated.

Disproportionate widening of the upper contours in the P–A view may be accentuated in the reclining position. Normal aortic pulsations in the presence of diminished pulsations in the rest of the cardiac contour should suggest the diagnosis. Differentiation from generalized cardiac enlargement is sometimes difficult. In adults effusion of less than 300 ml in volume usually cannot be recognized.

9.2. ADHESIONS. Adhesions between visceral and parietal layers of the pericardium are impossible to visualize. Adhesions between the pericardium and pleura may cause a systolic retraction of visible pleura or pulmonary tissue. Adhesions between the pericardium and the diaphragm, ribs, sternum, or vertebrae may be demonstrable with proper rotation of the patient. Pericardial adhesions may prevent the heart from shifting with changes in position but this feature may also be observed with unusually large hearts. An added linear shadow of increased density may rather infrequently be observed within the cardiac shadow adjacent to the border. This is due to a thickened pleuropericardial adhesion. When the pericardium is adherent to the mediastinal structures or vertebrae, apparent elevation of the heart may be observed when the diaphragm descends with deep inspiration.

Pulsations at the site of adhesion may be diminished, although the uninvolved portions of the heart may pulsate with normal or increased amplitude (adhesive pericarditis). Cardiac enlargement frequently occurs in such cases of adhesion to the chest wall or to the spine.

9.3. CONSTRICTION. Dense adhesions may envelop the greater portion of the entire heart as a glove envelops the hand, or only certain portions of the heart may be affected. These pericardial scars hamper diastolic expansion and may also influence systolic contraction. Over a period of time, a diminution in cardiac size and the development of a more vertical position may occur. Diminished pulsations are difficult to substantiate because of the great variability in the extent and degree of constriction in different patients. Roentgenkymograms offer a graphic representation of diminution of or complete absence of pulsations over a portion of the heart. They may also show a shortened period of diastolic relaxation as well as a plateau-type curve in the later portions of diastole.

9.4. CALCIFICATION. Calcification of the pericardium is recognized by dense, linear, sometimes wave-like, shadows following the borders of the heart. It is frequently seen better in the oblique positions (Figs. 25, 26). Calcification of the pericardium may partly or completely encircle the base of the heart in the region of the atrioventricular groove, and may extend over the upper part of the right ventricle. In some cases enlargement of the right and left atria results. The clinical picture of pericardial constriction may ensue even though the heart is evidently enlarged.

9.5. CYSTS. Localized protrusions of the cardiac silhouette may be due to an encapsulated pericardial effusion, to herniation or diverticulum, or to fluid within a cyst. It usually is ovoid or semicircular in shape, it is not opacified on angiocardiography, and its pulsations are transmitted from the contiguous portion of the heart. The definitive diagnosis usually is made at operation or at necropsy.

10. Aorta

10.1. ELONGATION AND DILATATION. Elongation of the aorta (Figs. 27A, B, 28A, B, C, D) occurs in association with increased arterial pressure or with increased blood flow through it. Under such circumstances the aorta becomes longer than normal between its fixed origin at the base of the heart and the dia-

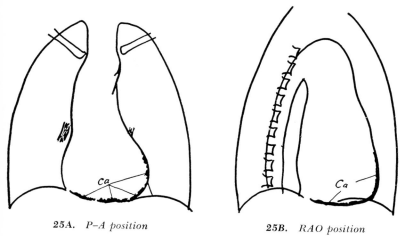

25A. *P–A position*   **25B.** *RAO position*

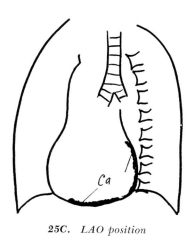

25C. *LAO position*

Figure 25. *Diffuse type of pericardial calcification. Small heart, no demonstrable chamber enlargement, calcification of contours noted in all positions.*

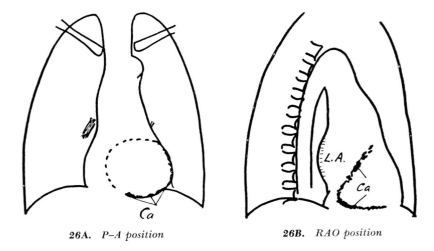

26A. *P–A position* **26B.** *RAO position*

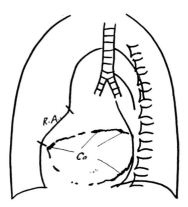

26C. *LAO position*

Figure 26. Atrioventricular ring type of pericardial calcification. The calcification is noted in some contours but not in others. In the RAO position it frequently seems to be linear or L-shaped. In the LAO position linear or punctate calcific densities may be noted within the heart density rather than at the contours. The heart is slightly or moderately enlarged, chiefly the atria.

phragm. There is usually an associated dilatation due to stretching of the wall. Elongation with dilatation also occurs as a result of loss of elasticity due to arteriosclerosis and to intrinsic disease of the aortic wall such as syphilitic aortitis. Detailed visualization of the entire thoracic aorta and its brachiocephalic branches is best achieved by angiocardiography.

a. *Ascending portion of the aortic arch.* The immediate supraventricular portion is hidden by the overlying right auricle and cannot be visualized except by angiocardiography. Elongation of the upper portion of the ascending aorta is best seen in the LAO and P–A positions. In the former position the vertical course of the ascending limb is changed to an anterior convexity; in the latter position the transverse portion of the arch is elevated to or above the level of the clavicles, the aortic knob protrudes far into the left lung field, and the lower portion of the trachea is pushed to the right by the horizontal portion of the arch.

It is difficult to ascertain dilatation of the ascending portion of the arch apart from elongation. Except when the density of the aorta is greatly increased or in the rare instances when calcification is found within its walls, measurement in both oblique positions is deceptive because of the adjacent position of the superior vena cava.

b. *Transverse portion of the aortic arch.* Elongation and dilatation are best observed in the LAO position. The curve of the arch is wider, with increased separation of the ascending and descending limbs. The dilated transverse portion of the arch may be sufficiently dense to render it visible even within the increased illumination of the trachea. In the P–A view the aortic indentation upon the esophagus is deepened, and the diameter of the lumen at this point can be accurately measured from the esophagus to the outer margin of the aortic knob. This diameter, however, is clinically unimportant. Pulling of the esophagus posteriorly and to the left below the aortic indentation

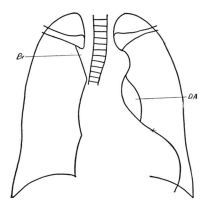

Figure 27A. *Elongation, dilatation, and tortuosity of the aorta and brachiocephalic vessels (Br). Note the increased curvature of the ascending aorta, the prominent aortic knob, and the tortuous descending portion of the arch (D.A.). The lower portion of the trachea is pushed to the right by this elongated and dilated aorta.*

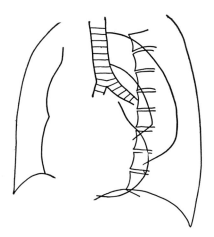

Figure 27B. *Same in the LAO position. The elongation and tortuosity cause an apparent, but not real, buckling or angulation since the course of the aorta turns in a direction away from the observer.*

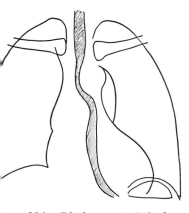

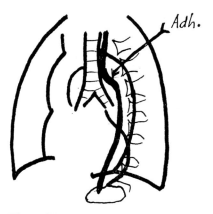

Figure 28A. Displacement of the barium-filled esophagus to the left. Elongation of the transverse portion of the aortic arch pulls the adherent esophagus away from its usual relation to the left atrium. When this is present, the barium-filled esophagus no longer may be used as a guide to left atrial enlargement.

Figure 28B. Same in the LAO position. Arrow points to the common site of adhesion (Adh.). The descending aorta is no longer prevertebral but is now paravertebral. The barium-filled esophagus is pulled away from its usual normal relationship to the left atrium.

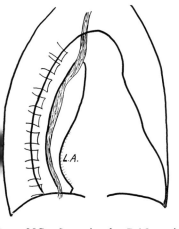

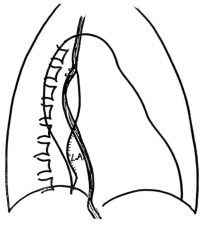

Figure 28C. Same in the RAO position. The barium-filled esophagus is pulled posteriorly because of its aortic adhesions. This simulates posterior displacement by an enlarged left atrium, which in this instance actually is enlarged, but not sufficiently so to indent or displace the esophagus.

Figure 28D. A similar case in the RAO position. The esophagus is pulled posteriorly above, then pushed anteriorly below by the tortuous thoracic aorta. Nevertheless, left atrial enlargement can be identified, but without the aid of the barium-filled esophagus.

(Figs. 28A, B, C, D) is due to the normal adhesions between the esophagus and an elongated aorta. Such pulling must be differentiated from displacement caused by an enlarged left atrium.

c. *Descending limb of the aortic arch and the thoracic aorta.* Participation of this portion in generalized elongation of the aortic arch results in tortuosity. In the LAO position a sinuous curvature or an apparent buckling may appear. Dilatation of the descending aorta is frequently seen in elderly individuals. In adults the density of the shadow of the descending aorta makes it readily visualized in the RAO position. It appears in the retrocardiac space and is distinguishable from the greater densities of the heart and spinal column, especially during deep inspiration. In aortic insufficiency the descending aorta is rendered more clearly visible, even in children.

Elongation and dilatation of the descending aorta results in a prominent curve with a convexity to the left, seen in the P–A view lying below the aortic knob and frequently extending beyond the hilus. Farther down, this density can often be followed within the cardiac shadow. Frequently, the entire aorta is diffusely dilated. The aortic shadow then has a fusiform or spindle-shaped contour.

10.2. calcification. Calcification of the aorta occurs most frequently in transverse and descending portions. In the P–A position calcified plaques in the transverse portion are viewed tangentially and are noted most readily in the aortic knob. Calcification confined to the ascending aorta has been considered as diagnostic of syphilitic aortitis.

10.3. hypoplasia. Hypoplasia of the aorta may occur as a solitary congenital anomaly. Relative hypoplasia is not infrequently seen in mitral stenosis and in some congenital anomalies when the volume of blood flow within the aorta is diminished. The diagnosis may be made on fluoroscopy when the ascending and descending limbs of the aortic

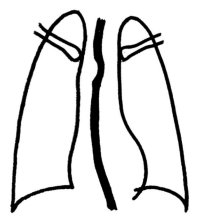

Figure 29A. *Right aortic arch. High crossing (usually as a solitary lesion; infrequently in association with other serious congenital lesions). Note the aortic indentation in the esophagus from the right.*

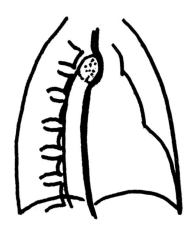

Figure 29B. *Same in the RAO position. Note the compression of the esophagus from behind by the high aortic crossing to the left. In those with right aortic descent, there is no such compression.*

arch are unusually close together. It may be confirmed by angiocardiography.

10.4. RIGHT AORTIC ARCH. The features of this congenital anomaly are shown in Figure 29A, B.

10.5. COARCTATION. The radiologic characteristics are: a rounded, enlarged left ventricle; elongated ascending aorta; widened innominate and subclavian arteries; absent aortic knob; erosion of the ribs; visualization of the constriction (Fig. 30A, B, C).

11. Aneurysm of the Aorta

11.1. SACCULAR. Only a localized ballooning or bulge should be called an aneurysm (Fig. 31A, B). Diagnosis of aneurysm is justified only when the mass is seen to be a part of the shadow of the aorta as viewed from all directions. The mass may show expansile or transmitted pulsations. The absence or presence of pulsations, however, cannot be used as a final diagnostic criterion. Calcification within the wall of the aneurysm is often present.

Aneurysm of the ascending and transverse portions of the aorta may displace and constrict the trachea and bronchi and may erode adjacent bony structures. Huge aneurysmal sacs may obscure large portions of the thorax. A positive differentiation from pleural effusion or intrathoracic neoplasm may be difficult. Angiocardiography may be expected to differentiate between an aneurysm and an adjacent mediastinal mass. In rare instances opacification is hindered by a narrowed orifice or by thrombi within the sac.

11.2. FUSIFORM. A fusiform aneurysm is impossible to differentiate from marked dilatation of the aorta except by angiocardiography.

11.3. DISSECTING HEMATOMA. The hematoma resulting from the rupture of the intima may extend within the media into the great vessels of the neck, up and down the aortic arch, and

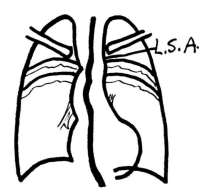

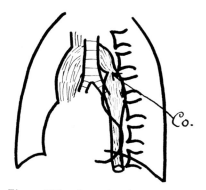

Figure 30A. *Coarctation of the aorta. The left ventricle is rounded and enlarged. There is an absence of the aortic knob in the presence of an elongated ascending aorta and widened innominate and left subclavian arteries. Erosion of the ribs is present. L.S.A., left subclavian artery.*

Figure 30B. *Same in the LAO position. Note the coarcted site (Co.).*

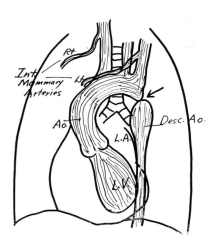

Figure 30C. *Angiocardiogram of same in the LAO position. The site of constriction, poststenotic dilatation, and some of the collateral vessels are demonstrated.*

367

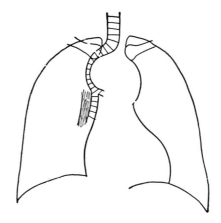

Figure 31A.   *Aneurysm of the transverse portion of the aortic arch.*

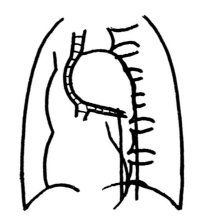

Figure 31B.   *Same in the LAO position.*

may extend into the abdominal aorta (Fig. 32; 3.6; 21.4.1). There is widening of the involved portions of the aorta and brachiocephalic vessels, which often is diagnostic only if films made before dissection are available for comparison.

Angiocardiography may indicate localized or diffuse thickening of the aortic wall at the site of the dissection, or an irregular or abrupt narrowing of the aortic lumen. Less frequently, contrast substance may appear within a false arterial passageway.

12. Widening of the Brachiocephalic Arteries

Elongation and dilatation of the right innominate artery is recognized by a triangular shadow extending upward and outward from the upper right contour of the ascending aorta (Fig. 12). Its prominence is enhanced by upward displacement of the elongated and dilated ascending aorta.

Widening of the left subclavian artery may be recognized

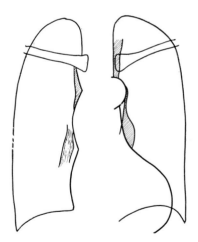

Figure 32. *Dissecting aneurysm of the aorta. The shaded portions represent areas of dissection within the walls of the aorta and the brachiocephalic vessels. Comparison with previous films is valuable.*

by a vertical density extending upward above the region of the aortic knob just to the left of the sternum, and later arching to the left. The most common circumstance for such widening is in association with coarctation of the aorta (Fig. 30A).

13. Dilatation of the Superior Vena Cava

Normally, the superior vena cava may be visible in the P–A view, although the curve of the ascending aorta is the more prominent. With increase in venous pressure, the superior vena cava may appear as a vertical shadow of variable width parallel to the sternum and extending above or lateral to the ascending aorta (Fig. 22A).

14. Pulmonary Artery

14.1. DILATATION OF THE TRUNK AND PRIMARY BRANCHES. Dilatation of the trunk is seen in the P–A view as a bulge with convexity to the left that appears below the aortic knob (Fig. 33A). Dilatation of the primary branches of the left pulmonary artery is seen in the LAO position as a shadow of increased width and density obliquely crossing the left bronchus (Fig. 33C). The shadow emerges from a centrally placed density due to the bifurcation of the trunk of the pulmonary artery. Markedly increased density occurs most often in the presence of emphysema and, if the density is of extreme degree, sclerosis of the pulmonary artery may be inferred. Calcified plaques may be present with pulmonary hypertension.

14.2. DILATATION OF THE SECONDARY OR HILAR VESSELS. The chief components of the hilar shadows are the secondary branches of the pulmonary artery. In the P–A view these are usually better visualized on the right. The air space of the right lower lobe bronchus emphasizes the cardiac density me-

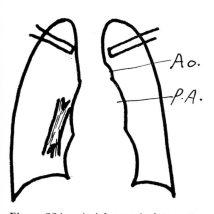

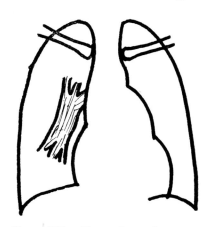

Figure 33A. *Atrial septal defect. In the early or less severe stages, the pulmonary artery trunk may be prominent even though the hilar branches of the pulmonary artery are within normal width limits. The left ventricle characteristically is small; there is no left atrial enlargement.*

Figure 33B. *More advanced stage of atrial septal defect. The pulmonary artery trunk is more prominent, the hilar branches wider, and characteristic increase in pulsatile amplitude may be noted (hilar dance). The lungs are hypervascular.*

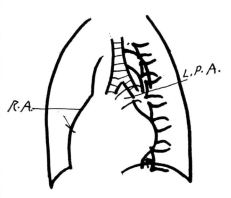

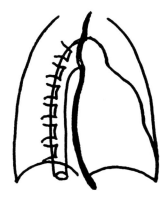

Figure 33C. *Same in the LAO position. Note the small left ventricle and the enlarged right ventricle and right auricle.*

Figure 33D. *Same in the RAO position. No left atrial enlargement.*

371

dially and the descending branch of the pulmonary artery laterally. On the teleroentgenogram the normal width of the shadow of the upper portion of the right descending branch varies from 9 to 14 mm in adults. Dilatation of the secondary branches of the pulmonary artery is best noted in the P–A view.

Expansile pulsations of small amplitude are normally observed in the hilar branches of the pulmonary artery. A marked increase in pulsations, accompanied by a rhythmic increase and decrease in density (hilar dance), is seen when the pulse pressure in the pulmonary artery is increased, as with large left-to-right intracardiac shunts and with pulmonary valvular or annular incompetency.

14.3. NARROWING OF THE PULMONARY ARTERY AND ITS BRANCHES. Such narrowing may be demonstrated in pulmonic or infundibular stenosis (Figs. 34, 35; 4.13; 15.6, 15, 27).

15. Pulmonary Fields

Pulmonary manifestations of heart failure are common. The blood vessels, parenchyma, and pleura may be involved.

15.1. HILAR DILATATION. Pulmonary hypertension and/or increased flow (Figs. 36A, C, E, H, 37A) is indicated by increased width of the secondary branches of the pulmonary artery. In the presence of diffuse stasis, the shadows of the secondary branches of the pulmonary artery may increase or diminish in size with increase or decrease of cardiac insufficiency.

15.2. PULMONARY STASIS. *Chronic diffuse pulmonary stasis* is manifested by increased density of the entire lung field, with contrast especially poor at the base. This density is due to vascular engorgement, interstitial and alveolar edema, and desquamated alveolar epithelium. Chronic stasis may at times be localized to one or more lobes, or to portions of such lobes,

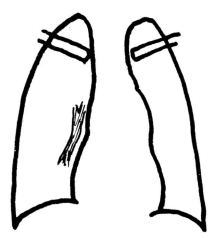

Figure 34A. *Pulmonic (valvular) stenosis with poststenotic dilatation of the trunk not extending to the hilar branches of the pulmonary artery. Pulmonary hypovascularity.*

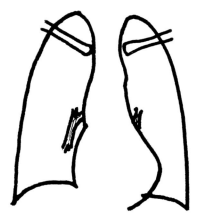

Figure 34B. *Pulmonic (infundibular) stenosis. There is no prominent pulmonary artery segment as in Fig. 34A; instead there is concavity as in Fig. 35B. Note that the hilar branches of the pulmonary artery are small; the lungs are hypovascular.*

373

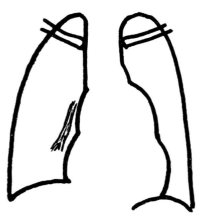

Figure 34C. *Pulmonic stenosis plus atrial septal defect or patent foramen ovale. The pulmonary artery trunk is prominent beyond the pulmonic stenosis (poststenotic dilatation). Note that this dilatation does not extend to the hilar branch of the pulmonary artery. The lungs are unusually hypovascular.*

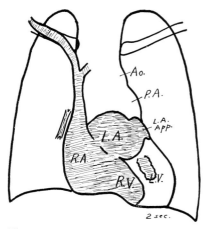

Figure 34D. *Angiocardiogram of pulmonic (valvular) stenosis plus atrial septal defect in the P–A position.*

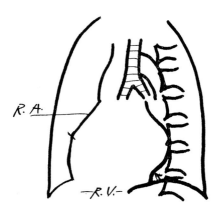

Figure 34E. *Same in the LAO position. Note right ventricular and right atrial enlargement. The arrow points to the elevation of the interventricular groove, increasing the diaphragmatic length of the right ventricle.*

374

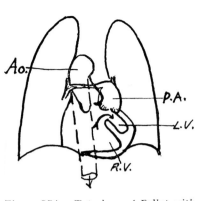

Figure 35A. *Tetralogy of Fallot with valvular pulmonic stenosis, poststenotic dilatation which does not, however, extend to the secondary (hilar) branches, with diminished pulmonary arterial outflow. The interventricular septal defect is noted below the aortic valve, with the arrow denoting the flow from R.V. (right ventricle). The aorta, fairly large, crosses over the right bronchus with right descent and low crossing (aortic arrow).*

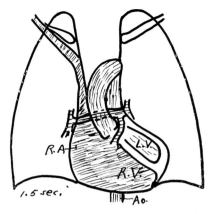

Figure 35B. *Angiocardiogram of the heart in tetralogy of Fallot (infundibular plus valvular stenosis). The blunted appearance of the lowermost left contour is due to right ventricular enlargement, which also displaces the interventricular septum and the left ventricle upward and backward. Although the shunt of blood through the septal defect is from the right to the left ventricle, opacification of the latter may be good, fair, or even poor.*

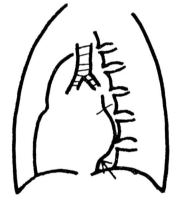

Figure 35C. *Same in the LAO position. The increased size of the right ventricle and the right atrium are seen here. The left ventricle is displaced posteriorly and upward above the arrow that denotes the interventricular groove.*

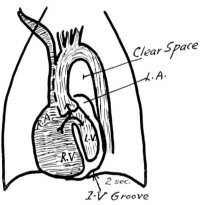

Figure 35D. *Angiocardiogram of same in the LAO position. The pulmonary artery is not opacified; the space below the aortic arch is clear.*

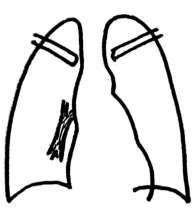

Figure 36A. *Interventricular septal defect. The left ventricle may be only slightly enlarged, as in this instance, or more so. The hilar branches of the pulmonary artery may not be dilated, as here, or they may be dilated in association with pulmonary hypervascularity. The pulmonary artery trunk, however, generally is fairly prominent.*

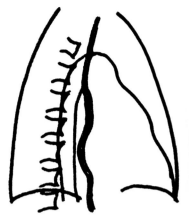

Figure 36B. *Same in the LAO position. Note the slight but definite left atrial enlargement, even though the left ventricular enlargement (Fig. 36A) was only slight.*

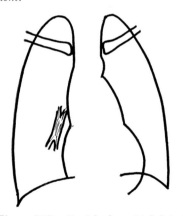

Figure 36C. *Ventricular septal defect. Substantial left-to-right shunt. Moderate to marked left ventricular enlargement, and slighter left atrial enlargement. Hilar pulmonary arterial dilatation. Pulmonary hypervascularity.*

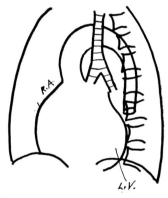

Figure 36D. *Same in the LAO position. With more marked degrees of left-to-right shunting and the consequent pulmonary hypertension, right-sided involvement occurs. Here note the right atrial enlargement secondary to that of the right ventricle.*

376

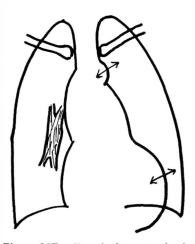

Figure 36E. *Ventricular septal defect plus aortic insufficiency secondary to prolapse of an aortic cusp into the defect. Marked enlargement of the left ventricle and lesser enlargement of the left atrium. The bidirectional arrows here indicate increased amplitude of aortic and left ventricular pulsations.*

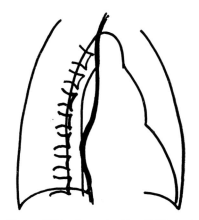

Figure 36F. *Same in the RAO position.*

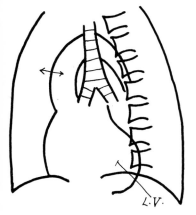

Figure 36G. *Same in the LAO position.*

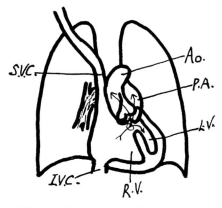

Figure 36H. *Angiocardiogram of Eisenmenger variety of ventricular septal defect. Pulmonary resistances are high enough to cause predominant flow from the right to the left ventricle. The right ventricle is enlarged as well as hypertrophied. The arrows indicate flow from the right ventricle (R.V.) to the left ventricle (L.V.), into the pulmonary artery (P.A.), through the septal defect into the aorta (Ao.). S.V.C. and I.V.C. indicate superior and inferior vena cava. The pulmonary artery trunk and hilar branches are dilated. Normally there is also an increase in pulmonary vascularity.*

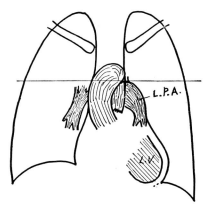

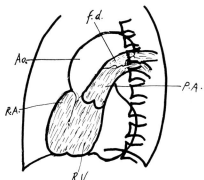

Figure 37A. *Angiocardiogram in patent ductus arteriosus. Note the elevation of the left pulmonary artery (L.P.A.) and the reopacification of the pulmonary arteries from the aorta.*

Figure 37B. *Angiocardiogram of same in the LAO position with the right-sided structures opacified. Note the filling defect (f.d.) in the pulmonary artery (P.A.) from the nonopacified aortic flow via the ductus.*

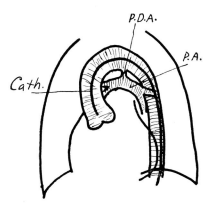

Figure 37C. *Aortogram of same, demonstrating the flow of opacified substance introduced into the aorta by means of a catheter (Cath.) through the ductus into the pulmonary artery.*

simulating inflammatory involvement. *Acute diffuse pulmonary stasis* may be indicated by radiating densities extending from hilar regions in a butterfly-like pattern. A diffuse stippled or miliary infiltration throughout the lungs may be due to minute areas of fibrosis and alveolar collapse. This may occur after chronic diffuse stasis disappears.

15.3.   PLEURAL INVOLVEMENT.   This is manifested by effusion or thickening either along the chest wall or in the interlobar fissures. Pleural effusions may be generalized or localized and are frequently seen in the interlobar spaces.

Part V | The Electrocardiographic Diagnosis

30 / Criteria for Electrocardiographic Techniques

1. General

Changes in the electrocardiogram occur in variable degree with change in posture, after meals, after smoking, after exercise, and with the use of drugs. The position of the body at the time the recording is made should be stated in the report. The preferred position of the patient is recumbent. The reclining table should be long enough and wide enough to support all extremities. To eliminate shivering, the temperature of the room in which the records are made should be comfortable. For precise, comparative work the patient should be in the basal state at each recording.

2. Bipolar Extremity Leads

Bipolar extremity leads record the differences in potential between two extremities when each is connected to one of the input terminals of the recording device. A lead such as this, in which both electrodes are distant from the heart, is described as bipolar. The difference in potential between the left arm and the right arm is designated as lead I, between the left leg and the right arm as lead II, and between the left leg and the left arm as lead III. In each instance the connections to the galvanometer are to be made in such a way that positivity of the first-named extremity with respect to the second results in an upward deflection in the finished record.

In taking these leads, the sensitivity of the recording instrument should be so adjusted that introduction of 1 mv in the circuit results in a deflection of 1 cm. In practice, this reference voltage, or "standardization," should be recorded at the beginning and at the end of each lead.

The electrodes may be placed on any part of the arms or of the left leg in making these leads, as long as they are below the shoulders in the former and below the inguinal fold anteriorly and the gluteal fold posteriorly in the latter. Any other placement of the electrodes made necessary by deformed or missing extremities must be noted on the record.

The electrodes may be any of several types provided that a low resistance can be obtained between the surface of the electrode and the skin, and provided that the material is of low resistance and displays no condenser properties. A convenient electrode to use on the extremities is one of German silver, 3.5 cm × 5.0 cm, that is held in place by an elastic band and that makes contact with the skin through a conducting jelly.

Electrodes and their contacts with the lead wires of the recording device must be kept scrupulously clean. The entire circuit from patient to machine must be inspected frequently for defects.

3. Unipolar Extremity Leads

The potential of any extremity may be obtained by connecting its electrode (exploring electrode) to one input terminal of the recording device. The other input terminal is connected to an indifferent electrode, preferably one with a potential as close as possible to the mean potential of the body during the cardiac cycle. Such an electrode can be constructed by connecting the right arm, the left arm, and the left leg to a central terminal, each through a fixed, noninductive resistance of

5000 or more ohms. It is imperative that the resistances between each extremity and the central terminal be equal. A galvanometric lead in which the central terminal is used as the indifferent electrode is described as unipolar.

Augmentation, whereby the resulting deflections are one and one-half times as large as their true size, may be accomplished by severing the connection between the central terminal and the extremity being studied.

In recording the extremity potentials, either in the ordinary unipolar or in the augmented way, the electrocardiograph is to be adjusted so that a deflection of 1 cm in the finished record corresponds to a potential difference of 1 mv. Any increase in sensitivity of the instrument made necessary by small deflections should be clearly recorded on the curve, preferably at the beginning and at the end of the lead. Connections to the galvanometer are to be made in such a way that relative positivity of the exploring electrode will cause an upright deflection in the electrocardiogram.

When made in the ordinary way, the records from the right arm, the left arm, and the left leg are to be designated by the symbols V_R, V_L, and V_F, respectively. When the records have been augmented, each of these symbols should be preceded by a lower case letter, a, as follows: aV_R, aV_L, aV_F.

4. Thoracic Leads

The exploring or precordial electrode should be circular and 3 cm or less in diameter. In children under 10 years the diameter should be 1.5 cm or less. It is desirable that multiple precordial leads be taken and that the position of the precordial electrode be indicated by a subscript after the lead according to the following plan:

> Subscript 1 shall be used for a lead from the right sternal margin at the fourth intercostal space; subscript 2 for a lead from the left sternal margin at the fourth intercostal space; subscript 4 for a lead from the fifth

intercostal space where it is crossed by the midclavicular line; subscript 3 for a lead from a point midway between points 2 and 4; subscript 5 for a lead from the junction of the left anterior axillary line with the horizontal level of position 4. Subscripts 6, 7, and 8 shall be used for leads on the same horizontal level but at the left midaxillary line (6), the left posterior axillary line (7), and the left midscapular line (8), respectively. When additional leads are made from the right side of the thorax, their location shall be indicated by Arabic subscripts as for the left side and followed by the letter R (for right). A lead from the fifth intercostal space in the right midclavicular line thus will bear the designation V_{4R}.

If vertical deviations in the placing of the electrodes are made for any reason, the level of reference should be a rib (and adjacent halves of the intercostal spaces) *at its junction with the sternum*. The rib is indicated by an Arabic numeral, and this numeral precedes the designation of the lead; e.g., $3V_4$ indicates a lead at the level of the third left sternocostal junction above the usual precordial location of lead V_4.

For routine purposes leads should be made from at least three areas widely distributed over the precordium. The combination of locations 1, 3, and 5 have been found useful, although leads from six or more positions are more informative and therefore preferable.

The indifferent or distant contact is to be placed on the central terminal. Leads obtained in this way are designated by the letter V followed by a subscript determined by the location of the exploring electrode as described above.

In taking precordial leads, connections to the recording device are to be made as described for the unipolar extremity leads so that relative positivity of the exploring electrode is represented by an upward deflection in the finished record.

In taking precordial leads with large deflections, it will be found convenient to adjust the electrocardiograph so that a deflection of 0.5 cm in the finished record corresponds to a potential difference of 1 mv. The sensitivity should be clearly indicated on the curve by recording at its beginning and at its end the effect of introducing a potential difference of 1 mv into the galvanometric circuit.

5. Esophageal Leads

The exploring or esophageal electrode is usually a small cylinder, approximately 3 mm × 4 mm, made of noncorrosive material. It is connected by insulated wire of approximately 100 cm in length to a clip or jack to which an input terminal of the galvanometer may be attached readily. Several "ring electrodes" insulated from each other at distances of 2.5 to 5.0 cm may be arranged along a small-bore tube similar to a stomach tube. With this electrode multiple leads may be made from several esophageal levels without moving the tube.

The depth of an electrode in the esophagus is measured from the external nares. In adults the exploring electrode is usually close to the heart at levels between 30 cm and 55 cm from the external nares. Placement and localization are best accomplished with the aid of a fluoroscope.

The central terminal is used as an indifferent electrode as described for other unipolar leads. Response of the electrocardiograph to the introduction of a potential difference of 1 mv must be adjusted to the size of the deflections to be recorded, and must be clearly shown on each lead made.

The leads obtained are designated by the symbol V followed by the subscript E and an Arabic number indicating the distance of the electrode from the external nares, e.g., V_{E23}, V_{E58}.

6. Vectorcardiograms

There is at present no agreement on the technique to be used in recording the vectorcardiogram. On theoretical grounds, orthogonal lead systems that incorporate approximate corrections for the electrical inhomogeneity of the body and the eccentric position of the heart are to be preferred.

31 / Nomenclature for Electrocardiographic Deflections*

1. The symbols P, T_P, QRS, T, and U are to be used to represent the deflections or groups of deflections encountered in the electrocardiogram. Criteria for the use of these symbols apply to all leads, unipolar and bipolar, normal and abnormal.

2. The P wave is normally the gradual initial deflection of any group, and may be a summit or a depression. The level of reference from which its voltage is measured is the isoelectric level (T–P or U–P interval). If it displays turning points on either side of its reference level, it is described as diphasic. If the initial turning point is above this level, it is said to be of the plus-minus (+ −) type, and if below, it is said to be of the minus-plus (− +) type.

In esophageal and intracardiac leads the P wave will usually be composed of multiple, rapid deflections not unlike the QRS group of leads from the body surface. It is recommended that the same symbols and criteria of application be used as for the initial ventricular group (see par. 5 below) but that the symbol for each atrial deflection be followed by the subscript P, e.g., Q_P, R_P, S_P, R'_P, S'_P, R''_P, S''_P. Furthermore, the level

* Modified from "Recommendations for standardization of electrocardiographic leads," by a committee of the American Heart Association, *Circulation* 10:565, 1954.

of reference of these deflections, as for the P wave itself, is to be the isoelectric line.

3. The T_P wave may be found in the P–R segment, that part of the trace between the end of the P wave and the beginning of QRS. It usually continues through the QRS interval. If discernible in body surface leads, it is a shallow deflection usually below but sometimes above its level of reference, the isoelectric line. In esophageal and intracardiac leads it is often of larger amplitude and may be diphasic. When there is atrioventricular block, an $S–T_P$ segment preceding and a low summit U_P following the T_P may be identified in such leads.

4. In the majority of electrocardiograms the QRS complex is superimposed on the T_P deflection. For this reason the level of reference from which the voltage of QRS is measured should be the level at which the first of the QRS components begins. The voltage of an upward QRS deflection is the vertical distance between the upper edge of the trace at the beginning of the QRS interval and the upper edge of the trace at the apex of the deflection. The voltage of a downward deflection is the vertical distance between the lower edge of the trace at the beginning of the QRS interval and the lower edge of the trace at the nadir of the deflection.

5. In order to indicate how the QRS complex should be subdivided for the purpose of assigning symbols to its parts, it should be borne in mind that the first deflection begins at the onset of the QRS interval when the trace first leaves the reference level. From this point the trace rises or falls to a turning point where the direction of its motion is reversed. It may pass through a second and third turning point or even more, causing notches, before crossing to the opposite side of the reference level.* At this crossing the first deflection ends

* When the trace is descending, it crosses the reference level at the instant when its lowest margin reaches a position below that which it occupied at the beginning of the QRS interval. When the trace is ascending, it crosses the reference level at the instant when its upper margin reaches a position above that which it occupied at the beginning of the QRS interval.

and the second begins. The second deflection, necessarily opposite in direction to the first, must display one turning point
and may display many; it does not end until the trace crosses
the reference level for the second time. There may be a deflection which begins at the second crossing and ends at the S–T
junction. No part of the QRS complex that does not cross the
reference level should be considered a separate deflection. If
the S–T junction is displaced in a direction opposite to the
turning point of the last deflection of QRS, that portion of
QRS that lies between this point and the S–T junction should
be considered a part of the last deflection.

The earliest QRS deflection that lies above the reference
level should be labeled R. Any downward deflection that precedes R should be labeled Q. The first of any downward deflections that may follow R should be labeled S. The first of
any upward deflections that may follow S should be labeled
R', and the first of any downward deflections that may follow
R' should be labeled S'. If it is necessary to label still later
deflections of the QRS group, the symbols R'', S'', and so on
should be used in accordance with the same principles. When
R is absent and the QRS complex consists of a single downward deflection, this deflection should be labeled QS. In statistical studies QS, Q, and S deflections should be considered
separately. For the purpose of roughly indicating the size of
the components of the QRS group relative to each other, the
upper case letters Q, R, and S may be used for larger deflections and the lower case letters q, r, and s for smaller deflections.

A deflection is "notched" when it displays more than one
turning point on the same side of the reference level. A deflection is slurred when it displays a distinct and local thickening on either limb or at its apex, owing to a sudden and
pronounced change in the slope of the curve.

When the form of the QRS complex varies from moment
to moment because of the effect of respiratory movements on
the position of the heart or for some similar reason, the classification of this complex should be determined by the variety

of complex which is most abundant or, if no type is numerically predominant, by the outline of the complexes which are of intermediate form. Small QRS complexes (largest deflection less than 0.5 mv) that display more than three components or multiple slurring and notching should be classed as "small and bizarre" or "vibratory."

6. The term S–T *junction* (or J) should be used to indicate the point or shoulder that marks the end of the QRS complex, the point where the steep slopes of the QRS deflections are more or less abruptly replaced by the more gradual slopes that precede or comprise the first limb of the T wave. In many electrocardiograms the S–T junction is followed by a nearly horizontal or gently sloping segment which lies on, above, or below the reference level and ends with the onset of a much steeper slope that rises or falls to the apex of T. The term S–T *segment* is used for this part of the ventricular complex when it exists, even though electrophysiologically it is the earliest part of the T deflection. When there is no point between the S–T junction and the apex of T at which a sharp change in the slope of the trace occurs, this part of the ventricular complex should be called the *first limb of the T wave*. When the term *S–T segment* is used without reference to some particular electrocardiogram or to some particular class of electrocardiograms, it should be understood to refer merely to that part of the ventricular complex that immediately follows the S–T junction.

The reference level for the measurement of the displacement of the S–T *junction* should be the T_p level. The level of reference for the measurement of the S–T *segment,* the T wave, and the U wave should be the isoelectric level when this can be determined; otherwise it should be the level of the trace at the beginning of the QRS interval.

7. The term *diphasic T waves* should be applied to those final ventricular deflections that present two distinct turning points, one on each side of the level of reference, as described for the P waves (see par. 2 above).

Other terms used in describing the T wave are *notched*

when two apices are noted in the same direction separated by a movement of the curve toward the base line; *rounded apex* when the usual pointed apex is replaced by a curve; *coved* when the S–T segment is convex upward but does not cross the line of reference and is followed by an inverted T wave.

32 / Nomenclature for Electrocardiographic Interpretation

10.2. Right deviation of the electrical axis of QRS
10.3. Left deviation of the electrical axis of T
10.4. Right deviation of the electrical axis of T
10.5. Deviation of the electrical axis of QRST (ventricular gradient)
10.6. Left deviation of the electrical axis of P
10.7. Right deviation of the electrical axis of P

11. DEFLECTIONS

11.0. Normal deflections
11.1. High voltage of P wave
11.2. Low voltage of P wave
11.3. Broad P wave
11.4. High voltage of QRS
11.5. Low voltage of QRS
11.6. Broad Q wave
11.7. Elevation of S-T junction (J)
11.8. Depression of S-T junction (J)
11.9. High voltage of T wave
11.10. Low voltage of T wave
11.11. Unusual U wave
11.12. Electrical alternans

12. SPATIAL VECTORCARDIOGRAM

12.1. P form
12.2. QRS form
12.3. Junction of QRS form and T form
12.4. T form

13. MISCELLANEOUS

13.1. Other conditions not listed above

33 / Criteria for Electrocardiographic Interpretation*

1. Sinus Mechanisms

1.0. NORMAL SINUS RHYTHM. The P wave is upright in leads I (except in dextrocardia), II, V_F, in the anterior and left anterolateral thoracic leads, and in the juxtaventricular and subventricular esophageal leads. Deviations from this rule may be encountered occasionally with unusual structure, size, or position of the atria. The P wave occurs regularly at a rate of 60 to 100 per minute (Fig. 1). It is followed by the ventricular deflections, QRST, except when the ventricular muscle is absolutely refractory or when there is a high grade of atrioventricular block.

1.1. SINUS TACHYCARDIA. This is the same as normal sinus rhythm except that the rate exceeds 100 per minute.

1.2. SINUS BRADYCARDIA. This is the same as normal sinus rhythm except that the rate is less than 60 per minute.

1.3. SINUS ARRHYTHMIA. This is the same as normal sinus rhythm except that the P waves, followed by the ventricular

---

* Specific electrocardiographic interpretations that are useful in making the anatomic cardiac diagnosis are included in the appropriate portions of Part I, Chapters 3 and 4.

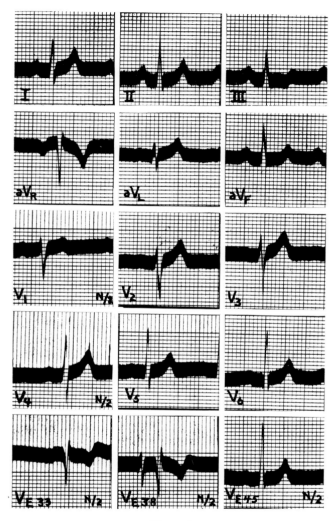

Figure 1

deflections, occur at irregular intervals. The arrhythmia is usually phasic and related to respiration, the cycles as a rule being longer in expiration (Fig. 2). Arbitrarily, the duration of cycle lengths must vary by 10 percent or more for the rhythm to be called sinus arrhythmia.

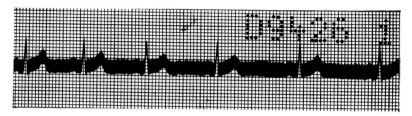

Figure 2

1.4. SINUS ARREST. In a sinus rhythm there is periodic failure of impulse formation. A P wave and its accompanying ventricular deflections fail to appear at the expected time. The pause that results is usually slightly shorter, but may be longer, than two normal cycles (Fig. 3).

1.5. SINO–ATRIAL BLOCK. In a sinus rhythm there is periodic failure of excitation of the atria by a sinus impulse. The dropped beats may occur sporadically, the resulting pause having the precise duration of two normal cycles, or may occur in regularly recurring patterns after every second, third, or

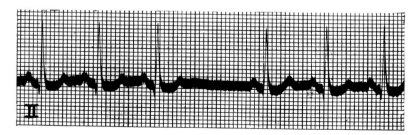

Figure 3

later normal beat. Phasic variations in the length of P-P cycles ascribed to progressive lengthening of sino-atrial conduction, analogous to what occurs in incomplete atrioventricular block (**33**.7.2), may be observed.

2. Atrial Mechanisms

2.1. ATRIAL PREMATURE SYSTOLE.   The premature beat compared with the sinus beats has the following characteristics in

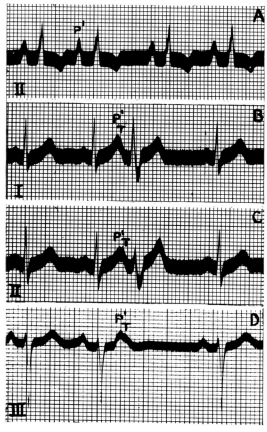

Figure 4

399

at least one lead: a P wave different in form; a P-R interval that is usually as long or longer, but infrequently shorter; a ventricular complex that may be the same (Fig. 4A), somewhat different (slightly aberrant, Fig. 4B), quite different (markedly aberrant, Fig. 4C), or absent (blocked atrial premature systole,* Fig. 4D). The cycle preceding and the cycle following the premature systole usually have a combined length of less than two normal cycles. The premature systole may depress the rate of the sino-atrial node temporarily. The cycle preceding and the cycle following the premature beat may have a combined length equal to or longer than two normal cycles. When an atrial premature systole regularly follows each normal systole, the electrocardiogram is said to show coupled beats (Fig. 5).

2.2. ATRIAL TACHYCARDIA. There is a rapid and regular succession of P waves different in form from the P waves of the basic sinus rhythm. The QRS group may be normal (Fig. 6),

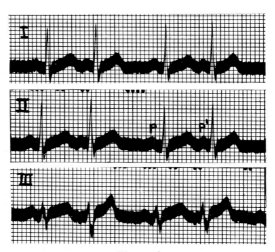

Figure 5

* This term is inaccurate in that the ventricular response rather than the atrial premature systole is blocked. Nevertheless, it is so generally used that it has been retained.

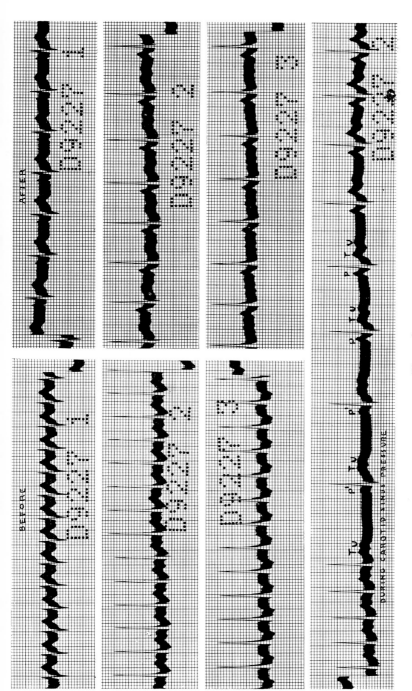

Figure 6

slightly aberrant, or markedly aberrant. When it is markedly aberrant, differentiation from a ventricular tachycardia is difficult. Frequently, the P wave coincides with the T wave of the preceding complex, thus making differentiation from other supraventricular tachycardias difficult (33.3.5). The atrial deflections in general are best seen in leads from the right sternal edge (Fig. 7), from the esophagus, or from within the atrium.

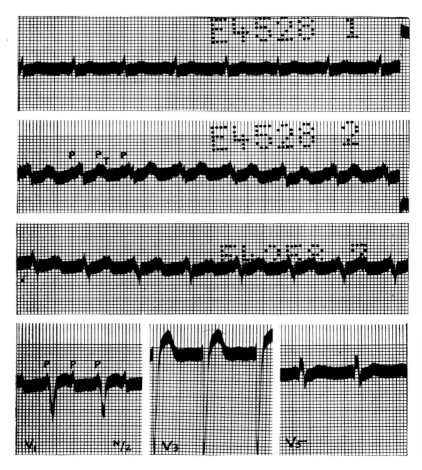

Figure 7

Ventricular deflections may be half as frequent as atrial deflections (1:2 ventricular response, Fig. 7) or even less frequent (1:3, 1:4 ventricular response [33.7.1–3]). In most instances the rate of the atria is between 160 and 280 per minute.

2.3. ATRIAL FLUTTER. Atrial activity is represented in the electrocardiogram by regular, continuous oscillations (P waves) which are uniform except where distorted by ventricular deflections (Fig. 8). These oscillations are recorded best in leads II, III, and V_F, where they are ascribed to an inverted P wave followed by a prominent upright T_P wave. They are also recorded well in lead V_1 and in juxta-atrial leads where the P wave may assume a biphasic character. They occur at a rate ranging from 200 to 380 per minute. The ventricular deflections usually occur regularly at a rate slower than and in con-

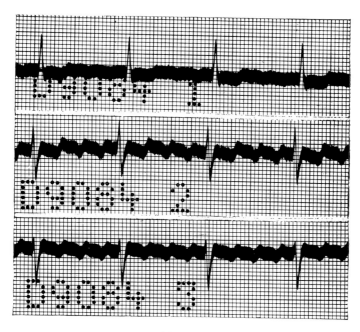

Figure 8

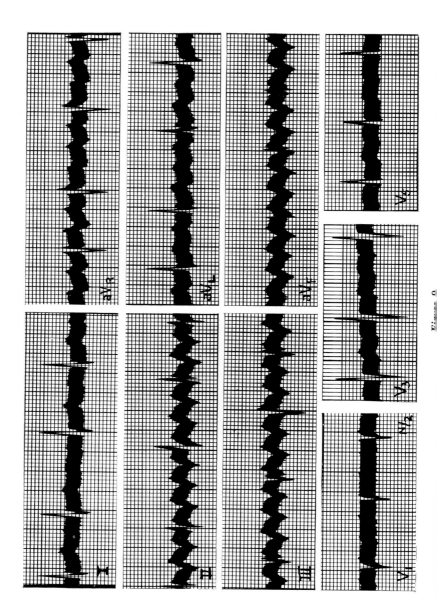

Figure 9.

stant ratio to the atrial rate, e.g., 1:2, 1:3, 1:4. At times, these ratios change in the same tracing. The ventricular rhythm is then irregular (Fig. 9). Rarely, the ratio is 1:1, and such electrocardiograms are usually indistinguishable from other supraventricular tachycardias (33.3.5). Differentiation from an atrial tachycardia with a rapid atrial rate and atrioventricular block is often difficult and at times impossible.

2.4. ATRIAL FIBRILLATION. Atrial activity is represented by irregular, variable deflections (f waves, Fig. 10) which have a rate in the neighborhood of 450 per minute. These are usually best recorded in esophageal leads, in lead V_1, or in intra-

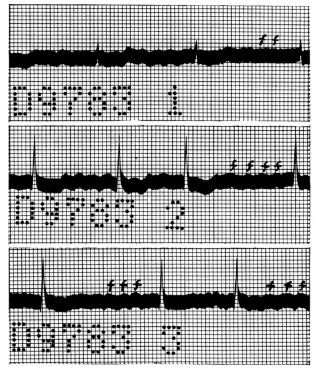

Figure 10

405

atrial leads (Fig. 11, V_{RA}). The ventricular deflections occur at irregular intervals except when there is complete atrioventricular block, or when there is a tachycardia arising in a lower center (atrioventricular dissociation).

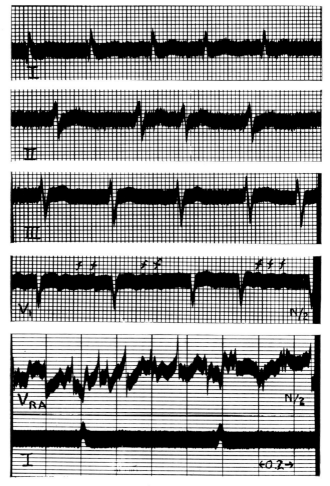

Figure 11

2.5. WANDERING PACEMAKER.   When the rate slows in a sinus arrhythmia, the pacemaker may change its location within the sino-atrial node or from the sino-atrial node to the atrioventricular node. The former shift is recognized by relatively minor changes in the shape of the P wave; the latter, by complete inversion of the P wave in leads II, III, and V_F and by shortening or reversal of the P-R interval (Fig. 12). When the pacemaker is in the atrioventricular node, the P wave may precede, coincide with, or follow the QRS complex. During the change from a sino-atrial to an atrioventricular nodal rhythm, there may be several P waves transitional in form (fusion P waves).

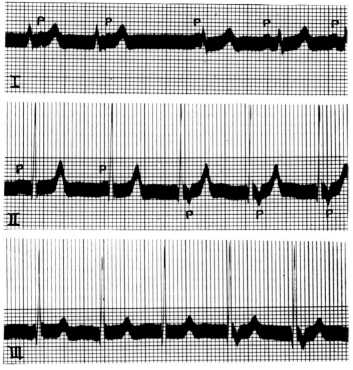

Figure 12

2.6. ATRIAL STANDSTILL. There is no evidence of electrical activity in the atria in any lead. The ventricles are controlled by a lower center.

3. Atrioventricular (A-V) Nodal Mechanisms

3.1. ATRIOVENTRICULAR (A-V) NODAL PREMATURE SYSTOLE. The P wave is characteristically inverted in leads II, III, and V_F and may occur before, during, or after the QRS deflections, depending upon whether excitation reaches the atria before, at the same time, or after it has reached the ventricles. The ventricular deflections are supraventricular in type but in most instances are slightly aberrant. The cycle preceding and the cycle following the premature systole have a total duration of usually less than two normal cycles (Fig. 13).

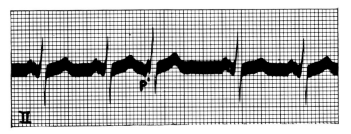

Figure 13

Rarely, a premature systole of this type fails to involve the atria because of retrograde block or because the atria are refractory. These chambers then continue to respond to a pacemaker at a higher level and the P waves are not altered in shape. The combined duration of the cycle preceding and the cycle following the abnormal beat is equal to two normal cycles. Such beats are indistinguishable from bundle of His premature systoles. They may be interpolated (33.4.3).

3.2. ATRIOVENTRICULAR (A-V) NODAL RHYTHM. A succession of regular systoles arises from the atrioventricular node at a rate usually between 40 and 80 per minute (Fig. 14). The electrocardiographic characteristics of each beat may be one of the several described for a premature systole from the A-V node (Fig. 13). Rarely, when QRS precedes the negative P wave, a second QRS may follow it. This phenomenon is called "reciprocal rhythm," is ascribed to re-entry of the impulse from the A-V node to the ventricles, and may be repetitive.

3.3. ATRIOVENTRICULAR (A-V) NODAL TACHYCARDIA. Same as atrioventricular nodal rhythm, except that the rate is over 100 per minute and may be as fast as 270 per minute (Fig. 15). In certain records the P waves cannot be recognized and the rhythm cannot with certainty be differentiated from other forms of supraventricular tachycardia. In other records there is retrograde block and the basic atrial rhythm is undisturbed. The latter are sometimes called bundle of His tachycardias.

3.4. ATRIOVENTRICULAR (A-V) NODAL ESCAPE. A single delayed

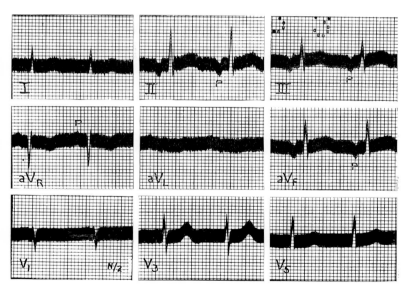

Figure 14

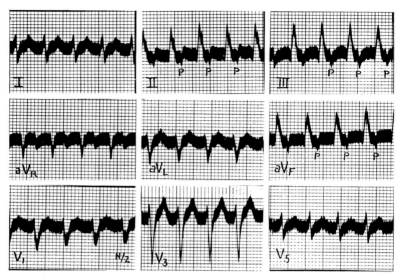

Figure 15

impulse emanates from the atrioventricular node when the
rate of excitation of the ventricles by an atrial pacemaker falls
below the inherent rate of impulse formation in the atrioventricular node. The escaped complex has the features of an
A-V nodal premature systole except that it is not premature
and the ventricular complex usually shows no aberration (Fig.
16A). If the atrial muscle has been excited by an impulse from
the sino-atrial node before the new center escapes, or if there
is retrograde block, the only abnormality will appear as a
delayed ventricular complex, the normal P wave coming before (Fig. 16B), with, or after the QRS group. When this
occurs, it cannot be said whether the new center is in the A-V
node or in the common bundle. The more inclusive term
ventricular escape is then used to describe it (33.4.2).

3.5. SUPRAVENTRICULAR TACHYCARDIA. The term *supraventricular tachycardia* is a collective one which includes all rapid
rhythms arising in the sino-atrial node, atrium, A-V node, or

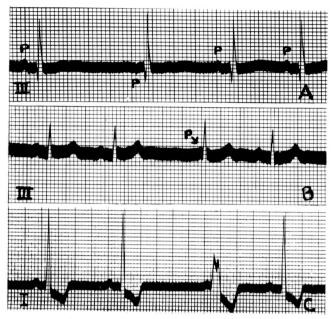

Figure 16

common bundle. It is a rhythm with a rate of over 100 per minute and ventricular complexes of supraventricular type but without distinguishable atrial deflections.

4. Ventricular Mechanisms

4.1. VENTRICULAR ESCAPE. A single impulse emanates from an ectopic focus in the common bundle or below its bifurcation when the rate of excitation of the ventricles by higher centers (S-A node, atria, A-V node) falls below the inherent rate of the ectopic center. The ventricular cycle terminated by the escaped beat is longer than the usual ventricular cycle. When the escaped center is in the common bundle, the electrocardiogram shows a delayed supraventricular complex with

411

no retrograde P wave because of retrograde block (see **33.3.4**
and Fig. 16B). When the escaped center is below the bifurcation of the common bundle, the QRS complex is aberrant
(Fig. 16C). Aberrant QRS complexes may also occur with the
escaped center in the common bundle when there is an associated bundle-branch block.

4.2.   IDIOVENTRICULAR RHYTHM.*   A succession of three or
more ventricular escaped beats occurs. These may arise in a
focus above (Fig. 17A) or below (Fig. 17B) the bifurcation of
the common bundle. The ventricular rate is usually between
30 and 40 beats per minute; it may be slower or faster but
rarely exceeds 50 beats per minute except in children or in

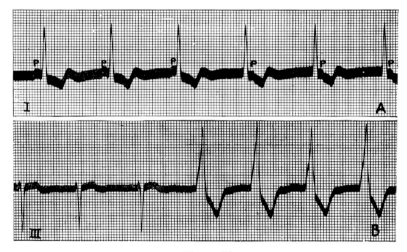

Figure 17

* An apparent discrepancy and a real overlap will be noted here between the terms *supraventricular* (**33.3.5**) and *idioventricular* (**33.4.2**). Actually the former term is descriptive of the appearance of QRS only; the
latter implies a separate pacemaker for the ventricles as compared to the
atria. This double approach, descriptive and physiologic, is unfortunate
but well fixed by usage.

response to drugs. During idioventricular rhythm there is atrioventricular dissociation (33.5), the atrial pacemaker being in the sino-atrial node, in the atrioventricular node, in an ectopic atrial focus, in the atrial muscle as a whole (flutter or fibrillation), or there may be no atrial activity (standstill). The atrial deflections bear no fixed or physiologic relation to the ventricular deflections. Idioventricular rhythm is seen most commonly in complete atrioventricular block. A special form of idioventricular rhythm occurs in ventricular parasystole (33.4.7).

4.3. VENTRICULAR PREMATURE SYSTOLE.   A premature beat arises from a center in the ventricles below the bifurcation of the common bundle. The QRS deflections are abnormally wide, notched, and slurred, and are followed by a T wave which usually is opposite in direction to the main QRS deflection. Because of retrograde block, the rhythm of the atria is not disturbed. For this reason the combined length of the cycle preceding and the cycle following the premature systole is equal to two normal cycles, and the long pause following this systole is said to be compensatory (Fig. 18A). This pause may not be compensatory if retrograde conduction occurs and disturbs the atrial rhythm. The pause also may not be compensatory if the atrial impulse occurring after the premature beat reaches the ventricles when they are no longer refractory from that beat. In this event the premature systole is truly an extrasystole, or "interpolated" premature systole (Fig. 18B). When a ventricular premature systole regularly follows each normal systole, the electrocardiogram is said to show "coupled beats," "coupling," or "bigeminal rhythm." Premature beats arising from the same focus usually follow preceding beats by a constant time interval (fixed coupling time).

4.4. VENTRICULAR TACHYCARDIA.   A succession of three or more ventricular premature systoles occurs usually at a rate ranging from 150 to 250 beats per minute. The rhythm is regular, but slight irregularity of the R-R intervals may be

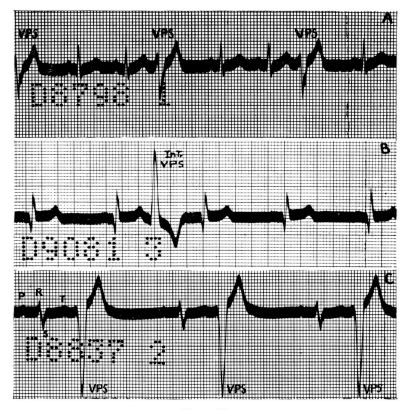

Figure 18

found. The form of the QRS complexes may also vary slightly.
The atrial rhythm often cannot be recognized (Fig. 19). If it
is recognized, it may be found to be a sinus or other atrial
rhythm. Atrioventricular dissociation (33.5) is present unless,
as occurs rarely, there is retrograde conduction and the atria
respond to the ventricles in a 1:1, 1:2, or smaller ratio. In such
instances P waves, inverted in leads II, III, and V_F, will be
seen at the appropriate intervals. In some unusual instances
successive ventricular beats are characterized by a principal
wave that deflects first in one, then in the other direction

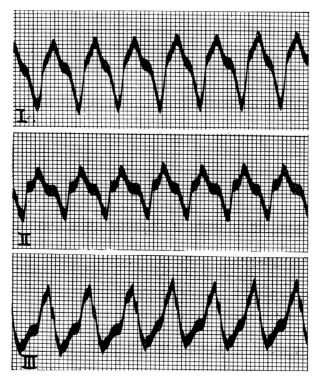

Figure 19

from the baseline. Such are said to display bidirectional ventricular tachycardia (Fig. 20).

4.5.   VENTRICULAR FIBRILLATION.   There are large continuous oscillations of the trace that are irregular in form and rate. Atrial deflections usually cannot be identified (Fig. 21) in leads from the surface of the body.

4.6.   VENTRICULAR PARASYSTOLE.   A ventricular center fails to be discharged by the dominant supraventricular pacemaker. The resulting "parasystolic" impulses, generated at an inher-

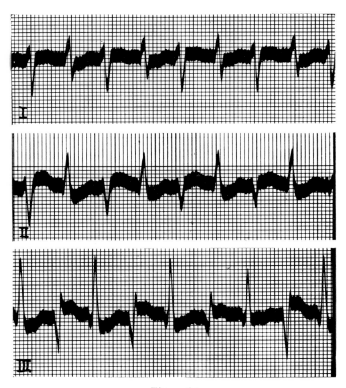

Figure 20

ent rate, activate the ventricles whenever the latter are not refractory from activation by the supraventricular pacemaker. The QRS complexes of parasystolic origin are ventricular in form. They occur irregularly and follow the supraventricular beats at irregular intervals. All intervals between parasystolic beats are simple multiples of a shortest interparasystolic interval. Usually the parasystolic rate is slower than the rate of the dominant pacemaker; occasionally it is faster. Rarely, a parasystolic center may be located in the atria, in the atrioventricular node, or in the bundle of His. Its manifest activity may be continuous or intermittent.

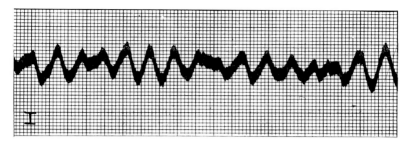

Figure 21

5. Atrioventricular Dissociation*

There is independent beating of the atria and of the ventricles. It is initiated when the rate of excitation of the ventricles by an atrial pacemaker is slower than the rate of a pacemaker in the atrioventricular node, bundle of His, or ventricles. It is perpetuated by the refractoriness of the atrioventricular junction. Atrioventricular dissociation is characterized electrocardiographically by the absence of a fixed or physiologic relation between atrial and ventricular deflections. The atria are usually activated by the sino-atrial node, the ventricles by the atrioventricular node. However, atrioventricular dissociation may occur during any other atrial or ventricular arrhythmia. The rates of the atria and ventricles depend on the location of the pacemakers activating these structures. The ventricular and atrial rhythms (except atrial fibrillation) are usually regular. But when an impulse from either the atrial or ventricular pacemaker reaches the atrioventricular junction during its nonrefractory phase, antegrade or retrograde conduction may take place, causing a QRS complex or retrograde P wave to appear prematurely (ventricular capture [Fig. 22] or atrial capture).

* The generic term *atrioventricular dissociation* and its simple definition are preferred to *interference dissociation* or *atrioventricular dissociation with interference* because of the ambiguity of the latter terms. The term *interference beats* is avoided for the same reason.

417

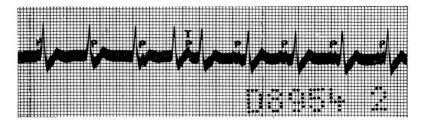

Figure 22

6. Mechanisms of Undetermined Origin

6.1. PREMATURE SYSTOLE OF UNDETERMINED ORIGIN. There is a premature beat not satisfying criteria for the diagnosis of atrial premature systole, atrioventricular nodal premature systole, bundle of His premature systole, or ventricular premature systole.

6.2. TACHYCARDIA OF UNDETERMINED ORIGIN. There is a rhythm with a rate of over 100 beats per minute not satisfying criteria for the diagnosis of sinus tachycardia, atrial tachycardia, atrioventricular nodal tachycardia, atrial fibrillation, atrial flutter, bundle of His tachycardia, or ventricular tachycardia.

7. Atrioventricular Conduction

7.0. P-R INTERVAL, NORMAL. The longest P-R interval* found in the bipolar or unipolar extremity leads is regarded as indicating the P-R interval. It is measured from the beginning of the P wave to the beginning of QRS whether this be repre-

---

* The longest P-R interval is not necessarily the correct one, but because it does not usually differ from the latter by more than 0.01 sec., and because it is easy to measure, it is preferred. The most exact approximation to the true P-R interval is obtained by measuring the longest time between the beginning of P and the end of QRS in the six bipolar and unipolar extremity leads, and subtracting from this the longest QRS interval found in these leads.

418

sented by a Q wave or an R wave. With normal heart rates its upper limit in adults in 0.20 sec.; in adolescents, ages 14 to 17 years, 0.18 sec.; and in children under 14 years of age, 0.16 sec. In precordial leads its maximum duration may be longer.

7.1.   INCOMPLETE A-V BLOCK (PROLONGED A-V CONDUCTION TIME). There is prolongation of A-V conduction characterized by a P-R interval longer than the maxima given for the normal P-R interval.

7.2.   INCOMPLETE A-V BLOCK WITH DROPPED BEATS.   There is periodic failure of A-V conduction. Some of the atrial deflections are not followed by ventricular complexes ("dropped beats"). Dropped beats may occur sporadically or in regularly recurring patterns (after every second, third, or fourth atrial deflection [Fig. 23B]). The P-R intervals of the conducted beats may be normal or prolonged. Often the cycles preceding a dropped beat show progressive prolongation of the P-R interval (Fig. 23A).

7.3.   COMPLETE A-V BLOCK.   No impulses reach the ventricles from the atria. The ventricles are activated by a pacemaker located below the block, either in the bundle of His or below its bifurcation. The ventricular pacemaker may shift from one location to another, resulting in QRS complexes of varying form. Rarely, the idioventricular rhythm may be interrupted by a supraventricular impulse when in a sino-atrial rhythm the P wave falls near the end of the ventricular T wave. The phenomenon is attributed to the supernormal phase of A-V conduction and may result in occasional retrograde as well as forward conduction through the junctional tissues in the presence of A-V block.

8. Intraventricular Conduction

8.0.   QRS INTERVAL, NORMAL.   The longest QRS interval found in the bipolar or unipolar extremity leads is the pre-

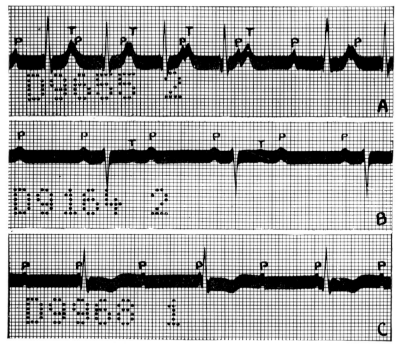

Figure 23

ferred measurement since normal standards for these leads are well established. It is measured from the beginning (Q or R) to the end of the QRS group. Its upper limit is 0.10 sec. in adults; 0.09 sec. in children from 5 to 14 years of age; 0.08 sec. in children under 5 years. In precordial leads its maximum duration is slightly longer.

8.1. DELAYED INTRINSICOID (RS) DEFLECTION, LEFT. In leads from the left side of the precordium (V_5 and V_6), the time measured from the beginning of QRS to the peak of the R wave exceeds 0.05 sec.

8.2. DELAYED INTRINSICOID (RS OR R′S′) DEFLECTION, RIGHT. In leads from the right side of the precordium (V_1 and V_2), the time measured from the beginning of QRS to the peak of the R wave exceeds 0.03 sec. When there is a second R wave (R′) in these leads, the peak of this wave is used as the point of measurement if R′S′ exceeds RS in size.

8.3.   QRS INTERVAL, PROLONGED.   The QRS interval is between 0.10 and 0.12 sec. Such prolongation may be caused by hypertrophy, by infarction, by electrolytic disturbances, by incomplete block of one or the other bundle branch, or by unknown factors.

Many records will not display features of QRS sufficiently characteristic to indicate which of these causes underlies the prolonged QRS interval. It is suggested that all these curves be classified simply as QRS interval, prolonged. Furthermore, it is likely that incomplete block of the right bundle branch and probably of the left bundle branch can exist with a QRS interval of 0.1 sec. or less. When either is suspected, it is suggested that the record be classified under category 13.1 (miscellaneous).

8.4.   QRS INTERVAL, PROLONGED, INTERMITTENT.   This term is applied to electrocardiograms displaying a normal sinus or other regular supraventricular rhythm, a constant P-R interval, and QRS groups that are of normal duration and prolonged (as defined above), as a rule alternately but occasionally irregularly or progressively. When the basic rhythm is atrial fibrillation, the QRS interval may be normal in length only after a long diastolic pause.

8.5.   BUNDLE-BRANCH BLOCK, LEFT.   The QRS interval is 0.12 sec. or more, and the components of QRS are notched and slurred. In leads I, V_L, sometimes in V_F, and in leads from the extreme left side of the precordium and left side of the thorax, the initial deflection is usually an R wave which is notched or slurred. In these same leads the peak of the R wave or one of its prominent notches occurs relatively late in the QRS interval. The S-T segment is most often displaced in a direc-

421

tion opposite to the principal QRS deflection, and the T wave usually also points in this direction. The appearance of QRS in other leads depends principally on the average direction of the electrical axis of QRS (Figs. 24, 25).

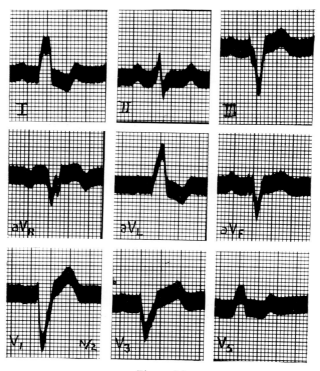

Figure 24

It is fairly certain that hypertrophy of the left ventricle can of itself occasionally cause a QRS interval of 0.12 sec. or more. These records will differ from the usual ones due to left bundle-branch block in that Q waves will be present in lead I and in the leads from the left arm and from the left side of the precordium, and the QRS deflections of the bipolar ex-

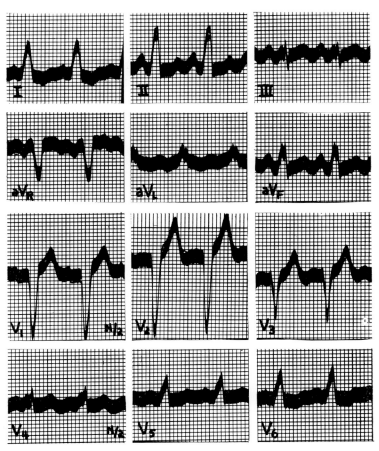

Figure 25

tremity leads usually will be quite high and relatively free from notching and slurring (33.8.7).

8.6. BUNDLE-BRANCH BLOCK, RIGHT. The QRS interval is 0.12 sec. or over. The characteristic finding is the occurrence of a late, usually large R or R′ in lead V_1, sometimes in leads V_2 and V_3, and occasionally in leads farther to the right (V_{3R},

423

V_{4R}). Preceding this there is usually a small rs. A record consisting of a deep Q and a broad, slurred R wave is often obtained in lead V_R. Usually in lead I and in leads from the left side of the precordium there is a narrow R wave of variable size and a broad, slurred S wave.

The electrical axis of QRS, chamber hypertrophy, and other factors determine a variety of types which are recognized by the characteristics of the ventricular complex in the bipolar and unipolar extremity leads (Figs. 26, 27). An infrequent form is one that resembles left bundle-branch block in these leads except for the presence of a Q wave or S wave of variable dimensions in leads I and V_L (Fig. 28).

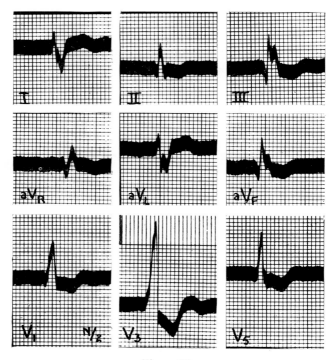

Figure 26

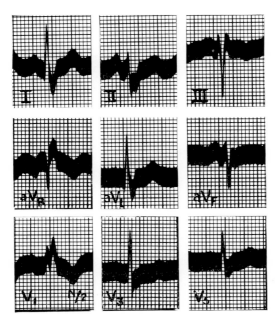

Figure 27

8.7. INTRAVENTRICULAR BLOCK, UNCLASSIFIED. This group includes all electrocardiograms with a QRS interval of 0.12 sec. or more that do not fit into any of the above classes. It is suggested that records with a wide QRS interval ascribed to hypertrophy alone and records variously described as showing arborization block, focal block, peri-infarction block, "bilateral" bundle-branch block, and other types of block be placed in this category until the mechanisms involved in each are clarified.

8.8. INTRAVENTRICULAR BLOCK, INTERMITTENT. This term is applied to electrocardiograms displaying a normal sinus or other regular supraventricular rhythm, a constant P-R interval, and QRS groups that are variably normal and abnormal (0.12 sec. or more) in width. This usually occurs alternately (Fig. 29A), but occasionally irregularly (Fig. 29B) or progres-

425

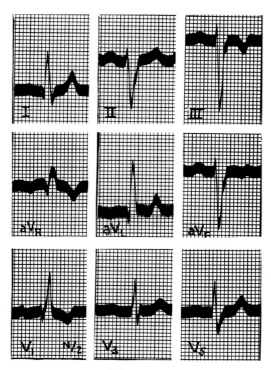

Figure 28

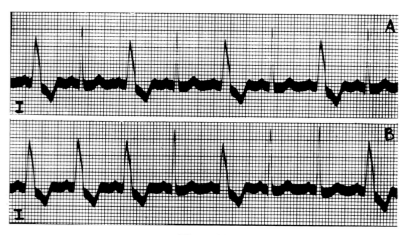

Figure 29

sively. When the basic rhythm is atrial fibrillation, the QRS interval may be normal in length only after a long diastolic pause. This term is intended to include intermittent bundle-branch block.

8.9.   ANOMALOUS ATRIOVENTRICULAR EXCITATION.* The record is characterized in one or several of the bipolar and unipolar extremity leads by a slurring or notching of the earliest QRS deflection. This additional component of QRS (anomalous component, delta wave) is caused by a premature excitation of some part of the ventricular muscle in an anomalous fashion. By virtue of this component's prematurity the P-R segment appears to be shortened or absent, the P-R interval abbreviated, and the QRS interval prolonged (Fig. 30).

The direction of excitation and the location of the anomalously excited portion of the ventricle determine whether the principal QRS deflection, particularly in leads from the right side of the precordium, will be positive or negative. Similar factors determine secondary displacement of the S-T segment and deviation of the T wave in a direction opposite to the principal QRS deflection.

Records are seen in which both anomalous and normal QRS complexes occur alternately or intermittently (Fig. 31).

9. Electrical Systole

9.1.   Q-T INTERVAL, PROLONGED. The Q-T interval is measured from the beginning of QRS to the end of the T wave. The longest interval found in any lead from the body surface is regarded as most nearly correct. It varies with the rate of the heart beat. A correction for rate can be made by the easily used formula, $Q\text{-}T = K \sqrt{\text{cycle length}}$. The Q-T interval may be regarded as prolonged if K exceeds 0.425.

The Q-T interval may be shortened by drugs, electrolyte

---

* Although this type of electrocardiogram is not believed to be the result of defective intraventricular conduction, it is placed under this category because of the considerable broadening of the QRS interval which is present.

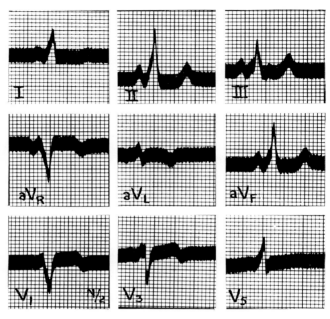

Figure 30

imbalance (hypercalcemia), and unknown factors. Criteria for the lower limit of normal are not established.

10. Electrical Axes*

10.0. NO DEVIATION OF THE ELECTRICAL AXIS OF QRS. By regarding summits as positive and depressions as negative, the

---

* The term *electrical axis* refers to the mean manifest electrical potential in space responsible for a designated deflection or deflections. Since potential has both size and direction, it may be treated as a vectorial quantity. Because it occurs in space, it has frontal, sagittal, and transverse components. Its length is measured usually in microvolt-seconds (μvs); its direction in terms of an angle it makes with one of the orthogonal coordinates. Most of the criteria are concerned with its frontal projection and the angle this makes with the horizontal (angle alpha); available data on its sagittal and transverse components are inadequate for quantitative criteria at this time. In the definitions given in 33.10.0, 1, and 2, the smaller polar angle between the limits of the angle alpha given is the one that applies.

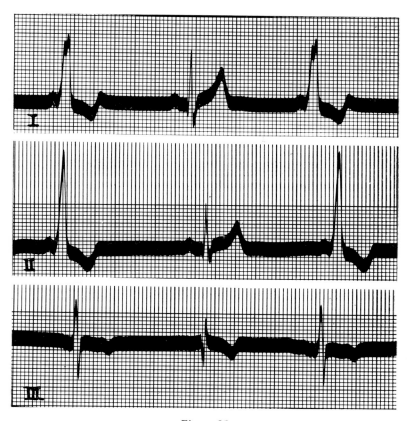

Figure 31

algebraic sum of the areas of the QRS deflections of the three bipolar leads and of lead V_F is positive, of lead V_R negative, and of lead V_L negative, zero, or positive. If this value is zero in lead I or zero in lead III, the record is also regarded as showing no deviation of the electrical axis provided that the value is positive in the remaining two bipolar extremity leads. This is equivalent to an angle alpha* of $+30°$ to $+90°$ (Fig. 32A).

* See footnote on page 428.

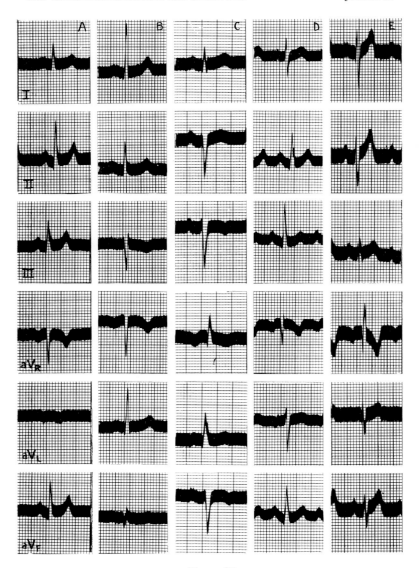

Figure 32

Usually the electrical axis of QRS is directed not only downward and to the left but backward as well. The backward direction manifests itself by a "transitional QRS"* in a precordial lead to the left of the midline anteriorly. The area of QRS deflections in anterior precordial leads to the right of the transitional QRS is negative and to its left positive.

In the frontal plane the average size of the electrical axis of QRS is 22 microvolt-seconds (μvs) in adults and 17 μvs in children under 15 years.

The area of the deflections may be estimated by inspection, but can be measured more precisely planimetrically.

10.1. LEFT DEVIATION OF THE ELECTRICAL AXIS OF QRS. The algebraic sum of the areas of Q, R, and S is positive in leads I and V_L, and negative in lead III. It is negative in leads V_F and II as well if the degree of deviation is marked.† With extreme deviation this value is positive in lead V_R and zero in lead I. The definition delimits an angle alpha of $+29°$ to $-90°$ (Figs. 32B and C). Usually with this direction in the frontal plane, the axis of QRS is deviated well backward, as manifested by a shift of the transitional zone to the left.

10.2. RIGHT DEVIATION OF THE ELECTRICAL AXIS OF QRS. The algebraic sum of the areas of Q, R, and S in leads I, V_R, and V_L is negative. With a greater degree of deviation to the right, this value may also be negative in leads II, III, and V_F, and positive in lead V_R. The definition delimits an angle alpha of $+91°$ to $-91°$ (Fig. 32D, E). In the sagittal plane the axis

* A transitional QRS in the precordial leads is defined as one having combined characteristics of leads recorded on either side of it. The algebraic sum of the areas of its deflections is close to zero.

† The Committee is aware that the quadrants of the rectilinear coordinates in the frontal plane are mislabeled in sign in contrast to mathematical custom. It is aware, too, that "deviation to the left" is maximal when the angle alpha is 0°. However, the electrocardiographic custom of regarding records with an angle alpha between 0° and $-90°$ (mathematical quadrant I) as displaying moderate to marked left deviation of the axis is so universal and ingrained that a change does not seem desirable.

may be directed backward or forward, the distinction being made on the appearance of the thoracic leads.

10.3. LEFT DEVIATION OF THE ELECTRICAL AXIS OF T. The angle alpha of the electrical axis of T is between $+29°$ and $-90°$. The angle is determined from the area and direction of the T wave in various leads as described for QRS (33.10.1).

10.4. RIGHT DEVIATION OF THE ELECTRICAL AXIS OF T. The angle alpha of the electrical axis of T is between $+91°$ and $-91°$. The angle is determined from the area and direction of the T wave in various leads as described for QRS (33.10.2).

10.5. DEVIATION OF THE ELECTRICAL AXIS OF QRST (VENTRICULAR GRADIENT). The electrical axis of QRST is treated as a vector sum of the electrical axes of QRS and T. Its mean length in the frontal plane in terms of the area of the ventricular deflections is approximately 46 microvolt-seconds (μvs). Its direction in the frontal plane is determined in the normal subject by the direction of the electrical axis of QRS, from which it usually does not differ by more than $30°$ in either direction. When the difference between the two is greater than $30°$, deviation of the ventricular gradient is said to exist.

10.6. LEFT DEVIATION OF THE ELECTRICAL AXIS OF P. The angle alpha of the electrical axis of P is between $+29°$ and $-90°$. The angle is determined from the area and the direction of the P wave in various leads as described for QRS (33.10.1).

10.7. RIGHT DEVIATION OF THE ELECTRICAL AXIS OF P. The angle alpha of the electrical axis of P is between $+91°$ and $-91°$. The angle is determined from the area and direction of the P wave in various leads as described for QRS (33.10.2).

11. Deflections*

11.0. NORMAL DEFLECTIONS. The range of normal values of atrial and ventricular deflections as determined in normal subjects in the age groups newborn to 1 year, 1 year to 10 years, 10 years to 20 years, and 20 years and over are shown in Tables I, II, III, and IV.

11.1. HIGH VOLTAGE OF P WAVE. The voltage of the P wave, measured in one direction from the isoelectric level, exceeds 0.25 mv in any of the bipolar extremity leads (I, II, III), in any of the precordial leads (V_1 to V_6), or in any of the augmented unipolar extremity leads (aV_R, aV_L, aV_F).

11.2. LOW VOLTAGE OF P WAVE. The voltage of the P wave, measured in one direction from the isoelectric level, is less than 0.05 mv in all of the commonly recorded surface leads, or in all those available.

11.3. BROAD P WAVE. The width of the P wave measured at its base exceeds 0.10 sec. in the bipolar or unipolar extremity leads. A P wave with a duration of 0.12 sec. or more in these leads is regarded by some as evidence of intra-atrial block.

11.4. HIGH VOLTAGE OF QRS. The voltage is regarded as high when the largest QRS deflection on one side of the reference level (end of the P-R segment) exceeds 2.0 mv in any of the bipolar or augmented unipolar extremity leads, or 4.0 mv in any of the usually recorded precordial leads.

* For practical reasons, the criteria for some of these definitions are somewhat arbitrary. Therefore the definitions may include values which are at variance with the range shown in the tables of normal values. The Committee recognizes that standards based on measurement of separate components of the electrocardiogram may be less reliable than standards based on measurements of relationships between the initial and final ventricular deflections. Similar considerations limit the validity of anatomic-electrocardiographic correlations based on these standards (see **3, 4**).

433

Table 1. *Normal Children, Newborn to 1 Year, Supine. Size of the Electrocardiographic Deflections in the Bipolar Extremity, Augmented Unipolar Extremity, and Precordial Leads Is Given in Tenths of a Millivolt**

Lead	P				Q				R				S				RS				S-T				T			
	No. Cases	Min.	Max.	Mean	No. Cases	Min.	Max.	Mean	No. Cases	Min.	Max.	Mean	No. Cases	Min.	Max.	Mean	No. Cases	Min.	Max.	Mean	No. Cases	Min.	Max.	Mean	No. Cases	Min.	Max.	Mean
I	158	−1.0	2.5	0.94	164	0	3.0	1.15	165	0	17.0	5.58	165	0	15.0	4.34	—	—	—	—	195	−0.1	0.1	—	143	−2.0	6.0	2.23
II	158	0	2.5	1.63	165	0	5.5	1.95	165	1.0	25.0	10.04	165	0	8.5	2.99	—	—	—	—	197	−0.1	0.2	—	143	0	7.0	2.84
III	158	−1.0	2.0	0.80	164	0	9.0	3.26	164	1.0	24.0	8.91	164	0	6.5	2.18	—	—	—	—	197	−0.2	0.2	—	143	−3.0	5.0	0.73
aVR	158	−2.5	1.5	−1.09	165	0	13.0	5.92	165	0	9.0	2.32	165	0	18.0	7.45	—	—	—	—	197	−0.1	0.1	—	143	−5.0	2.0	−2.39
aVL	153	−1.5	1.5	0.22	164	0	5.5	1.34	165	0	10.0	3.33	165	0	16.0	5.23	—	—	—	—	197	−0.1	0.1	—	143	−1.5	3.5	0.97
aVF	158	−1.0	3.0	1.17	165	0	6.0	2.36	165	1.5	21.5	8.15	165	0	7.5	2.29	—	—	—	—	197	−0.05	0.2	—	143	−2.0	5.0	1.68
V₁	155	−1.0	2.5	0.69	137	0	0	0	137	3.0	29.0	13.61	123	0	28.0	8.57	142	3.0	50.0	22.73	161	−0.2	0.1	—	126	−8.0	6.0	−2.65
V₂	186	0	2.5	1.13	137	0	0	0	137	3.0	43.0	19.98	121	1.0	42.0	18.35	162	3.0	66.0	40.14	159	−0.2	0.2	—	125	−9.0	9.0	−2.84
V₃	117	0	3.0	1.44	114	0	3.0	1.09	114	5.5	40.0	20.49	112	1.0	39.0	17.72	116	(18.0)†	73.0	38.71	116	−0.2	0.25	—	116	−7.0	6.0	−1.37
V₄	161	0	2.0	1.05	139	0	3.0	1.32	139	3.0	37.0	21.21	123	0	42.0	12.88	146	4.0	63.0	31.73	157	−0.1	0.2	—	123	−7.0	6.5	2.46
V₅	122	0	2.0	1.14	118	0	5.5	2.09	118	3.0	34.0	14.49	119	0	30.0	7.00	121	5.0	48.0	21.89	121	—	0.2	—	122	−4.0	7.0	2.93
V₆	141	0	2.0	0.84	119	0	5.0	1.64	138	0	24.0	8.00	138	0	30.0	2.72	161	3.0	34.0	12.17	161	—	0.1	—	125	−3.0	6.0	2.27

* Based on normal series studied by Ziegler.

† 6 months–1 year age group only.

Table II. *Normal Children, 1 to 10 Years, Supine. Size of the Electrocardiographic Deflections in the Bipolar Extremity, Augmented Unipolar Extremity, and Precordial Leads Is Given in Tenths of a Millivolt**

Lead	P				Q				R				S				RS				S-T				T			
	No. Cases	Min.	Max.	Mean	No. Cases	Min.	Max.	Mean	No. Cases	Min.	Max.	Mean	No. Cases	Min.	Max.	Mean	No. Cases	Min.	Max.	Mean	No. Cases	Min.	Max.	Mean	No. Cases	Min.	Max.	Mean
I	225	0.5	2.5	1.04	227	0	2.5	1.11	223	1.5	17.0	6.75	225	0	8.0	2.88	—	—	—	—	227	−1.0	1.0	—	223	1.0	6.5	2.53
II	224	0	3.0	1.63	228	0	5.4	1.55	223	2.0	28.0	12.21	223	0	6.5	2.38	—	—	—	—	227	−1.0	2.0	—	223	0	7.0	3.25
III	224	−1.5	2.0	0.62	227	0	8.0	2.50	223	1.0	23.0	7.99	223	0	9.0	1.70	—	—	—	—	228	−1.0	1.0	—	223	−3.0	4.0	0.52
aV$_R$	293	−2.0	0	−1.56	347	0	14.0	5.70	342	0	6.5	1.60	342	0	19.5	7.77	—	—	—	—	227	−1.0	1.0	—	292	−6.0	−0.2	−2.79
aV$_L$	293	−1.0	2.0	0.32	347	0	4.0	0.84	342	0	11.8	3.15	342	0	11.0	3.72	—	—	—	—	227	−1.0	1.0	—	292	−4.0	4.0	1.10
aV$_F$	293	−0.6	2.0	1.03	347	0	5.0	1.33	342	0.5	21.0	9.30	342	0	14.0	1.61	—	—	—	—	227	−1.0	1.0	—	292	−1.0	6.0	1.84
V$_1$	198	−1.0	2.5	0.72	203	0	0	0	198	0.4	20.0	7.15	197	0	36.5	11.02	103	6.5	46.5	28.85	134	−1.0	2.0	—	197	−6.0	3.0	−2.86
V$_2$	201	−0.6	2.0	0.92	204	0	0	0	192	2.0	28.0	12.90	196	3.0	44.0	18.31	101	9.0	61.0	37.45	133	−1.0	2.5	—	197	−8.5	6.0	−1.91
V$_3$	182	0.1	2.0	0.80	185	0	1.0	0.44	181	4.0	42.0	14.00	180	0	36.0	13.66	87	14.0	60.0	32.17	118	0	2.5	—	191	−13.0	12.5	1.30
V$_4$	200	0	1.5	0.73	203	0	6.0	1.21	199	4.0	50.0	20.16	199	0	26.0	7.53	102	13.0	61.0	32.94	133	0	2.0	—	199	−4.0	14.5	4.54
V$_5$	188	0	1.5	0.62	190	0	8.0	1.53	186	6.0	40.0	18.97	186	0	15.0	3.62	88	15.0	47.0	23.89	88	−1.0	1.2	—	186	0	12.0	4.51
V$_6$	197	0	1.5	0.61	201	0	5.0	1.47	196	5.0	23.0	11.94	195	0	13.0	1.23	102	5.0	26.0	14.74	93	−1.0	1.0	—	196	0	8.5	3.41
V$_7$	28	0	1.0	0.50	28	0	3.0	0.78	28	5.5	20.0	11.13	28	0	5.5	1.29	—	—	—	—	28	0	0.8	—	28	0.7	6.5	3.50
V$_{3R}$	28	−0.8	1.5	0.57	28	0	2.0	0.09	28	1.3	9.9	4.18	28	0	19.5	5.51	—	—	—	—	28	0	0.6	—	28	−4.8	0.9	−1.77
V$_{4R}$	28	−0.4	1.5	0.44	28	0	2.0	0.09	28	1.0	4.8	2.80	28	0	10.5	8.67	—	—	—	—	28	0	0.4	—	28	−4.9	−1.0	−1.59

*This table is based on normal series studied by Ziegler; Switzer and Besoain; Kneese de Melo; and Yu, Joos, and Katsampes.

Table III. *Normal Adolescents, 10 to 20 Years, Supine. Size of the Electrocardiographic Deflections in the Bipolar Extremity, Augmented Unipolar Extremity, and Precordial Leads Is Given in Tenths of a Millivolt**

Lead	No. Cases	P			Q			R			S			T		
		Min.	Max.	Mean	Min.	Max.	Mean	Min	Max.	Mean	Min.	Max.	Mean	Min.	Max.	Mean
I	124	0.2	1.5	0.74	0	2.5	0.30	1.3	13.0	5.26	0	6.8	1.40	0.2	5.0	2.32
II	124	0	2.1	1.01	0	2.8	0.37	2.9	20.0	9.66	0	6.3	1.59	0.2	6.5	2.89
III	124	-1.0	1.8	0.43	0	4.6	0.50	0.7	15.8	6.05	0	9.0	1.18	-1.19	3.9	0.65
aV$_R$	214	-1.75	-0.2	-1.03	0	13.7	2.68	0	8.0	1.39	0	17.0	4.94	-5.2	-0.1	-2.36
aV$_L$	214	-1.0	1.4	0.29	0	4.2	0.34	0	10.1	2.24	0	14.2	2.51	-2.5	3.6	0.87
aV$_F$	214	-0.8	2.2	0.74	0	3.8	0.42	1.0	21.0	8.22	0	4.9	0.99	-0.5	5.4	1.76
V$_1$	138	-0.2	2.2	0.77	0	1.5	0.01	0.4	16.7	5.29	0	26.6	11.99	-3.5	7.5	0.22
V$_2$	139	-0.2	2.0	0.78	0	0	0	0.5	23.5	8.16	2.6	45.5	15.81	-3.8	14.1	2.19
V$_3$	138	0	1.8	0.73	0	0.7	0.01	1.6	26.0	10.15	0.9	31.1	12.76	-3.7	13.5	3.39
V$_4$	139	0	1.5	0.62	0	4.4	0.21	3.1	31.6	13.98	0.2	22.2	8.27	-2.8	12.6	4.43
V$_5$	139	0	1.2	0.55	0	3.1	0.49	4.2	29.0	13.56	0	15.1	3.03	0.1	10.5	3.71
V$_6$	138	0	1.0	0.50	0	4.2	0.66	3.5	25.0	11.44	0	11.3	1.74	0	7.8	3.04
V$_7$	24	0.2	0.8	0.4	0	2.5	0.9	5.0	16.0	15.0	0	5.4	0.9	0.7	5.0	2.4
V$_{3R}$	24	—	1.2	0.7	0	0	0	1.5	8.0	3.8	0	16.0	7.6	-3.6	1.8	-1.1
V$_{4R}$	24	—	1.0	0.4	0	1.5	—	0.7	5.5	2.3	1.0	9.5	5.4	-2.4	1.1	-1.1

*This table is based on normal series studied by Vaquero, Limón, and Limón; Switzer and Besoain; Kneese de Melo; Yu, Joos, and Katsampes.

Table IV. *Normal Adults, 20 Years and Over, Supine. Size of the Electrocardiographic Deflections in the Bipolar Extremity, Augmented Unipolar Extremity, and Precordial Leads Is Given in Tenths of a Millivolt**

Lead	P				Q				R				S				RS or QR				S-T				T			
	No. Cases	Min.	Max.	Mean	No. Cases	Min.	Max.	Mean	No. Cases	Min.	Max.	Mean	No. Cases	Min.	Max.	Mean	No. Cases	Min.	Max.	Mean	No. Cases	Min.	Max.	Mean	No. Cases	Min.	Max.	Mean
I	475	0	2.5	0.69	505	0	2.0	0.27	505	0.7	19.4	5.51	505	0	6.4	1.27	63	3.0	20.6	8.54	100	-0.3	0.9	0.11	505	-0.5	5.6	2.20
II	475	0	3.0	1.07	505	0	4.0	0.38	505	0.5	28.0	9.41	505	0	8.2	1.36	63	8.0	32.0	15.14	100	-1.0	1.0	0.21	505	0	8.0	2.67
III	475	-0.8	2.0	0.56	505	0	4.0	0.48	505	0	22.0	5.56	505	0	13.0	1.29	63	3.2	25.0	10.62	100	-0.6	0.8	0.04	505	-2.0	5.5	0.77
V_R	32	-1.0	-0.5	-0.63	62	0	8.0	2.48	62	0	3.0	0.90	62	0	11.0	3.01	62	3.5	12.0	6.50	32	0	0	0	62	-4.0	-0.5	-1.65
V_L	32	-0.5	0.5	0.07	62	0	1.5	0.16	62	0	7.0	1.21	62	0	7.0	2.04	62	0.5	8.5	3.37	32	0	0	0	62	-1.0	1.5	0.29
V_F	32	0	2.0	0.72	62	0	2.0	0.30	62	0	15.0	6.82	62	0	6.5	0.74	62	3.5	16.5	7.77	32	0	0	0	62	0	4.5	1.10
aV_R	411	-1.5	-0.1	-0.79	552	0	16.8	2.38	552	0	4.1	0.94	552	0	15.7	3.76	—	—	—	—	—	—	—	—	479	-5.5	-0.2	-2.40
aV_L	411	-1.0	1.4	0.51	552	0	3.5	0.27	552	0	10.1	2.61	552	0	11.3	1.35	—	—	—	—	—	—	—	—	479	-4.0	6.0	0.78
aV_F	411	-1.8	1.7	0.74	552	0	3.0	0.38	552	0	20.0	4.73	552	0	7.1	0.81	—	—	—	—	—	—	—	—	479	-0.6	5.2	1.85
V_1	371	-1.1	2.2	0.57	567	0	0	0	567	0	15.5	3.09	567	0.8	26.2	9.44	63	6.6	35.0	14.99	33	0	0.5	0.01	542	-4.0	12.2	0.84
V_2	371	-0.7	2.0	0.60	594	0	0	0	594	0	23.0	5.96	594	0	39.2	14.09	63	13.0	55.0	26.82	33	0	1.0	0.09	542	-2.6	18.0	4.70
V_3	371	-0.5	2.0	0.61	567	0	1.5	0.01	567	0.7	54.6	8.93	567	0	27.5	9.51	63	11.1	54.6	24.12	33	0	2.0	0.20	542	-2.0	21.0	5.16
V_4	371	-0.2	2.3	0.60	594	0	4.0	0.13	594	1.8	46.0	13.78	594	0	28.8	5.93	63	9.0	51.6	26.16	33	0	1.0	0.03	542	-0.5	17.0	5.05
V_5	371	0	2.4	0.56	567	0	3.4	0.43	567	0.4	33.6	12.01	567	0	16.1	1.96	63	10.0	36.4	19.31	33	0	0	0	542	0	11.0	3.83
V_6	371	0	1.8	0.54	564	0	2.7	0.44	564	2.0	22.6	9.68	564	0	14.3	1.00	33	7.0	24.5	13.93	33	0	0	0	512	0	6.9	2.80
V_c†	—	—	—	—	30	0	0	0	30	2.0	12.8	5.81	30	0	16.2	6.09	30	5.5	24.2	11.91	—	—	—	—	30	0.2	5.2	2.55

* The table is based on normal series studied by Kossmann and Johnston; Kossmann and Goldberg; Wilson and Nyboer; Deeds and Barnes; Vaquero, Limón, and Limón; Myers, Klein, Stofer, and Hiratzka; Sokolow and Friedlander; Kneese de Melo.

† Ve, lead from tip of the ensiform cartilage.

11.5. LOW VOLTAGE OF QRS. The voltage is regarded as low when the largest QRS deflection on one side of the reference level (end of the P-R segment) is less than 0.5 mv in all of the bipolar extremity leads and augmented unipolar extremity leads, and less than 1.5 mv in all of the usually recorded precordial leads. The term is to be used only when the criteria are met in all of the leads, or in all those available.

11.6. BROAD Q WAVE. The duration of the initial depression of the QRS group is 0.04 sec. or greater. The definition does not apply if the only QRS deflection is downward (QS).

11.7. ELEVATION OF S-T JUNCTION (J). The elevation of the junction compared to the reference level (end of the P-R segment) exceeds 0.1 mv in the bipolar extremity leads, or 0.075 mv in the augmented unipolar extremity leads, or 0.2 mv in the usually recorded precordial leads.

11.8. DEPRESSION OF S-T JUNCTION (J). The depression of the junction compared to the reference level (end of the P-R segment) exceeds 0.1 mv in the bipolar extremity leads or in the usually recorded precordial leads, or 0.075 mv in the augmented unipolar extremity leads.

11.9. HIGH VOLTAGE OF T WAVE. The voltage of the T wave, measured in one direction from the reference level, exceeds 0.7 mv in any of the bipolar extremity leads, or 0.5 mv in any of the augmented extremity leads, or 2.0 mv in any of the precordial leads.

11.10. LOW VOLTAGE OF T WAVE. The voltage of the highest T wave measured in one direction from the reference level is less than 0.1 mv in all of the extremity leads, and less than 0.2 mv in all of the usually recorded precordial leads. The term is to be used only when the criteria are met in all of the leads, or in all those available.

11.11.   UNUSUAL U WAVE.   A prominent or inverted deflection immediately after the T wave is present in any of the usually recorded leads from the external surface of the body.

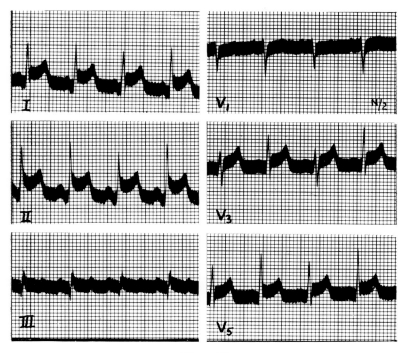

Figure 33

11.12.   ELECTRICAL ALTERNANS.   In a normal sinus or other supraventricular rhythm or tachycardia, variations in the form of the ventricular complexes occur in alternate beats without variations in the duration of the QRS interval. Most often the variation in form involves QRS and T (Fig. 33); rarely, T alone is affected.

439

12. Spatial Vectorcardiogram

12.1. P FORM. Abnormal in direction, shape, or area.

12.2. QRS FORM. Abnormal in direction, shape, or area.

12.3. JUNCTION OF QRS FORM AND T FORM. Abnormally displaced.

12.4. T FORM. Abnormal in direction, shape, or area.

13. Miscellaneous

13.1. OTHER CONDITIONS NOT LISTED ABOVE.

Index

443

phlebitis without, 152–153
of pulmonary arteries, 33, 269–270
and vasospasm, secondary, 130
venous
blood-clotting mechanism and, 149–150
intimal damage and, 148–149
multiple factors, 150
venous stasis and, 150
Thrombus
antemortem and postmortem, 287–288
arterial embolism and, 140
"ball," 286
"globoid," 286
marantic, 286
stasis, 286
Toxemia of pregnancy, 13–14
Toxic agent, heart disease and, 21
Toxoplasmosis, myocardial, 293
Trabeculae carneae, 235
Transitional QRS, 431
Transposition, of great vessels
complete, 93–94
corrected, 78–79
incomplete, 94
Trauma
arterial, 144
arterial thrombosis and, 137
arteriovenous fistula and, 144
of coronary artery, 36
of heart, 61
heart disease and, 21
hemodynamic, 41
to pericardium, 67
and vasospasm, secondary, 130
Treponema pallidum, 255
Trichinosis, 292–293
Tricuspid
annular incompetency, 104
atresia, 91–92
stenosis, 91–92
valve
atresia, 196–198
disease, 46–47
downward displacement of, 77, 89–90

Ebstein's malformation, 198–199
hypoplasia, 196
insufficiency, 46–47
stenosis, 46–47, 196
Truncus arteriosus
partial persistent, 195, 214
persistent, 194–195
signs, 82
Trypanosoma cruzi, 293
Tuberculosis
of endocardium, 281
granulomatous pericarditis and, 307–308
thrombosis of pulmonary artery and, 269
of valve, 281
Tubular hypoplasia of aortic arch, 216
Tumors
atrial myxomas, 17
in conduction system, 317
lymphatic, 157
of myocardium, congenital, 297
of pericardium, 310
signs and symptoms, 16–17

Ulceration, and atherosclerosis of aorta, 262–263
Unipolar extremity leads, 384–385
Unknown cause, of heart disease, 21–22
Uremia, 22

Valsalva, sinus of, aneurysm of, 71–72
Valves
annular sclerosis and, 281–282
aortic (*see* Aortic valve)
aortic stenosis, congenital, and, 72
atheroma of, 282–283
ball-valve
obstructions, 108–109, 286
thrombus, 39
deformity, 41–43
miscellaneous structural diseases, 40
mitral (*see* Mitral valve)